Geriatric Emergency Care

Editors

MAURA KENNEDY
SHAN W. LIU

CLINICS IN
GERIATRIC MEDICINE

www.geriatric.theclinics.com

Consulting Editor
G. MICHAEL HARPER

November 2023 • Volume 39 • Number 4

ELSEVIER

1600 John F. Kennedy Boulevard • Suite 1800 • Philadelphia, Pennsylvania, 19103-2899

http://www.theclinics.com

CLINICS IN GERIATRIC MEDICINE Volume 39, Number 4
November 2023 ISSN 0749–0690, ISBN-13: 978-0-443-18373-7

Editor: Taylor Hayes
Developmental Editor: Anita Chamoli

Clinics in Geriatric Medicine (ISSN 0749-0690) is published quarterly by Elsevier Inc., 360 Park Avenue South, New York, NY 10010-1710. Months of issue are February, May, August, and November. Business and Editorial Offices: 1600 John F. Kennedy Blvd., Suite 1800, Philadelphia, PA 191023-2899. Periodicals postage paid at New York, NY, and additional mailing offices. Subscription prices are $312.00 per year (US individuals), $748.00 per year (US institutions), $100.00 per year (US & Canadian student/resident), $340.00 per year (Canadian individuals), $946.00 per year (Canadian institutions), $444.00 per year (international individuals), $946.00 per year (international institutions), and $195.00 per year (international student/resident). Foreign air speed delivery is included in all *Clinics* subscription prices. All prices are subject to change without notice. POSTMASTER: Send address changes to *Clinics in Geriatric Medicine*, Elsevier Health Sciences Division, Subscription Customer Service, 3251 Riverport Lane, Maryland Heights, MO 63043. **Telephone: 1-800-654-2452 (U.S. and Canada); 314-447-8871 (outside U.S. and Canada). Fax:** 314-447-8029. **E-mail:** journalscustomerservice-usa@elsevier.com **(for print support)** or journalsonlinesupport-usa@elsevier.com **(for online support).**

Reprints. For copies of 100 or more, of articles in this publication, please contact the Commercial Reprints Department, Elsevier Inc., 360 Park Avenue South, New York, New York 10010-1710. Tel.: 212-633-3874; Fax: 212-633-3820, E-mail: reprints@elsevier.com.

Clinics in Geriatric Medicine is covered in *MEDLINE/PubMed (Index Medicus), EMBASE/Excerpta Medica, Current Contents/Clinical Medicine (CC/CM),* and the *Cumulative Index to Nursing & Allied Health Literature.*

Contributors

CONSULTING EDITOR

G. MICHAEL HARPER, MD, AGSF, CMD
Professor of Medicine, University of California, San Francisco, Staff Physician, San Francisco VA Medical Center, San Francisco, California, USA

EDITORS

MAURA KENNEDY, MD, MPH
Chief, Division of Geriatric Emergency Medicine, Massachusetts General Hospital; Assistant Professor of Emergency Medicine, Harvard Medical School, Boston, Massachusetts, USA

SHAN W. LIU, MD, SD
Director, Geriatric Emergency Medicine Fellowship, Massachusetts General Hospital; Associate Professor of Emergency Medicine, Harvard Medical School, Boston, Massachusetts, USA

AUTHORS

KEVIN J. BIESE, MD
Vice Chair Academic Affairs and Clinical Associate Professor, Department of Emergency Medicine, University of North Carolina, Department of Medicine, Center for Aging and Health, University of North Carolina at Chapel Hill, Chapel Hill, North Carolina, USA

JASON BOWMAN, MD
Assistant Professor, Department of Emergency Medicine, Harvard Medical School, Brigham and Women's Hospital; Department of Psychosocial Oncology and Palliative Medicine, Dana Farber Cancer Institute, Boston, Massachusetts, USA

KYLE R. BURTON, MD, MPP
Emergency Medicine Physician, Department of Emergency Medicine, Johns Hopkins Hospital, Baltimore, Maryland, USA

LAUREN CAMERON-COMASCO, MD
Assistant Professor, Department of Emergency Medicine, Beaumont Hospital, Royal Oak, Michigan, USA

ANITA N. CHARY, MD, PhD
Assistant Professor, Department of Emergency Medicine, Baylor College of Medicine, Department of Medicine, Section of Health Services Research, Baylor College of Medicine, Houston, Texas, USA

SCOTT M. DRESDEN, MD, MS
Associate Professor, Department of Emergency Medicine, Center for Healthcare Studies and Outcomes Research, Northwestern University Feinberg School fo Medicine, Chicago, Illinois, USA

NATALIE M. ELDER, MD, PharmD
Assistant Professor, Emergency Medicine, University of Vermont, Burlington, Vermont, USA

ALYSSA ELMAN, MSW
Department of Emergency Medicine, Weill Cornell Medical College/NewYork-Presbyterian Hospital, New York, New York, USA

NAOMI GEORGE, MD, MPH
Assistant Professor, Division of Critical Care Medicine, Department of Emergency Medicine, University of New Mexico School of Medicine, Albuquerque, New Mexico, USA

CAMERON J. GETTEL, MD, MHS
Assistant Professor, Department of Emergency Medicine, Yale School of Medicine, Center for Outcomes Research and Evaluation, Yale School of Medicine, New Haven, Connecticut, USA

ELIZABETH M. GOLDBERG, MD, ScM
Associate Professor, Department of Emergency Medicine, School of Medicine, University of Colorado, Anschutz Medical Campus, Aurora, Colorado, USA

ELAINE GOTTESMAN, MSW
Department of Emergency Medicine, Weill Cornell Medical College/New York-Presbyterian Hospital, New York, New York, USA

JIN H. HAN, MD, MSc
Associate Professor of Emergency Medicine, Department of Emergency Medicine, Vanderbilt University Medical Center, Geriatric Research, Education, and Clinical Center, Tennessee Valley Healthcare System, Nashville, Tennessee, USA

SUSAN N. HASTINGS, MD, MHS
Professsor, Center of Innovation to Accelerate Discovery and Practice Transformation (ADAPT), Durham VA Health Care System, Department of Medicine, Duke University School of Medicine, Geriatric Research, Education, Clinical Center, Durham VA Health Care System, Center for the Study of Human Aging and Development, Duke University School of Medicine, Department of Population Health Sciences, Duke University School of Medicine, Durham, North Carolina, USA

SEAN F. HEAVEY, MD
Geriatric Emergency Medicine Fellow, Department of Emergency Medicine, University of California Davis, Sacramento, California, USA

MATTHEW A. HOWARD III, MD
Professor and Chair, Department of Neurosurgery, University of Iowa, Iowa City, Iowa, USA

KAORI ITO, MD, PhD, FACS, FCCM
Associate Professor, Department of Emergency Medicine, Division of Acute Care Surgery, Teikyo University School of Medicine, Tokyo, Japan

JOHN KELLETT, MD
Department of Emergency Medicine, Odense University Hospital, University of Southern Denmark, Odense, Denmark

JENNIFER L. KOEHL, PharmD, BCPS
Emergency Medicine Clinical Specialist, Department of Pharmacy, Emergency Medicine, Massachusetts General Hospital, Boston, Massachusetts, USA

SANGIL LEE, MD, MS
Associate Professor of Emergency Medicine, Department of Emergency Medicine, University of Iowa Carver College of Medicine, Iowa City, Iowa, USA

ANGEL LI, MD, MBA
Department of Emergency Medicine, The Ohio State University, Columbus, Ohio, USA

PHILLIP D. MAGIDSON, MD, MPH
Assistant Professor, Johns Hopkins Hospital, Johns Hopkins Bayview Medical Center, Baltimore, Maryland, USA

COLLEEN M. MCQUOWN, MD
Physician, Louis Stokes Veterans Affairs Medical Center, Cleveland, Ohio, USA

DON MELADY, MD, MSc(Ed)
Associate Professor, Department of Family and Community Medicine, Faculty of Medicine, University of Toronto; Director of the Geriatric Emergency Medicine Fellowship, Schwartz-Reisman Emergency Medicine Institute, Mount Sinai Hospital, Toronto, Ontario, Canada

CHRISTIAN H. NICKEL, MD
Emergency Department, University Hospital Basel, University of Basel, Basel, Switzerland

KEI OUCHI, MD, MPH
Associate Professor, Department of Emergency Medicine, Harvard Medical School, Brigham and Women's Hospital, Boston, Massachusetts, USA

THIDATHIT PRACHANUKOOL, MD
Assistant Professor, Department of Emergency Medicine, Faculty of Medicine, Ramathibodi Hospital, Mahidol University, Bangkok, Thailand; Department of Emergency Medicine, Harvard Medical School, Brigham and Women's Hospital, Boston, Massachusetts, USA

TONY ROSEN, MD, MPH
Assistant professor, Department of Emergency Medicine, Weill Cornell Medical College/New York-Presbyterian Hospital, New York, New York, USA

MARGARET E. SAMUELS-KALOW, MD, MPhil, MSHP
Associate Professor, Department of Emergency Medicine, Massachusetts General Hospital, Boston, Massachusetts, USA

JOHN G. SCHUMACHER, MA, PhD
Professor and Co-Director of the Doctoral Program in Gerontology, Department of Sociology, Anthropology, and Public Health, University of Maryland, Baltimore County (UMBC), Department of Epidemiology and Public Health, Secondary Appointment, School of Medicine, University of Maryland, Baltimore, Maryland, USA

KALPANA N. SHANKAR, MD, MSc, MSHP
Adjunct Assistant Professor, Department of Emergency Medicine, Brigham and Women's Hospital, Boston, Massachusetts, USA

EMILY K. TSIVITSE, PhD, APRN, AGPCNP
Postdoctoral Fellow, Louis Stokes Veterans Affairs Medical Center, Cleveland, Ohio, USA

KATREN R. TYLER, MD
Clinical Professor of Emergency Medicine, University of California Davis, Sacramento, California, USA

Contents

Older patients are more vulnerable to acute illness or injury because of reduced physiologic reserve associated with aging. Therefore, their assessment in the emergency department (ED) should include not only vital signs
and their baseline values but also changes that reflect physiologic reserve,
such as mobility, mental status, and frailty. Combining aggregated vitals
sign scores and frailty might improve risk stratification in the ED. Implementing these changes in ED assessment may require the introduction
of senior-friendly processes to ensure ED treatment is appropriate to the
older patients' immediate discomfort, personal goals, and likely prognosis.

Nonspecific complaints such as generalized weakness and fatigue are
common in older adults presenting to an emergency department. These
complaints may be caused by acute or chronic medical problems, or
they may be exacerbated or caused by socioeconomic risks factors. Acute
causes may be related to serious medical conditions requiring prompt
treatment. A thorough history and physical examination in conjunction
with an interdisciplinary approach allows emergency departments to identify acute conditions as well as geriatric syndromes and unmet home
needs, such as food insecurity and caregiver burden. A whole-health system approach should be used for safe transitions of care.

Of 4 older adults, 1 will fall each year in the United States. Based on 2020
data from the Centers of Disease Control, about 36 million older adults fall
each year, resulting in 32,000 deaths. Emergency departments see about
3 million older adults for fall-related injuries with falls having the ability to
cause serious injury such as catastrophic head injuries and hip fractures.
One-third of older fall patients discharged from the ED experience one
of these outcomes at 3 months.

Trauma in the older adult will increasingly become important to emergency physicians hoping to optimize their patient care. The geriatric patient population possesses higher rates of comorbidities that increase their risk for trauma and make their care more challenging. By considering the nuances that accompany the critical stabilization and injury-specific management of geriatric trauma patients, emergency physicians can decrease the prevalence of adverse outcomes.

This article covers the epidemiology of delirium and the overlapping condition of altered mental status and encephalopathy that is relevant to those who practice in the emergency department.

Elder mistreatment is experienced by 5% to 15% of community-dwelling older adults each year. An emergency department (ED) encounter offers an important opportunity to identify elder mistreatment and initiate intervention. Strategies to improve detection of elder mistreatment include identifying high-risk patients; recognizing suggestive findings from the history, physical examination, imaging, and laboratory tests; and/or using screening tools. ED management of elder mistreatment includes addressing acute issues, maximizing the patient's safety, and reporting to the authorities when appropriate.

Three-quarters of patients over the age of 65 visit the emergency department (ED) in the last six months of their lives. Approximately 20% of hospice residents have ED visits. These patients must decide whether to receive emergency care that prioritizes life support, which may not achieve their desired outcomes and might even be futile. The patients in these end-of-life stages could benefit from early palliative care or hospice consultation before they present to the ED. Furthermore, early integration of palliative care at the time of ED visits is important in establishing the goals of the entire treatment.

Emergency department (ED) care for persons living with dementia (PLWD) involves the identification of dementia or cognitive impairment, ED care which is sensitive to the specific needs of PLWD, effective communication with PLWD, their care partners, and outpatient clinicians who the patient and care-partner know and trust, and care-transitions from the emergency department to other health care settings. The recommendations in this article made based on wide-ranging heterogeneous studies of various

Older adults experiencing social isolation and impairments in functional status or cognition represent unique populations that are particularly at risk during ED-to-community transitions of care and may benefit from targeted intervention implementation. Future efforts should target optimizing screening techniques to identify those at risk, developing and validating patient-centered outcome measures, and using policy and reimbursement levers to include transitional care management services for older adults within the ED setting.

This article introduces core topics in health equity scholarship and provides examples of how diversity, equity, and inclusion impact the aging population and emergency care of older adults. It offers strategies for promoting diversity, equity, and inclusion to both strengthen the patient–clinician therapeutic relationship and to address operations and systems that impact care of the geriatric emergency department patient.

CLINICS IN GERIATRIC MEDICINE

ISSUES OF RELATED INTEREST

Medical Clinics of North America
https://www.medical.theclinics.com/
Primary Care: Clinics in Office Practice
https://www.primarycare.theclinics.com/
Emergency Medicine Clinics
https://www.emed.theclinics.com

THE CLINICS ARE AVAILABLE ONLINE!
Access your subscription at:
www.theclinics.com

Foreword

Dr Nascher Would Be Pleased

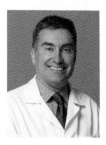

G. Michael Harper, MD
Consulting Editor

Clinicians have not always recognized that caring for older adults requires specialized knowledge and skills. Although the term "geriatrics" first appeared in print well over 100 years ago, it took most of the twentieth century for Geriatric Medicine to gain a foothold as a distinct medical specialty. Dr Ignatz Leo Nascher, an Austrian American pharmacist and physician, coined the term in a 1909 article published in the *New York Medical Journal*.[1] He realized that old age, which he called senility, "is a distinct period of life" and that older people require a unique approach to care just as children do. Over time the study of aging became a distinct field of research, and new models to care for older adults eventually began to emerge. However, it wasn't until 1988, nearly 80 years after Nascher's landmark article, that the US Accreditation Council for Graduate Medical Education (ACGME) accredited the first clinical geriatrics fellowship programs, and the first certifying examination in geriatric medicine was offered jointly by the American Board of Internal Medicine and the American Board of Family Medicine.

The story of Geriatric Emergency Medicine is not unlike that of Geriatric Medicine except that it unfolded on a comparatively accelerated timeline. Much like Dr Nascher, visionary pioneers in Emergency Medicine observed that older adults requiring emergency care also would benefit from a new and different clinical model. As Dr Teresita Hogan and her colleagues put it in a 2023 article published in the *Journal of Geriatric Emergency Medicine*, "The standard emergency approach that excels in the young, fails in older patients."[2] In 1990, the term "Geriatric Emergency Medicine" made its print debut in *Emergency Medicine Clinics of North America*, a sister publication to this one, in an issue that was dedicated to the subject.[3] Over the following 30 years, progress occurred at a stunning rate with the publication of the first Geriatric Emergency Medicine textbook in 1996, creation of geriatric core competencies for emergency medicine residents in 2010, and accreditation of the first Geriatric Emergency Departments by the American College of Emergency Physicians in 2018.[4]

Clin Geriatr Med 39 (2023) xiii–xiv
https://doi.org/10.1016/j.cger.2023.07.001
0749-0690/23/© 2023 Published by Elsevier Inc.

That brings me to this outstanding issue of *Clinics in Geriatric Medicine*, our third issue since 2013 devoted to Geriatric Emergency Medicine, and expertly curated by our guest editors, Drs Maura Kennedy and Shan W. Liu. This issue updates important topics covered in previous issues like falls, pain management, elder mistreatment, and delirium while providing new insights about frailty and dementia care. For those who want to bring age-friendly care to their emergency department, there is an article describing what it takes to do so. If Dr Nascher were alive today, he would read this issue with amazement and delight to see what one simple word, "geriatrics," has grown to become.

G. Michael Harper, MD
Professor of Medicine
University of California
San Francisco
4150 Clement Street, Box 181G
San Francisco, CA 94121, USA

E-mail address:
Michael.Harper@ucsf.edu

REFERENCES

1. Nascher IL. NY Med J 1909;90:358–9.
2. Hogan TM, Gerson LW, Sanders AB. The History of Geriatric Emergency Medicine. J Geriatr Emerg Med 2023;4(1):1–21. https://doi.org/10.17294/2694-4715.1044.
3. Adams J, Wolfson AB. Ethical issues in geriatric emergency medicine. Emerg Med Clin North Am 1990;8:183–92.
4. Carpenter CR, Melady D, Krausz C, et al. Improving Emergency Department Care for Aging Missourians: Guidelines, Accreditation, and Collaboration. Missouri medicine 2017;114:447–52.

Preface

Geriatric Emergency Medicine: The Need Has Never Been Greater

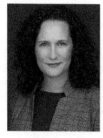 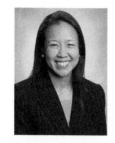

Maura Kennedy, MD, MPH   Shan W. Liu, MD, SD
Editors

The *Clinics in Geriatric Medicine* first published an issue on geriatric emergency medicine a decade ago. Since that original issue in 2013, the field of geriatric emergency medicine has grown tremendously,[1] as has the need for expertise and training in geriatric emergency care.[2] With the aging of the population, we have seen a significant increase in emergency department (ED) visits by older adults, including growing numbers of ED visits for geriatric-specific conditions, such as falls.[3,4] Since the publication of the most recent geriatric emergency medicine issue of *Clinics in Geriatric Medicine* in 2018, we experienced a global pandemic that disproportionately affected the older population in terms of morbidity and mortality. Years later, we are still seeing the COVID-19 pandemic's impact on older adults, including diminished function and functional reserve, loneliness, and anxiety.[5–7] Globally, EDs are experiencing high levels of crowding, exacerbated by the COVID-19 pandemic, impacting the care provided older adults in the ED.[8]

Giving us hope is the tremendous growth we have seen in the field of geriatric emergency medicine and the recognition of this important field. The geriatric ED guidelines had just been published at the time of the first geriatric emergency issue of *Clinics in Geriatric Medicine*. Now over 400 EDs across five countries have received geriatric ED accreditation from the American College of Emergency Physicians.[1] The knowledge base for geriatric emergency care has grown substantially due to contributions from researchers focusing on geriatric emergency care, including the Geriatric Emergency Care Applied Research (GEAR) network.[9] Efforts to translate knowledge into practice is occurring globally, including the Geriatric Emergency Department Collaborative toolkits,[10] international efforts to update the Geriatric ED guidelines using the GRADE approach, the Silver Book II guidelines from the British Geriatric Society,[11]

Clin Geriatr Med 39 (2023) xv–xvii
https://doi.org/10.1016/j.cger.2023.06.003
0749-0690/23/© 2023 Published by Elsevier Inc.

and the European Society for Emergency Medicine posters project.[12] Education in geriatric emergency medicine has also expanded with growing numbers of geriatric emergency medicine fellowships,[2] online geriatric emergency medicine curricula for medical students and residents,[13] and Webinars and online curricula for emergency clinicians available through the Geriatric Emergency Department Collaborative[14,15] and geriatric emergency medicine organizations across the world.

This 2023 geriatric emergency medicine issue of the *Clinics of Geriatric Medicine* updates prior issues and moves the field forward in several ways. The first article is a novel one, looking at physiologic reserve and frailty from the ED perspective. The delirium article has been updated to include information on delirium prevention in the ED setting. The article "Optimizing the Care of Persons with Dementia in Emergency Department," which focuses on the emergency care of persons with dementia, leverages new research from the GEAR network. Given the growth in accredited geriatric EDs, a full article has been dedicated to developing a geriatric ED. Finally, we conclude the issue with a new article exploring the important topic of diversity, equity, and inclusion through the lens of geriatric emergency care.

This work stands on the shoulders of those geriatric emergency medicine leaders who established the field and mentored so many who are now leading the field and mentoring the next generation of leaders. We dedicate this issue to the founding leaders of this field and to our colleagues who stepped forward to combat a global pandemic, who fight to dismantle racism and ageism, and who strive to improve the emergency care of older adults worldwide.

Maura Kennedy, MD, MPH
Department of Emergency Medicine
Massachusetts General Hospital
55 Fruit Street
Boston, MA 02114, USA

Shan W. Liu, MD, SD
Department of Emergency Medicine
Massachusetts General Hospital
55 Fruit Street
Boston, MA 02114, USA

E-mail addresses:
mkennedy8@partners.org (M. Kennedy)
sliu1@mgh.harvard.edu (S.W. Liu)

REFERENCES

1. Hogan TM, Gerson LW, Sanders AB. The history of geriatric emergency medicine. J Geriatr Emerg Med 2023;4(1):1–21. https://doi.org/10.17294/2694-4715.1044.

2. Rosen T, Liu SW, Cameron-Comasco L, et al. Geriatric emergency medicine fellowships: current state of specialized training for emergency physicians in optimizing care for older adults. AEM Educ Train 2020;4(S1):S122–9. https://doi.org/10.1002/aet2.10428.

3. Santangelo I, Ahmad S, Liu S, et al. Examination of geriatric care processes implemented in level 1 and level 2 geriatric emergency departments. J Geriatr Emerg Med 2022;3(4). https://doi.org/10.17294/2694-4715.1041.

4. Shankar KN, Liu SW, Ganz DA. Trends and characteristics of emergency department visits for fall-related injuries in older adults, 2003-2010. West J Emerg Med 2017;18(5):785–93. https://doi.org/10.5811/WESTJEM.2017.5.33615.
5. Hoffman GJ, Malani PN, Solway E, et al. Changes in activity levels, physical functioning, and fall risk during the COVID-19 pandemic. J Am Geriatr Soc 2022; 70(1):49–59. https://doi.org/10.1111/JGS.17477.
6. Kirkland SA, Griffith LE, Oz UE, et al. Increased prevalence of loneliness and associated risk factors during the COVID-19 pandemic: findings from the Canadian Longitudinal Study on Aging (CLSA). BMC Public Health 2023;23(1). https://doi.org/10.1186/S12889-023-15807-4.
7. Seifert A, Hassler B. Impact of the COVID-19 pandemic on loneliness among older adults. Front Sociol 2020;5:590935. https://doi.org/10.3389/FSOC.2020.590935/BIBTEX.
8. Kelen GD, Wolfe R, D'onofrio G, et al. Emergency department crowding: the canary in the health care system. *NEJM Catalyst Innovations in Care*. Delivery 2021; 2(5). https://doi.org/10.1056/CAT.21.0217.
9. Hwang U, Carpenter C, Dresden S, et al. The Geriatric Emergency Care Applied Research (GEAR) network approach: a protocol to advance stakeholder consensus and research priorities in geriatrics and dementia care in the emergency department. BMJ Open 2022;12:60974. https://doi.org/10.1136/bmjopen-2022-060974.
10. Geriatric Emergency Department Collaborative. Geriatric emergency department collaborative toolkits. Available at: https://gedcollaborative.com/resources/implementation-toolkits/. Accessed October 6, 2023.
11. Conroy S, Carpenter C, Banerjee J. Silver book II: quality care for older people with urgent care needs. 2021. Available at: https://www.bgs.org.uk/resources/resource-series/silver-book-ii. Accessed June 10, 2023.
12. European Society for Emergency Medicine, European Geriatric Medicine Society. Geriatric emergency medicine project. Available at: https://posters.geriemeurope.eu/info/geriem/. Accessed October 6, 2023.
13. Clerkship Directors in Emergency Medicine. M4 curriculum. Available at: https://www.saem.org/about-saem/academies-interest-groups-affiliates2/cdem/for-students/online-education/m4-curriculum. Accessed October 6, 2023.
14. Geriatric Emergency Department Collaborative. On-demand webinars. Available at: https://gedcollaborative.com/events/on-demand-webinars/. Accessed October 6, 2023.
15. Geriatric Emergency Department Collaborative. Online learning. Available at: https://gedcollaborative.com/online-learning/. Accessed October 6, 2023.

Assessing Physiologic Reserve and Frailty in the Older Emergency Department Patient: Should the Paradigm Change?

Christian H. Nickel, MD[a],*, John Kellett, MD[b]

KEYWORDS

- Frailty • Clinical frailty scale • NEWS • Aggregated vital sign score • Prognostication
- Undertriage

KEY POINTS

- Vital signs in older adults are neither sensitive nor specific for the prediction of severe illness, ICU admission, or death.
- Inappropriate interpretation of vital sign changes may result in undertriage, which may result in delayed or inadequate treatment of older patients in the emergency department.
- Mental status, mobility, and frailty can improve the assessment of an older adults' severity of illness.
- A number of tools are available for use in the emergency department to assess for frailty and physiologic reserve.

INTRODUCTION

Since 1990, patients aged 85 years and older have been the fastest growing segment of the population.[1] Older adults are key service users of the emergency department (ED). Unfortunately, this has only been reflected recently in training programs for emergency providers.[2–5] Furthermore, despite publication of the Geriatric Emergency Department Guidelines 10 years ago, most EDs do not currently adhere to these guidelines.[6]

As we age, our physiology is constantly changing at structural, functional, and molecular levels, and the maximal function of our vital organs declines. This physiologic decline in maximum organ performance is roughly linear and parallel for all our major organs; it starts early in life and proceeds at about 1.5% per year.[7] However, variations

[a] Emergency Department, University Hospital Basel, University of Basel, Petersgraben 2, Basel CH-4031, Switzerland; [b] Department of Emergency Medicine, Odense University Hospital, University of Southern Denmark, Denmark
* Corresponding author.
E-mail address: christian.nickel@usb.ch
Twitter: @replynickel (C.H.N.)

Clin Geriatr Med 39 (2023) 475–489
https://doi.org/10.1016/j.cger.2023.05.004
0749-0690/23/© 2023 Elsevier Inc. All rights reserved.

in this rate between individuals and between different organs in the same individual can result in some of us aging at a faster rate than our chronological age or some of our organs failing ahead of others. All these changes are variable from patient to patient and in combination often create a complex clinical picture that must be interpreted accurately in the acutely ill older patient, which changes are acute and recoverable and which are permanent and at best can only be ameliorated. Therefore, it is important to differentiate between "biological age" and "chronological age."[8,9] For most of us, decline in physiologic reserve does not prevent us from doing everything we want or need to do until we are over 70 years of age, and it is usually not until the last 2 years or so of life that causes significant morbidity. Paradoxically, despite the secular increase in life expectancy, this period of morbidity before death has become compressed and may be further compressed by promoting lifestyle and other interventions.[10]

VITAL SIGN INTERPRETATION IN OLDER EMERGENCY DEPARTMENT PATIENTS

Vital signs are the cheapest and most easily available objective measure of illness or injury severity in the ED; the five traditional vital signs of respiratory rate, temperature, pulse rate, blood pressure, and oxygen saturation are indicators of hypoperfusion and hypoxaemia, which are the final common pathways of clinical deterioration and death.[11] Changes in vital signs are compensatory and represent the body's attempt to restore circulatory homeostasis, which depends on its physiologic reserve that diminishes with age. **Table 1** outlines the important physiologic changes associated with aging.

Unfortunately, there is no consensus on what vital sign values are normal, and textbooks report significant variations in their "normal" resting ranges.[12] Moreover, overreliance on the "values" of vital signs reduces the patient to a series of numbers, so that treatment is often simplistically directed at returning values to within the normal range. The UK National Early Warning Score (NEWS) was based on an aggregated vital sign score designed to predict death within 24 hours regardless of patient age and assigns a score of zero to vital sign values with the lowest risk of death within 24 hours[13]; it could be argued that these "least likely to die within 24 hours" values could be considered "normal." However, age considerably influences the ability of NEWS to predict mortality after 24 hours, and a severe underestimation in-hospital mortality risk is observed in patients aged 80 years and older.[14] Furthermore, although patients hospitalized with "normal" vital signs have a low risk of imminent death, they make up a significant fraction of all in-hospital deaths.[15] Therefore, estimating risk with traditional vital signs alone is inaccurate in older patients[16] who may present to the ED with "normal" values even if they have severe illness or injury. As they are neither sensitive nor specific for the prediction of severe illness, intensive care unit (ICU) admission, or death in older adults, vital sign values in older patients should be interpreted with caution.[17] Inappropriate interpretation of vital sign changes may result in undertriage which may result in delayed or inadequate treatment of older ED patients[18]; consideration of vital signs has been shown to increase the level of acuity assessed at triage, which was especially so in the case of older patients.[19] However, although vital sign changes are important for many triage decisions, several other factors should be considered before deciding if a vital sign adequately captures a patient's severity of illness.

FACTORS TO CONSIDER IN ADDITION TO VITAL SIGN CHANGES
Mental Status

The brain is a priority organ whose function must be defended at all costs. Therefore, any change in mental function should be looked and taken seriously. Although

Table 1
Physiologic changes of aging (selection)

Cardiovascular System	Clinical Implications
Heart: Diminished coronary artery flow,[122] secondary to coronary artery disease, increased arterial wall thickness, increased pulse pressure Increase in collagen, inflammation, fat deposition, and decreased myocyte number Reduced response to β-adrenergic stimulation[123] *Myocardium*[124]: Preserved systolic function, alterations in left ventricular diastolic function (reduced early diastolic filling, increased late diastolic filling) *Arterial wall*[124]: Increased intimal thickness, reduced compliance Decline in autonomic sensitivity[125]	Increased risk for cardiac ischemia Abnormal EKG in more than 50% of patients aged 65 y and older. Bundle branch block, left axis deviation, prolonged PR and QT intervals.[126] Arrhythmias more common in higher age groups.[127] Resting heart rate increased, maximal heart rate decreased.[128] Blunted heart rate response to stressors; consequence is heart relying on increasing preload and stroke volume for increase in cardiac output, that is, sensitive to hypovolemia. Older heart dependent on the Frank–Starling mechanism to maintain stroke volume Increased systolic blood pressure (50% in patients aged 60 y and older), increased afterload, reduced cardiovascular reserve as well as increased the risk of heart failure. High prevalence of orthostatic hypotension
Lung: Decreased compliance, decreased respiratory muscles, diaphragm weakness, decreased response to hypoxemia and hypercapnia[129] Decrease in diffusion capacity of about 5% per decade after age 40 y	Reduced ventilatory response to both hypercapnia and hypoxia (by approximately 50%).[130] Decreased respiratory reserve; patients often appear "normal" during respiratory decline,[129] but decompensate rapidly[131]
Kidney: Decrease in glomerular filtration rate[132] starts at around age 30 y and continues to decline at a rate of about 1 mL per year[133] *Tubular dysfunction:* Reduced secretion of potassium and to a reduced reabsorption of sodium, calcium, and magnesium[133] Less tonicity of kidney medulla compared to younger adults. Reduction in the antidiuretic hormone effect resulting in a reduction in the water reabsorption capability[133]	Serum creatinine should remain normal with aging as loss of muscle is proportional to decreased glomerular filtration rate (GFR) Renal tubular system more vulnerable to hypoxia or toxic agents[133] Higher susceptibility to hyperkalemia in response to potassium sparing diuretics Reduction of water reabsorption capability making patients more susceptible to dehydration

advanced stage dementia and hyperactive delirium may be obvious, subtle alteration of mental status is often not noticed.[20,21] There are five components to mental status: arousal, memory, thought content, mood, and behavior. Abnormal levels of arousal is associated with mortality,[22,23] and patients with it on admission to hospital are common.[24–27] Changes in arousal are the most frequently monitored using a range of scales such as the Glasgow Coma Scale,[28] AVPU (Alert, responds to Verbal stimulus, responds to Painful stimulus and Unresponsive) scale, and the Richmond Agitation-Sedation Scale.[29] An "altered mental status" or a reduced level of arousal of acute onset, in the absence of trauma, is specific for delirium in older patients.[24,26,27,30] Conversely, the absence of a chief complaint of "altered mental status" does not mean that delirium is absent. It will be missed unless it is actively evaluated using a validated delirium assessment tool.[24] The Confusion Assessment Method (CAM score),[31] its modifications such as the rapid clinical test for delirium, 4 A test (4AT) score and brief confusion assessment method (bCAM,)[32] and several others have become the standard method of assessment.[33,34] A toolkit for delirium identification, prevention, and management has been created.[35] To date, however, there is a lack of ED-based interventional studies demonstrating delirium prevention and treatment in the ED, and few ED interventions have demonstrated to reduce delirium incidence and its duration.[33,36]

Mobility

Impaired mobility and functional capacity have long been recognized as a feature of serious acute illness, which was reported as prostration or "taking to the bed" in older texts.[37]

More recently, it was demonstrated in community-living older persons that bed rest increased steeply about 3 to 5 months before death.[38] "Taking to bed" may, therefore, be a sign of impending death, which should prompt consideration of end-of-life discussions.[38] In the past, bed rest was the recommended and often the only treatment of serious illness, and loss of functional capacity for albeit younger patients with severe acute illness was usually transient and recoverable. However, in 1947, Dr Richard Asher warned of "the dangers of going to bed"[39] as hospitalization itself can cause loss of function; during an acute hospitalization, older adults spend approximately 83% of their hospital stay in bed and 12% of their time in a chair.[40] Prolonged immobility while in hospital is associated with declines in muscle strength, muscle mass, and both cognitive and physical function.[41,42] Conversely, early physical and/or occupational therapy may be useful to shorten delirium duration.[43]

Gait, cognition, and falls are closely related,[44] and poor gait performance can be used as a predictor of dementia.[45] Gait speed is the time taken to walk 10 m measured by a stopwatch[46] and has been proposed as the "sixth vital sign."[47] Gait speed predicts hospitalization and the risk of decline in health and function in older people[48] and may also be used as a screening test for frailty in acutely ill older people[49–53] Slow gait speed (<0.8 m/s) has high sensitivity for identifying frailty.[53] Of note, the gait speed required to use pedestrian crossings in the United Kingdom is ≥ 1.2 m/s[54] Gait speed can also monitor the progression of frailty,[50,55] recovery from illness, and the need for support patients may require after discharge.[56,57] A reduction of 0.1 m/s in gait speed increases the risk of early mortality by 12%,[58] whereas a gait speed greater than 1 m per second (2.2 mph) identifies individuals who can probably live independently and are less likely to be hospitalized or suffer an adverse event if they are admitted.[57]

FRAILTY AS A "VITAL SIGN"

The inclusion of frailty as a "vital sign" in the ED has been suggested as a way to improve triage assessment of illness severity.[4,59–62] Frailty is a state of increased vulnerability to stressor events making older adults living with frailty prone to adverse outcomes such as falls, delirium, and disability as well as prolonged recovery and increased mortality.[63–66] Such stressors could be minor, for example, a change in medication, resulting in substantial deterioration of the usual state. Typical ED presentations of frail older adults are falls, acute confusion with fluctuating course (delirium), "nonspecific" symptoms such as weakness and fatigue, and fluctuating disability.[63,65,67,68]

There are two conceptual models of frailty: the phenotype model and the cumulative deficit model.[66,69] Fried and colleagues identify frailty by the presence of at least three of five phenotypic features: reduced grip strength, slow gait speed, recent weight loss, exhaustion, and low levels of physical activity.[66] The frailty phenotype model requires measurements of grip strength and gait speed. Such measurements might not be feasible in the ED, and self-reporting is frequently flawed.[70] Alternatively, Rockwood and colleagues defined frailty as cumulative deficits, which indicate biological age. This age-related health deficit accumulation is measured with the "frailty index," which is the number of deficits present, divided by the number of deficits that were counted.[71] The more health deficits there are, the greater the risk of adverse outcomes. In this model, no single feature is necessary for diagnosis, and an overall picture is built through summing deficits found on assessment.[69] Both conceptual models are in use and identify older adults at greater risk.[72] Frailty should not be confused with multi-morbidity.[73] Although these concepts are related, they are different entities[74]; comorbidity reflects those organs in an individual that have prematurely "failed" ahead of the rest of the body, whereas frailty is an indicator of "biological" age[8,9] and is, therefore, a better predictor of mortality than "chronological" age.[75]

WHY ASSESS FRAILTY IN THE EMERGENCY DEPARTMENT?

The key functions of the ED are to identify patients who cannot wait to be seen and vulnerable or frail older adults at risk of adverse outcomes such as repeated ED visits, hospitalization, disability, institutionalization, and death.[76–79] These patients should be accurately identified soon after their presentation and their needs expertly assessed so that additional resources are made available if required and to ensure their management is appropriate to their immediate discomfort, personal goals of care, and likely prognosis.[80]

HOW TO ASSESS FRAILTY OR VULNERABILITY IN THE EMERGENCY DEPARTMENT?

Many ED clinicians use their clinical judgment rather than screening tools to assess patient vulnerability and frailty.[81] However, compared with formal scales, clinical judgment may not be a reliable or accurate process,[82] as the assessment of frailty by clinical judgment can be subject to variation.[81] Furthermore, frailty is not a dichotomous "black or white" state; there are various degrees of frailty and these correspond with increasing risk of adverse outcomes.

The multidisciplinary comprehensive geriatric assessment (CGA) is the gold standard for identifying frail older patients[83]; however, it takes time to complete and is labor intensive. Therefore, quicker frailty assessment tools have been studied as alternatives that might be practical to use in the ED. For example, frailty can be easily assessed using the Clinical Frailty Scale (CFS) which is one of the most frequently used frailty measures in the urgent care setting[84] and been validated for use in the ED.[85–87] It is a 9-point scale with pictographs and clinical descriptions that help to assign scores ranging from very fit (score 1) to terminally ill (score 9). It has recently been updated to version 2.0 with revised level headings to address the caveat that the habitual health state of patients 2 weeks before acute illness should be assessed[88] (https://www.dal.ca/sites/gmr/our-tools/clinical-frailty-scale.html). The CFS is an independent predictor for hospital admission, in-hospital mortality, 1-month survival after ICU admission, survival 1 year after traumatic injury, outcomes after cardiopulmonary resuscitation, and predictor of hospital length of stay.[87,89–92] In addition, when assessed early in the ED, the CFS predicts 1-year all-cause mortality and predicts survival time in a graded manner.[93] This is important as the prediction windows of vital sign abnormalities and triage acuity estimates have short-lived validity and should not be used for long-term prognostication.[94]

Although the adoption of the CFS is feasible in the ED,[81] there is controversy regarding its ease of use.[95] Other vulnerability and frailty assessment tools are available, such as the Tilburg Frailty Indicator for community-dwelling older adults,[96] the Fatigue, Resistance, Ambulation, Illnesses and Loss of Weight Scale (validated in a late middle-aged African American population),[97] and the seven question tool of the Program on Research for Integrating Services of the Maintenance of Autonomy.[98] Some of these tools have been studied in the acute care setting[99,100] or have successfully been implemented in routine ED care.[5,101–103]

The Dutch Acutely Presenting Older Patient screener[61] uses seven functional and cognitive domains to predict the risk of functional decline and mortality within 3 months of ED presentation and is now widely used in Dutch EDs. It takes 2 minutes to complete and was demonstrated to potentially improve triage decisions.[101] External validation, however, demonstrated limited prognostic accuracy for adverse health outcomes up to 6 months after ED presentation.[104] The interRAI ED Contact Assessment is an assessment and clinical decision support tool that assesses various domains including function, cognition, and symptoms. It has been shown to predict long hospital lengths of stay and readmissions among older ED patients.[105] Although it can be used to identify 25% of older patients who need a CGA, only 5% of these patients assessed by CGA were subsequently referred for geriatric services by their treating physician.[106]

It remains controversial which frailty screening tool is the most suitable for the ED setting, as there are often barriers to implementation, such as concerns about increasing workload, and lack of clear evidence that using a screening tool is beneficial.[95] For example, a meta-analysis failed to show that using either the Identification of Seniors at Risk Tool or the Triage Risk Screening Tool meaningfully increased or decreased the risk of adverse outcomes.[103]

SHOULD FRAILTY ASSESSMENT BE PART OF THE EMERGENCY DEPARTMENT TRIAGE PROCESS?

Triage determines if a patient can wait to be seen or not, and the wait time depends on the patients' distress, their risk of imminent death or morbidity, and their need for time-dependent interventions and treatment (**Fig. 1**). Patients with normal physiologic reserve can often wait, as they are likely to recover from most acute illness/injury more time is available to consider treatment, which may not even be needed. In contrast, we believe that frail acutely ill/injured patients with reduced physiologic reserve should not wait as long, as their medical condition may be more likely to acutely decline making them less likely to recover as the effectiveness of any treatment is probably more time-dependent.

In practice, the risk of imminent death and morbidity and need to be evaluated immediately is initially made by rapid assessment of "acuity" and/or some generally accepted specific indicators such as unresponsiveness, apnoea, respiratory distress, fitting, toxin exposure, and so forth. These rapid intuitive assessments are then usually supplemented by vital sign measurements. Frailty and triage acuity seem to be complimentary measures[107,108] Specifically, in older ED patients, the CFS outperforms mortality prediction by the Emergency Severity Index (ESI).[87] As longer waiting time is a notable risk factor for older patients,[109] they should not wait, yet the ESI assigned 20% of frail patients aged 65 years and older to "can wait to be seen" triage levels (ie, ESI levels 3–5).[87] Either alone or in combination with an aggregated vital sign score, the CFS has been shown to be independently associated with 30-day mortality, even after adjustment for chronological age, a comorbidity index, and a history of

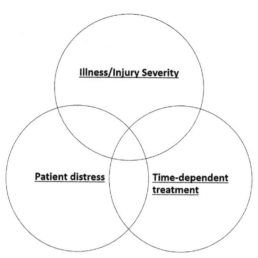

Fig. 1. The factors at triage that determine if a patient can wait and how they overlap.

dementia.[110] In acutely ill hospitalized patients, the association of frailty with mortality was found to be greatest in those with the most severe illness,[111] and in patients hospitalized in an internal medicine department those with the highest triage acuity levels on presentation had the highest mortality across all levels of frailty.[112] Therefore, as both frailty and illness/injury severity combined are strong, independent, and complementary predictors of adverse patient outcomes, we believe that they should both be part of the ED triage process of older patients.[86,87,113] Both the ESI and the CFS can be quickly determined with similar and little effort. It should be possible to do both routinely to prevent the undertriage of frail older patients.[18,87,114,115]

CAN FRAILTY ASSESSMENT CHANGE THE PROCESS OF EMERGENCY DEPARTMENT CARE?

For non-frail patients without acute illness, time is available for investigations to ensure the correct diagnosis is made. However, for patients living with frailty suffering from acute illness or injury, estimating their likely prognosis over the coming months and years is needed to ensure realistic goals of treatment are set and wise management decisions made. Recently, the Frailty-adjusted Prognosis in ED tool (FaP-ED), which predicts 30-day mortality combining by frailty and aggregated vital signs was developed to effectively capture "geriatric disease/injury severity" in a consecutive sample of older ED patients[62]; vital signs were aggregated using the NEWS, and frailty level was determined with the CFS (**Fig. 2**). These types of tool should not replace clinical judgment but rather support it; their prognostic estimates could quickly guide (resuscitative) decision-making that is appropriately aligned with what matters most to the patient.[87] Although frailty assessment in the ED should not lead to premature exclusion of management options or therapeutic nihilism, early frailty identification might help guide diagnostic testing and formulation of appropriate treatment plans as well as identifying those patients who might benefit from (components of) a CGA.[62]

Further ED-based frailty research should evaluate when and how frailty should be used to assess acute illness and injury severity, so that health care utilization and patient outcomes are improved.[116] Although a Cochrane review found that performing a CGA increased the chances of patients returning to independent living in their own

NEWS	1-2	3	4	5	6	7	8
9	1.9%	9.8%	6.1%	29.0%	31.0%	32.0%	51.0%
8	1.4%	7.7%	4.7%	24.0%	25.0%	26.0%	45.0%
7	1.1%	6.0%	3.7%	19.0%	21.0%	22.0%	38.0%
6	0.9%	4.7%	2.9%	15.0%	17.0%	17.0%	32.0%
5	0.7%	3.6%	2.2%	12.0%	13.0%	14.0%	27.0%
4	0.5%	2.8%	1.7%	9.7%	11.0%	11.0%	22.0%
3	0.4%	2.2%	1.3%	7.6%	8.4%	8.7%	18.0%
2	0.3%	1.7%	1.0%	5.9%	6.6%	6.8%	14.0%
1	0.2%	1.3%	0.8%	4.6%	5.1%	5.3%	11.0%
0	0.2%	1.0%	0.6%	3.6%	4.0%	4.2%	8.9%

CFS

Fig. 2. Prediction of older individuals' probability of 30-day mortality (FaP-ED tool) based on an aggregated vital sign score (the National Early Warning Score [NEWS]) and a measure of frailty (the Clinical Frailty Scale [CFS]).[62] Further information, including performance criteria are available at: https://sorenkabellnissen.shinyapps.io/FrailtyPrognosticationED/.

homes at 3 months, and fewer people were admitted to a nursing home at 1 year,[117] undertaking a complete CGA on every older ED patient is unrealistic. However, performing components of the CGA, such as addressing the 5 Ms (matters most, mind, mobility, medication, and multi-complexity) in the ED is likely to be beneficial for many older adults by preventing unnecessary hospital admissions, better outcomes if admitted hospital, and fewer readmissions.[118]

SUMMARY

ED processes need to be reconfigured to better identify acuity of illness in older ED patients. Older patients should be streamed through a rapid triage process that assesses their physiologic reserve, which does not require prolonged or detailed interrogation or investigation of patients, their carers, or their medical records but acknowledges and accommodates the patients' vulnerability. Inclusion of frailty assessments in conjunction with vital sign-based triage assessments may help ensure older patient receive timely appropriate care that aligns with their needs, goals, and values.[119–121]

CLINICS CARE POINTS

- Vital signs in older adults should not be interpreted without considering physiologic reserve.
- Measures of physiologic reserve include mental status, mobility, and frailty.
- The Clinical Frailty Scale may be the most feasible frailty scale for the emergency department (ED) setting.
- Combining aggregated vitals sign scores and frailty can improve risk stratification, the assessment of illness, or injury severity and prognostication in older ED patients.
- Senior friendly reconfiguration of ED processes should ensure that the management of frail older patients is appropriate to their illness severity, personal goals, and likely prognosis.

DISCLOSURES

C.H. Nickel: none. J. Kellett: Founder and major shareholder of Tapa Healthcare DAC, a start-up medical software company.

REFERENCES

1. Christensen K, Doblhammer G, Rau R, et al. Ageing populations: the challenges ahead. Lancet 2009;374:1196–208.
2. Lucke JA, Mooijaart SP, Heeren P, et al. Providing care for older adults in the emergency department: expert clinical recommendations from the European task force on geriatric emergency medicine. Eur Geriatr Med 2022;13:309–17.
3. Bellou A, Nickel C, Martín-Sánchez FJ, et al. The European curriculum of geriatric emergency medicine: a collaboration between the European society for emergency medicine (EuSEM) and the European union of geriatric medicine society (EUGMS). Emergencias 2016;28:295–7.
4. Mooijaart SP, Carpenter CR, Conroy SP. Geriatric emergency medicine-a model for frailty friendly healthcare. Age Ageing 2022;51.
5. Geriatric emergency department guidelines. Ann Emerg Med 2014;63:e7–25.
6. Shih RD, Carpenter CR, Tolia V, et al. Balancing vision with pragmatism: the geriatric emergency department guidelines-realistic expectations from emergency medicine and geriatric medicine. J Am Geriatr Soc 2022;70:1368–73.
7. Strehler BL, Mildvan AS. General theory of mortality and aging. Science 1960; 132:14–21.
8. Wick JY. Understanding frailty in the geriatric population. Consult Pharm 2011; 26:634–45.
9. Schuurmans H, Steverink N, Lindenberg S, et al. Old or frail: what tells us more? J Gerontol A Biol Sci Med Sci 2004;59:M962–5.
10. Fries JF, Bruce B, Chakravarty E. Compression of morbidity 1980-2011: a focused review of paradigms and progress. J Aging Res 2011;2011:261702.
11. Gilhooley C, Burnhill G, Gardiner D, et al. Oxygen saturation and haemodynamic changes prior to circulatory arrest: implications for transplantation and resuscitation. J Intensive Care Soc 2019;20:27–33.
12. Grant S. Limitations of track and trigger systems and the National Early Warning Score. Part 1: areas of contention. Br J Nurs 2018;27:624–31.
13. Prytherch DR, Smith GB, Schmidt PE, et al. ViEWS–Towards a national early warning score for detecting adult inpatient deterioration. Resuscitation 2010; 81:932–7.
14. Nissen SK, Candel BGJ, Nickel CH, et al. The impact of age on predictive performance of national early warning score at arrival to emergency departments: development and external validation. Ann Emerg Med 2021;79(4):354–63.
15. Holland M, Kellett J. A systematic review of the discrimination and absolute mortality predicted by the National Early Warning Scores according to different cutoff values and prediction windows. Eur J Intern Med 2022;98:15–26.
16. Schultz M, Rasmussen LJH, Carlson N, et al. Risk assessment models for potential use in the emergency department have lower predictive ability in older patients compared to the middle-aged for short-term mortality - a retrospective cohort study. BMC Geriatr 2019;19:134.
17. Lamantia MA, Stewart PW, Platts-Mills TF, et al. Predictive value of initial triage vital signs for critically ill older adults. West J Emerg Med 2013;14:453–60.
18. Grossmann FF, Zumbrunn T, Frauchiger A, et al. At risk of undertriage? Testing the performance and accuracy of the emergency severity index in older emergency department patients. Ann Emerg Med 2012;60:317–25.e3.
19. Cooper RJ, Schriger DL, Flaherty HL, et al. Effect of vital signs on triage decisions. Ann Emerg Med 2002;39:223–32.
20. Meagher DJ. Delirium: optimising management. Bmj 2001;322:144–9.

21. Hustey FM, Meldon SW. The prevalence and documentation of impaired mental status in elderly emergency department patients. Ann Emerg Med 2002;39: 248–53.
22. Francia E, Torres O, Laiz A, et al. Ability of physiological parameters versus clinical categories to predict mortality on admission to an internal medicine ward. Eur J Intern Med 2009;20:636–9.
23. Duckitt RW, Buxton-Thomas R, Walker J, et al. Worthing physiological scoring system: derivation and validation of a physiological early-warning system for medical admissions. An observational, population-based single-centre study. Br J Anaesth 2007;98:769–74.
24. Han JH, Wilber ST. Altered mental status in older patients in the emergency department. Clin Geriatr Med 2013;29:101–36.
25. Naughton BJ, Moran MB, Kadah H, et al. Delirium and other cognitive impairment in older adults in an emergency department. Ann Emerg Med 1995;25: 751–5.
26. Aslaner MA, Boz M, Çelik A, et al. Etiologies and delirium rates of elderly ED patients with acutely altered mental status: a multicenter prospective study. Am J Emerg Med 2017;35:71–6.
27. Bellelli G, Mazzone A, Morandi A, et al. The effect of an impaired arousal on short- and long-term mortality of elderly patients admitted to an acute geriatric unit. J Am Med Dir Assoc 2016;17:214–9.
28. Teasdale G, Jennett B. Assessment of coma and impaired consciousness. A practical scale. Lancet 1974;2:81–4.
29. Sessler CN, Gosnell MS, Grap MJ, et al. The Richmond Agitation-Sedation Scale: validity and reliability in adult intensive care unit patients. Am J Respir Crit Care Med 2002;166:1338–44.
30. Tieges Z, McGrath A, Hall RJ, et al. Abnormal level of arousal as a predictor of delirium and inattention: an exploratory study. Am J Geriatr Psychiatr 2013;21: 1244–53.
31. Inouye SK, van Dyck CH, Alessi CA, et al. Clarifying confusion: the confusion assessment method. A new method for detection of delirium. Ann Intern Med 1990;113:941–8.
32. Tieges Z, Maclullich AMJ, Anand A, et al. Diagnostic accuracy of the 4AT for delirium detection in older adults: systematic review and meta-analysis. Age Ageing 2021;50:733–43.
33. Carpenter CR, Hammouda N, Linton EA, et al. Delirium prevention, detection, and treatment in emergency medicine settings: a geriatric emergency care applied research (GEAR) network scoping review and consensus statement. Acad Emerg Med 2021;28:19–35.
34. Santangelo IA, Surriya, Liu Shan, et al. Examination of geriatric care processes implemented in level 1 and level 2 geriatric emergency departments. J Geriat Emerg Med 2023;3.
35. Kennedy M, Webb M, Gartaganis S, et al. ED-DEL: Development of a change package and toolkit for delirium in the emergency department. J Am Coll Emerg Physicians Open 2021;2:e12421.
36. Lee S, Chen H, Hibino S, et al. Can we improve delirium prevention and treatment in the emergency department? A systematic review. J Am Geriatr Soc 2022;70:1838–49.
37. Osler SW. The principles and practice of medicine. Designed for the use of practitioners and students of medicine. Fourth Edition. Edinburgh & London: Young J Pentland; 1901 1901.

38. Gill TM, Gahbauer EA, Leo-Summers L, et al. Taking to bed at the end of life. J Am Geriatr Soc 2019;67:1248–52.

39. Asher RA. The dangers of going to bed. Br Med J 1947;2:967.

40. Baldwin C, van Kessel G, Phillips A, et al. Accelerometry shows inpatients with acute medical or surgical conditions spend little time upright and are highly sedentary: systematic review. Phys Ther 2017;97:1044–65.

41. Falvey JR, Mangione KK, Stevens-Lapsley JE. Rethinking hospital-associated deconditioning: proposed paradigm shift. Phys Ther 2015;95:1307–15.

42. Béland E, Nadeau A, Carmichael PH, et al. Predictors of delirium in older patients at the emergency department: a prospective multicentre derivation study. Cjem 2021;23:330–6.

43. Jordano JO, Vasilevskis EE, Duggan MC, et al. Effect of physical and occupational therapy on delirium duration in older emergency department patients who are hospitalized. J Am Coll Emerg Physicians Open 2023;4:e12857.

44. Zhang W, Low LF, Schwenk M, et al. Review of gait, cognition, and fall risks with implications for fall prevention in older adults with dementia. Dement Geriatr Cogn Disord 2019;48:17–29.

45. Beauchet O, Annweiler C, Callisaya ML, et al. Poor gait performance and prediction of dementia: results from a meta-analysis. J Am Med Dir Assoc 2016; 17:482–90.

46. Peters DM, Fritz SL, Krotish DE. Assessing the reliability and validity of a shorter walk test compared with the 10-Meter Walk Test for measurements of gait speed in healthy, older adults. J Geriatr Phys Ther 2013;36:24–30.

47. Fritz S, Lusardi M. White paper: "walking speed: the sixth vital sign". J Geriatr Phys Ther 2009;32:46–9.

48. Studenski S, Perera S, Wallace D, et al. Physical performance measures in the clinical setting. J Am Geriatr Soc 2003;51:314–22.

49. Lewis ET, Dent E, Alkhouri H, et al. Which frailty scale for patients admitted via Emergency Department? A cohort study. Arch Gerontol Geriatr 2019;80:104–14.

50. Viccaro LJ, Perera S, Studenski SA. Is timed up and go better than gait speed in predicting health, function, and falls in older adults? J Am Geriatr Soc 2011;59: 887–92.

51. Podsiadlo D, Richardson S. The timed "Up & Go": a test of basic functional mobility for frail elderly persons. J Am Geriatr Soc 1991;39:142–8.

52. Woo J, Ho SC, Yu AL. Walking speed and stride length predicts 36 months dependency, mortality, and institutionalization in Chinese aged 70 and older. J Am Geriatr Soc 1999;47:1257–60.

53. Clegg A, Rogers L, Young J. Diagnostic test accuracy of simple instruments for identifying frailty in community-dwelling older people: a systematic review. Age Ageing 2015;44:148–52.

54. Asher L, Aresu M, Falaschetti E, et al. Most older pedestrians are unable to cross the road in time: a cross-sectional study. Age Ageing 2012;41:690–4.

55. Subbe CP, Jones S. Predicting speed at traffic lights–the problem with static assessments of frailty. Age Ageing 2015;44:180–1.

56. Peel NM, Kuys SS, Klein K. Gait speed as a measure in geriatric assessment in clinical settings: a systematic review. J Gerontol A Biol Sci Med Sci 2013;68: 39–46.

57. Peel NM, Navanathan S, Hubbard RE. Gait speed as a predictor of outcomes in post-acute transitional care for older people. Geriatr Gerontol Int 2014;14: 906–10.

58. Veronese N, Stubbs B, Volpato S, et al. Association between gait speed with mortality, cardiovascular disease and cancer: a systematic review and meta-analysis of prospective cohort studies. J Am Med Dir Assoc 2018;19:981–8.e7.
59. Cicutto LC. Frailty: is this a new vital sign? Chest 2018;154:1–2.
60. Mooijaart SP, Lucke JA, Brabrand M, et al. Geriatric emergency medicine: time for a new approach on a European level. Eur J Emerg Med 2019;26:75–6.
61. Blomaard LC, Speksnijder C, Lucke JA, et al. Geriatric screening, triage urgency, and 30-day mortality in older emergency department patients. J Am Geriatr Soc 2020;68:1755–62.
62. Kabell Nissen S, Rueegg M, Carpenter CR, et al. Prognosis for older people at presentation to emergency department based on frailty and aggregated vital signs. J Am Geriatr Soc 2022;71(4):1250–8.
63. Clegg A, Young J, Iliffe S, et al. Frailty in elderly people. Lancet 2013;381: 752–62.
64. Eeles EM, White SV, O'Mahony SM, et al. The impact of frailty and delirium on mortality in older inpatients. Age Ageing 2012;41:412–6.
65. Simon NR, Jauslin AS, Bingisser R, et al. Emergency presentations of older patients living with frailty: Presenting symptoms compared with non-frail patients. Am J Emerg Med 2022;59:111–7.
66. Fried LP, Tangen CM, Walston J, et al. Frailty in older adults: evidence for a phenotype. J Gerontol A Biol Sci Med Sci 2001;56:M146–56.
67. Joosten E, Demuynck M, Detroyer E, et al. Prevalence of frailty and its ability to predict in hospital delirium, falls, and 6-month mortality in hospitalized older patients. BMC Geriatr 2014;14:1.
68. Zhang Q, Zhao X, Liu H, et al. Frailty as a predictor of future falls and disability: a four-year follow-up study of Chinese older adults. BMC Geriatr 2020;20:388.
69. Rockwood K, Song X, MacKnight C, et al. A global clinical measure of fitness and frailty in elderly people. CMAJ (Can Med Assoc J) 2005;173:489–95.
70. Roedersheimer KM, Pereira GF, Jones CW, et al. Self-reported versus performance-based assessments of a simple mobility task among older adults in the emergency department. Ann Emerg Med 2016;67:151–6.
71. Rockwood K. Conceptual models of frailty: accumulation of deficits. Can J Cardiol 2016;32:1046–50.
72. Rockwood K, Howlett SE. Fifteen years of progress in understanding frailty and health in aging. BMC Med 2018;16:220.
73. Arendts G, Burkett E, Hullick C, et al. Frailty, thy name is. Emerg Med Australas 2017;29:712–6.
74. Villacampa-Fernández P, Navarro-Pardo E, Tarín JJ, et al. Frailty and multimorbidity: two related yet different concepts. Maturitas 2017;95:31–5.
75. Romero-Ortuno R, Kenny RA. The frailty index in Europeans: association with age and mortality. Age Ageing 2012;41:684–9.
76. Rothman MD, Leo-Summers L, Gill TM. Prognostic significance of potential frailty criteria. J Am Geriatr Soc 2008;56:2211–6.
77. Ensrud KE, Ewing SK, Cawthon PM, et al. A comparison of frailty indexes for the prediction of falls, disability, fractures, and mortality in older men. J Am Geriatr Soc 2009;57:492–8.
78. Cunha AIL, Veronese N, de Melo Borges S, et al. Frailty as a predictor of adverse outcomes in hospitalized older adults: a systematic review and meta-analysis. Ageing Res Rev 2019;56:100960.
79. Jørgensen R, Brabrand M. Screening of the frail patient in the emergency department: a systematic review. Eur J Intern Med 2017;45:71–3.

80. Graf CE, Zekry D, Giannelli S, et al. Efficiency and applicability of comprehensive geriatric assessment in the emergency department: a systematic review. Aging Clin Exp Res 2011;23:244–54.
81. Elliott A, Phelps K, Regen E, et al. Identifying frailty in the Emergency Department—feasibility study. Age Ageing 2017;46:840–5.
82. van Dam CS, Trappenburg MC, Ter Wee MM, et al. The prognostic accuracy of clinical judgment versus a validated frailty screening instrument in older patients at the emergency department: findings of the AmsterGEM study. Ann Emerg Med 2022;80:422–31.
83. Stuck AE, Siu AL, Wieland GD, et al. Comprehensive geriatric assessment: a meta-analysis of controlled trials. Lancet 1993;342:1032–6.
84. Elliott A, Hull L, Conroy SP. Frailty identification in the emergency department—a systematic review focussing on feasibility. Age Ageing 2017;46:509–13.
85. Serina P, Lo AX, Kocherginsky M, et al. The clinical frailty scale and health services use for older adults in the emergency department. J Am Geriatr Soc 2021; 69:837–9.
86. Elliott A, Taub N, Banerjee J, et al. Does the clinical frailty scale at triage predict outcomes from emergency care for older people? Ann Emerg Med 2021;77: 620–7.
87. Kaeppeli T, Rueegg M, Dreher-Hummel T, et al. Validation of the clinical frailty scale for prediction of thirty-day mortality in the emergency department. Ann Emerg Med 2020;76:291–300.
88. Fournaise A, Nissen SK, Lauridsen JT, et al. Translation of the updated clinical frailty scale 2.0 into Danish and implications for cross-sectoral reliability. BMC Geriatr 2021;21:269.
89. Wallis SJ, Wall J, Biram RW, et al. Association of the clinical frailty scale with hospital outcomes. QJM 2015;108:943–9.
90. Guidet B, de Lange DW, Boumendil A, et al. The contribution of frailty, cognition, activity of daily life and comorbidities on outcome in acutely admitted patients over 80 years in European ICUs: the VIP2 study. Intensive Care Med 2020;46: 57–69.
91. Braude P, Carter B, Parry F, et al. Predicting 1 year mortality after traumatic injury using the Clinical Frailty Scale. J Am Geriatr Soc 2022;70:158–67.
92. Mowbray FI, Manlongat D, Correia RH, et al. Prognostic association of frailty with post-arrest outcomes following cardiac arrest: a systematic review and meta-analysis. Resuscitation 2021;167:242–50.
93. Rueegg M, Nissen SK, Brabrand M, et al. The clinical frailty scale predicts 1-year mortality in emergency department patients aged 65 years and older. Acad Emerg Med 2022;29:572–80.
94. Bech CN, Brabrand M, Mikkelsen S, et al. Risk factors associated with short term mortality changes over time, after arrival to the emergency department. Scand J Trauma Resuscitation Emerg Med 2018;26:29.
95. van der Burgh R, Wijnen N, Visscher M, et al. The feasibility and acceptability of frailty screening tools in the Emergency Department and the additional value of clinical judgment for frailty detection. Eur J Emerg Med 2022;29:301–3.
96. Gobbens RJ, van Assen MA, Luijkx KG, et al. The Tilburg frailty indicator: psychometric properties. J Am Med Dir Assoc 2010;11:344–55.
97. Morley JE, Malmstrom TK, Miller DK. A simple frailty questionnaire (FRAIL) predicts outcomes in middle aged African Americans. J Nutr Health Aging 2012;16: 601–8.

98. Raîche M, Hébert R, Dubois M-F. PRISMA-7: a case-finding tool to identify older adults with moderate to severe disabilities. Arch Gerontol Geriatr 2008;47:9–18.

99. Apóstolo J, Cooke R, Bobrowicz-Campos E, et al. Predicting risk and outcomes for frail older adults: an umbrella review of frailty screening tools. JBI Evidence Synthesis 2017;15:1154–208.

100. Theou O, Squires E, Mallery K, et al. What do we know about frailty in the acute care setting? A scoping review. BMC Geriatr 2018;18:139.

101. Blomaard LC, Mooijaart SP, Bolt S, et al. Feasibility and acceptability of the 'Acutely Presenting Older Patient' screener in routine emergency department care. Age Ageing 2020;49:1034–41.

102. Heeren P, Devriendt E, Wellens NIH, et al. Old and new geriatric screening tools in a Belgian emergency department: a diagnostic accuracy study. J Am Geriatr Soc 2020;68:1454–61.

103. Carpenter CR, Shelton E, Fowler S, et al. Risk factors and screening instruments to predict adverse outcomes for undifferentiated older emergency department patients: a systematic review and meta-analysis. Acad Emerg Med 2015; 22:1–21.

104. van Dam CS, Trappenburg MC, Ter Wee MM, et al. The accuracy of four frequently used frailty instruments for the prediction of adverse health outcomes among older adults at two Dutch emergency departments: findings of the AmsterGEM study. Ann Emerg Med 2021;78:538–48.

105. Costa AP, Hirdes JP, Heckman GA, et al. Geriatric syndromes predict postdischarge outcomes among older emergency department patients: findings from the interRAI Multinational Emergency Department Study. Acad Emerg Med 2014;21:422–33.

106. Mowbray FI, Ellis B, Schumacher C, et al. The association between frailty and a nurse-identified need for comprehensive geriatric assessment referral from the emergency department. Can J Nurs Res 2023. 8445621221144667.

107. Romero-Ortuno R, Wallis S, Biram R, et al. Clinical frailty adds to acute illness severity in predicting mortality in hospitalized older adults: an observational study. Eur J Intern Med 2016;35:24–34.

108. Mowbray F, Brousseau AA, Mercier E, et al. Examining the relationship between triage acuity and frailty to inform the care of older emergency department patients: findings from a large Canadian multisite cohort study. Cjem 2020;22: 74–81.

109. Jones S, Moulton C, Swift S, et al. Association between delays to patient admission from the emergency department and all-cause 30-day mortality. Emerg Med J 2022;39:168–73.

110. Romero-Ortuno R, Wallis S, Biram R, et al. Clinical frailty adds to acute illness severity in predicting mortality in hospitalized older adults: an observational study. Eur J Intern Med 2016;35:24–34.

111. Engvig A, Wyller TB, Skovlund E, et al. Association between clinical frailty, illness severity and post-discharge survival: a prospective cohort study of older medical inpatients in Norway. Eur Geriatr Med 2022;13:453–61.

112. Pulok MH, Theou O, van der Valk AM, et al. The role of illness acuity on the association between frailty and mortality in emergency department patients referred to internal medicine. Age Ageing 2020;49:1071–9.

113. Ng CJ, Chien LT, Huang CH, et al. Integrating the clinical frailty scale with emergency department triage systems for elder patients: a prospective study. Am J Emerg Med 2023;66:16–21.

114. Grossmann FF, Zumbrunn T, Ciprian S, et al. Undertriage in older emergency department patients–tilting against windmills? PLoS One 2014;9:e106203.
115. Dreher-Hummel T, Nickel CH, Nicca D, et al. The challenge of interprofessional collaboration in emergency department team triage - an interpretive description. J Adv Nurs 2021;77:1368–78.
116. Lo AX, Kennedy M. Do we really need another risk prediction rule? Yes, we do. Acad Emerg Med 2022;29:678–80.
117. Ellis G, Gardner M, Tsiachristas A, et al. Comprehensive geriatric assessment for older adults admitted to hospital. Cochrane Database Syst Rev 2017;9: Cd006211.
118. Tinetti M, Huang A, Molnar F. The geriatrics 5M's: a new way of communicating what we do. J Am Geriatr Soc 2017;65:2115.
119. Skyttberg N, Vicente J, Chen R, et al. How to improve vital sign data quality for use in clinical decision support systems? A qualitative study in nine Swedish emergency departments. BMC Med Inf Decis Making 2016;16:61.
120. van Oppen JD, Coats TJ, Conroy SP, et al. What matters most in acute care: an interview study with older people living with frailty. BMC Geriatr 2022;22:156.
121. Phelps K, Regen E, van Oppen JD, et al. What are the goals of care for older people living with frailty when they access urgent care? Are those goals attained? A qualitative view of patient and carer perspectives. Int Emerg Nurs 2022;63:101189.
122. Benetos A, Waeber B, Izzo J, et al. Influence of age, risk factors, and cardiovascular and renal disease on arterial stiffness: clinical applications. Am J Hypertens 2002;15:1101–8.
123. Stratton JR, Cerqueira MD, Schwartz RS, et al. Differences in cardiovascular responses to isoproterenol in relation to age and exercise training in healthy men. Circulation 1992;86:504–12.
124. Oxenham H, Sharpe N. Cardiovascular aging and heart failure. Eur J Heart Fail 2003;5:427–34.
125. Chester JG, Rudolph JL. Vital signs in older patients: age-related changes. J Am Med Dir Assoc 2011;12:337–43.
126. Jones J, Srodulski ZM, Romisher S. The aging electrocardiogram. Am J Emerg Med 1990;8:240–5.
127. Aviles RJ, Martin DO, Apperson-Hansen C, et al. Inflammation as a risk factor for atrial fibrillation. Circulation 2003;108:3006–10.
128. Lakatta EG. Cardiovascular aging in health. Clin Geriatr Med 2000;16:419–44.
129. Darden DB, Moore FA, Brakenridge SC, et al. The effect of aging physiology on critical care. Crit Care Clin 2021;37:135–50.
130. Peterson DD, Pack AI, Silage DA, et al. Effects of aging on ventilatory and occlusion pressure responses to hypoxia and hypercapnia. Am Rev Respir Dis 1981;124:387–91.
131. Menaker J, Scalea TM. Geriatric care in the surgical intensive care unit. Crit Care Med 2010;38:S452–9.
132. Denic A, Lieske JC, Chakkera HA, et al. The substantial loss of nephrons in healthy human kidneys with aging. J Am Soc Nephrol 2017;28:313–20.
133. Musso CG. Geriatric nephrology and the 'nephrogeriatric giants'. Int Urol Nephrol 2002;34:255–6.

Nonspecific Complaints in Older Emergency Department Patients

Colleen M. McQuown, MD*, Emily K. Tsivitse, PhD, APRN, AGPCNP

KEYWORDS

- Emergency medicine • Nonspecific complaints • Caregiver • Multidisciplinary

KEY POINTS

- Nonspecific chief complaints are presenting symptoms for which there is no specific working diagnosis or symptoms from a specific body system or organ.
- Nonspecific chief complaints in older emergency department patients may be caused by acute or chronic medical conditions ranging from benign to life threatening.
- The most common specific diagnoses made in older adults with nonspecific chief complaints are infection, heart failure, and electrolyte disturbance.
- Although specific diagnoses can be made for many older patients with nonspecific chief complaints, often patients leave the emergency department with nonspecific diagnoses such as malaise, generalized weakness, or functional impairment.
- Patients who are discharged with a nonspecific diagnosis have a high risk for repeat emergency department visits and hospital admission.

INTRODUCTION

Older adults are frequent users of prehospital emergency services and emergency departments (ED) but are more likely to have nonspecific complaints (NSC) than younger patients.[1,2] In addition, nonacute physical, cognitive, or social needs may exacerbate acute medical problems prompting older adults or their caregivers to seek emergency care.[3–5] ED providers may find these older adult patients difficult to manage, given their complex care needs and sometimes vague symptom presentation.

Definition

NSC can be defined in numerous ways. NCS may be characterized by lack of fever and without signs or symptoms from a specific body system or organ.[6,7] Other definitions include conditions for which a specific working diagnosis cannot be found.[8] Some studies query "no specific complaint" or "other complaint" in the medical record

Louis Stokes Veterans Affairs Medical Center, 10701 East Boulevard. Cleveland, OH 44106, USA
* Corresponding author.
E-mail address: colleen.mcquown@va.gov

Clin Geriatr Med 39 (2023) 491–501
https://doi.org/10.1016/j.cger.2023.04.007
0749-0690/23/Published by Elsevier Inc.

or a list of complaints such as weakness, feeling unwell, general disability, and failure to thrive.[6,9,10] Others state NSC also includes "[the] absences of trauma, bleeding, fever, headache, chest pain, abdominal pain, dyspnea, cough, vertigo, nausea, vomiting, diarrhea, dysuria, swollen extremity, stroke-like symptoms, syncope, palpitations, skin lesions, allergic reaction, anxiety, psychotic symptoms, suicidal tendency, confusion, intoxication, or seizure."[11]

NSC can be further broken down to those with an underlying acute medical cause, those with an unresolved or untreated chronic cause, and those with a socioeconomic cause.[3,5,12] **Fig. 1**. Atypical presentation of disease may lead to vague complaints such as dizziness, generalized weakness, or altered behavior.[2] Chronic diseases may contribute to functional or cognitive decline.

Prevalence

In a recent systematic review, older adults present to the ED with NSC 6.4% to 14% of the time.[6] This review included a variety of NSC definitions, with some referenced studies looking at a focused group such as those with only a complaint of weakness or fatigue. NSC are more common in older adults than younger adults.[7,9,13] A 2022 study looking at the 6 most frequent chief complaint categories by age found that in patients age 18 to 74 years, no NSC made the top of the list, but in patients age 75 to 84 years 2 of the top 6 complaints were nonspecific (falls without injury/generalized weakness and collapse/dizziness) and in patients age 85 years and older 3 of the top 6 complaints were nonspecific (falls without injury/generalized weakness, collapse/dizziness, and confusion/altered behavior/drowsiness).[2] In that study older adults were also significantly more likely to have "social/prescription issue" as a chief complaint. Weakness and fatigue are more frequent complaints of older adults, increasing with age, with one study finding of 7.7% of patients 85 years and older versus 0.6% of patients younger than 45 years presenting with that same chief complaint.[2] A study of prehospital ambulance calls in patients 65 years and older found that 25% needed to be categorized as "other calls" because the complaint did not fall into the categories of cardiac, respiratory, gastrointestinal, injury/musculoskeletal, or neurologic.[14]

Given the multidimensionality that can influence NSC, older adults who present with NSC in the ED are seen as a diagnostic challenge and experience higher hospitalization rates, longer ED visits, and are often undertriaged despite their 3-fold increase of

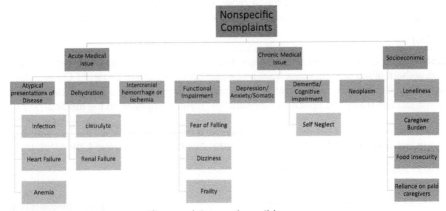

Fig. 1. Categories of nonspecific complaints and possible causes.

in-hospital deaths.[6,9,10,15] Resource use of the ED varies by study, with some finding use of diagnostic resources to be high among patients with NSC,[9] whereas another found NSC to be associated with high use of physician resources (longer patient-physician consultation, contact primary care, collect history) but not associated with more use of diagnostic resources.[13] These differences may reflect variations in study inclusion criteria.

Considerations

Geriatric psychosocial issues (ie, depression, loneliness) and socioeconomic disadvantage may contribute to the older adults' nonspecific complaints.[12,16] For example, somatic complaints such as pain, weakness, dizziness, and abnormal feeling can be a presentation of depression or anxiety in older adults.[17] Although 25% of geriatric ED patients present with depression, ED physicians have been shown to be poor identifiers of geriatric depression.[18] Social factors including isolation, poverty, and decrease in quality of life can contribute to depressed affect that may present in an atypical fashion for the older adult, resulting in nonspecific complaints. Elder mistreatment and self-neglect can also present with vague complaints or contribute to the development of NSC.[19] For instance, neglect might lead to dehydration or electrolyte disturbance presenting as generalized weakness, confusion, or falls.

Caregiver strain may influence the presentation of an older adult to the ED with NSCs. Burgdorf and colleagues found that community-dwelling disabled older adults were at greater risk of presenting to the ED if their caregiver provided more than 40 hours of care per week, providing help with complex tasks and physical strain when providing care, resulting in larger Medicare expenditures for these patients.[20] Although unpaid informal caregivers enable older adults to stay out of nursing homes and live a more independent life in the community, spousal dyads experiencing distress, strain, and sadness placed older adult patients at a 23% higher rate of ED visits.[21] High caregiver burden is associated with frequent ED use and hospitalization, even after controlling for medical factors.[4]

Caregivers with high fatigue and emotional distress may view the ED as a form of respite benefit, dropping their loved ones off for easier access to institutional care when skilled nursing facilities or hospice are not an option.[3] Reducing caregiver strain by assessing and better supporting those identified in need not only benefit the patients' health outcomes but also have potential to reduce ED utilization among this vulnerable subpopulation.[20] This chapter outlines the clinical considerations and consultations that should be considered in the ED evaluation and post-ED transition for older adult patients with NSC.

DISCUSSION
Geriatric Syndromes and Prehospital Factors Associated with Emergency Department Visits for Nonspecific Complaints

Multiple medical and nonmedical factors are common in patients with NSC. In one study, NSC were associated with higher Charlson Comorbidity Index and worse baseline functional status compared with specific complaints.[10] Another study found that NSCs that did not result in a specific diagnosis at the time of the ED visit was associated with visiting the ED 2 more times in 18 months.[5] This same qualitative study found that functional decline, fear of falling, fatigue, and loss of muscle strength were geriatric syndromes associated with ED visits.

Baseline physical dependence, frailty, and lower socioeconomic status are associated with frequent ED use in older adults and repeat ED visits regardless of chief complaint, highlighting the need to consider NSC along with specific complaints at the time of the ED visit.[4,12,22,23] Risk factors for repeat ED visits in discharged patients are often not related to their acute medical complaints but may need to be addressed at the time of the ED visit. These risk factors include nutritional problems, insomnia, frailty, functional decline, fear of falling, and caregiver strain.[4,5,22–24] Factors associated with ambulance versus self-transport in older adults included poor physical function, deficiency in activities of daily living (ADL), and worse social function.[1]

Older adults with NSC are at risk of being undertriaged at time of emergency medical service (EMS) or on arrival to the hospital, despite NSC being associated with increase in ED resources, length of stay, risk of hospitalization, and death.[6,7,9,13,25,26] One study found NSC at time of calling emergency services to be associated with EMS changing priority from low to high after arrival.[25] As ambulance services work on protocols based on chief complaint, having an NSC or "unclear problem" presents a prehospital challenge.[14] Patients with a prehospital NSC have higher mortality and are more likely to have a serious medical condition found after ED investigation than many specific complaints.[26,27] Given the high risk associated with NSC in older adults, prehospital protocols should be written to encourage transport to emergency facilities and consider serious conditions as differential diagnoses.

Polypharmacy and potentially inappropriate medication use are also a risk factor for NSC. One study found that 12.2% of NSC visits in the ED were found to be directly related to medication. Other studies found that patients with NSC took more medications than patients with specific complaints.[7,10] Taking medication for diabetes was associated with a higher chance of having NSC, whereas being on an antibiotic was associated with a lower chance of having NSC.[13]

EMERGENCY DEPARTMENT EVALUATION OF NONSPECIFIC COMPLAINTS

Adult failure to thrive, atypical presentation, frailty, or geriatric syndrome are other common concepts used to describe similar NSC presentations. Although some of these concepts have more defined screening tools and criteria than others, what all these terms have in common is a lack of clear consensus on "next steps" for workup and plan of care for the complex older adult as compared with standardized protocol that supports a specific complaint. To note, the clinician should not lump these terms together under one umbrella, thus perpetuating the lack of urgency but should stay vigilant in identifying symptoms that may be atypical presentation of a more serious underlying condition.

Creating a differential diagnosis list may pose as a challenge for the ED provider when an older adult presents with NSC. There is no specific management algorithm or guideline for treatment, and altered mental status may further contribute to difficulties in history taking. These seemingly nonurgent complaints require a more creative approach to diagnosis, given the subjective nature and often underestimated severity of illness. Therefore, investigation into both patient factors along with socioeconomic and community-based issues through a specific geriatric assessment should be a priority when working up an NSC patient.

Most NSC patients will present to the ED with normal vital signs and may never receive a formal diagnosis for their symptoms.[27] Peng and colleagues illustrated in an NSC sample of Swiss patients, only 46% received a correct ED diagnosis, and missed diagnoses were rarely corrected at discharge.[11] In addition, functional impairment, depression, or anxiety remained the most missed yet correct diagnoses, illuminating the need for deeper investigation of the social and emotional factors that may contribute to the presentation of nonspecific complaints.[11]

Although older adult patients may present with vague or atypical conditions, the ED provider should consider the most common primary ED discharge diagnoses for NSC including infectious disease, pneumonia, or urinary tract infection, followed by cardiovascular and neurologic diseases.[27,28] Other common diagnoses are electrolyte disorders, dehydration, anemia, intercranial hemorrhage, neoplasm, and gastrointestinal bleed[7,9,10,27,28] (**Fig. 2**). Initial workup for these diagnoses should be pursued followed by a more detailed examination including social and home factors and medication reconciliation.

Laboratory

In reference to the previously listed common diagnoses for NSC, Patzen and colleagues saw that in older adults who presented to the ED, overall clinical chemistry laboratories only contributed to 51% of the validated final diagnoses, whereas imaging contributed 18%.[29] Standard clinical chemistry including electrolytes, kidney and liver function, and standard hematology may serve as a good starting point and general

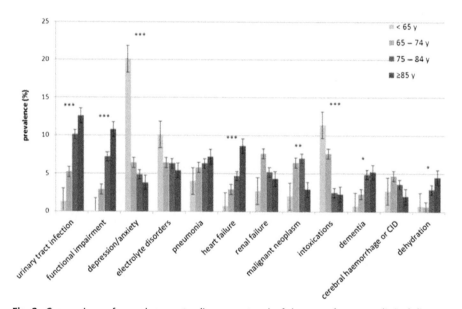

Fig. 2. Comparison of prevalence rates (in percentage) of the most frequent clinical diagnoses or clinical diagnostic groups in young (<65 years; N = 149), young-old (65–74 years; N = 172), middle-old (75–84 years; N = 445), and oldest old (≥85 years; N = 444) patients of our cohort in descending order. The prevalence of urinary tract infection ($P < .001$), functional impairment ($P < .001$), heart failure ($P < .001$), dementia ($P = .05$), and dehydration ($P = .02$) was considerably higher in older patients than in younger patients. The prevalence of depression/anxiety ($P < .001$) and intoxications ($P < .001$) was significantly higher in younger patients than in older patients. The prevalence of malignant neoplasm ($P = .009$) was significantly higher in young-old and middle-old patients than in young and oldest old patients. Significant differences are highlighted by asterisks (* $= P \leq .05$; ** $= P < .01$; *** $= P < .001$). CID, cerebral ischemic disease. (*From* Karakoumis J, Nickel CH, Kirsch M, et al. Emergency Presentations With Nonspecific Complaints-the Burden of Morbidity and the Spectrum of Underlying Disease: Nonspecific Complaints and Underlying Disease. *Medicine (Baltimore)*. 2015; 94(26):e840. https://doi.org/10.1097/MD.0000000000000840, as Figure 3 in original print. Journal is open access and article allows for creative commons license and distribution without permission.)

approach to narrowing down NSC symptoms. However, the ED provider may need to consider the subjective nature of the presentation and add additional laboratory tests to their discretion. Heart failure is a common cause of NSC,[28] but physical examination should be used to guide the need for laboratory evaluation for heart failure.

To note, in older adults, asymptomatic bacteriuria may be common and may lead to misdiagnosis of urinary tract infection. Reliance on laboratory criteria alone rather than in combination with patient symptom and history to define infection may mask the true underlying nature of the NSC.[30] Thus, further investigation into patient history and home-based factors may help paint a clearer picture of the true nature contributing to the patients' symptoms.

Imaging

Based on the most common NSC discharge diagnoses listed earlier, chest imaging for pneumonia and head CT for change in mental status may be warranted.

Social Work Consultation

Although many specific diagnoses are eventually found for older adults with NSC, socio-economic factors may play a significant role in the use of the ED.[1,10,28] In addition, many patients are not found to have a specific diagnosis related to an acute medical condition, rather problems functioning with chronic medical or physical conditions.[2,10,28] Still, others are found to have no specific diagnosis after ED evaluation.[6,10,28] Social work consultation while in the ED may present as a safety net for older adults who have fallen through the cracks and lack community care and resources. Social work can assist in assessing social and home-based care needs, which may attribute to the NSC presentation. Elder mistreatment and self-neglect may be associated with NSCs and can be screened by social work or other trained ED staff.[31]

Physical Therapy and Occupational Therapy Consultation

ED providers may benefit from reviewing with the older adult how they are able to perform ADL and instrumental ADLs (IADL) at home. Insight into the older adult's ability to perform self-care ADL tasks such as bathing, toileting, and transferring or more complex decision-making IADL tasks such as cooking, cleaning, and transportation may present as a key finding to narrowing down NSC diagnoses. The inability to complete ADL and IADL tasks may signify deconditioning and potential increase in fall risk.

Subsequently, older adults may benefit from a physical therapy/occupational therapy consult while in the ED when presenting with NSC.

Research has shown that older adults who receive physical therapy services in the ED after presenting with a fall were significantly less likely to have 30 and 60 days fall-related ED visits.[32]

Medication Review/Pharmacist Consultation

Polypharmacy has a high prevalence in older adults who present to the ED. In addition, older adults are more susceptible to drug-related problems, given the physiologic changes that occur with aging including loss of body mass or decreased kidney and liver function. In older adults, drug-related problems occur 12% of the time and have shown to be among the top 5 causes of nonspecific complaints when presenting to the ED.[33] Although drug-related issues may not always be considered in the differential diagnoses, this relationship has shown to attribute to 83% of the causes of acute morbidity.[33] Therefore, early detection of drug-related problems may help assist in treatment of NSC. To help with medication review and associated drug-related problems, the ED provider might consider a pharmacy consult. A pharmacology consult can conduct a more thorough medication review identifying unnecessary medications or medications deemed inappropriate for older adults as suggested by the American Geriatric Society BEERS Criteria guidelines.

EMERGENCY DEPARTMENT CARE TRANSITIONS FOR PATIENTS WITH NONSPECIFIC COMPLAINTS

There is no standard model for best discharge planning for the older adult. However, additional resources should be considered for optimizing effective postdischarge services. Having a chief NSC is associated with being discharged without a specific diagnosis.[9,34] As NSC have a high risk of return ED visit, arranging for post-ED care may be especially important. Barriers to care transition include new physical limitations, caregiver strain, and fear related to the NSC.[24]

Need For Safe Discharge

It is important to promote a whole-system approach using an interdisciplinary team planning including social work, pharmacist, case manager/coordinator, physical/occupational therapy, and ED provider. A family meeting may also be considered before discharge to coordinate future care needs (ie, transportation needs, medical equipment deliveries, encouraging the need for medication or lifestyle changes based on patient status, highlighting patient decompensation and need for increased family involvement in care if needed).

Simpson and colleagues showed that older adults who had an outpatient referral ordered before ED discharge (whether that be with orthopedic, family practice, urology and so forth) had lower odds of a 30-day ED readmission or 30-day unplanned hospital admission.[35] However, within the same cohort, less than half of the older adults attended their outpatient follow-up appointment[35]; this highlights the need to involve family and social work in the discharge planning procedures, to help emphasize attendance in follow-up appointments, and to make sure all home and community services that may interfere with the follow-up appointment can be addressed (ie, transportation, walking devices, wheelchair transfers).

Given the association of elder mistreatment and self-neglect with many NSC, ED providers should offer admission as needed for further investigation into the cause of NSC.[31] Adult protective services should be contacted if elder mistreatment or self-neglect is suspected. Safe dispositions should consider home resources, available caregivers, willingness to accept home services, and transportation.[31]

REFERRALS FOR HOME AND COMMUNITY SERVICE

Patient preferences should be taken into consideration when the older adult is being evaluated for discharge.[36] Coordinated referrals may be necessary for the older adult on discharge from the ED. Referrals for community services may include residential nursing care, household cleaning, or help with meal prep. Caregivers may exhibit signs of caregiver strain or burden while in the ED and may benefit from additional community services in providing care of the older adult.

Caregiver Support

With the growing aging population, increased attention and support for caregivers of community-dwelling older adults and the need for clinicians to better incorporate the needs of caregivers into the care planning will be required.

Caregiver literature suggests clinicians and health systems aim to better incorporate caregivers into the care team by identifying those caregivers at need and standardizing measurement of this assessment as well as using patient portals to improve information sharing.[20]

Follow-up with Primary Care or Geriatric Syndrome–Specific Clinic

Primary care providers are best positioned to connect caregivers with supportive resources and could tailor caregiver needs with additional training programs in the ambulatory care setting. In addition, because many patients are discharged without a specific diagnosis or may be discharged without having all NSC addressed, patients may benefit from a reevaluation clinic or planned acute care visit.[37]

Information gathered within the ED visit may elicit a need for a comprehensive geriatric assessment via a geriatric consult once the older adult is discharged from the ED. Comprehensive geriatric assessments have been shown to increase the likelihood of an older adult both surviving and being in his/her home within 12 months.[38] Post-ED discharge, follow-up phone calls and targeted geriatric care by a transitional care nurse or social worker has shown to reduce the risk of geriatric inpatient admission and lower Medicare expenditures, as illustrated by the GEDI WISE program (Geriatric Emergency Department Innovations in Care Through Workforce, Informatics, and Structural Enhancement).[39,40]

SUMMARY

NSC are a common ED presentation for older adults. These NSC may be related to atypical presentations of acute medical conditions, unresolved chronic medical problems, geriatric syndromes, and socioeconomic factors. The workup must be focused on ruling out acute medical conditions, while considering social determinates of health and comorbid conditions. A multidisciplinary approach can help identify and plan for geriatric syndromes, unmet home needs, caregiver support challenges, and ED revisit risk factors. Patients who are discharged benefit from prompt follow-up and care coordination.

CLINICS CARE POINTS

- Nonspecific complaints in the ED are often multifactorial and require a thorough history and physical examination to investigate.
- Atypical presentations of acute disease should always be considered when older patients present to the ED with vague complaints.
- Nonspecific complaints may originate from social determinates of health-related needs that may result in return ED visits or hospital admission if not addressed.
- Patients discharged without a specific diagnosis are at high risk for returning to the ED, so coordinating prompt primary care follow-up and transition of care should be a priority.

DISCLOSURE

Financial support for Emily Tsivitse was provided by the Veterans Affairs Quality Scholars (VAQS) postdoctoral program. There was no external funding.

REFERENCES

1. Shah MN, Glushak C, Karrison TG, et al. Predictors of emergency medical services utilization by elders. Acad Emerg Med 2003;10(1):52–8.

2. Ogliari G, Coffey F, Keillor L, et al. Emergency department use and length of stay by younger and older adults: nottingham cohort study in the emergency department (NOCED). Aging Clin Exp Res 2022;34(11):2873–85.
3. Jacobsohn GC, Hollander M, Beck AP, et al. Factors influencing emergency care by persons with dementia: stakeholder perceptions and unmet needs. J Am Geriatr Soc 2019;67(4):711–8.
4. Bonin-Guillaume S, Durand AC, Yahi F, et al. Predictive factors for early unplanned rehospitalization of older adults after an ED visit: role of the caregiver burden. Aging Clin Exp Res 2015;27(6):883–91.
5. Kolk D, Kruiswijk AF, MacNeil-Vroomen JL, et al. Older patients' perspectives on factors contributing to frequent visits to the emergency department: a qualitative interview study. BMC Publ Health 2021;21(1):1709.
6. Kemp K, Mertanen R, Laaperi M, et al. Nonspecific complaints in the emergency department- a systematic review. Scand J Trauma Resuscitation Emerg Med 2020;28:6.
7. Nemec M, Koller MT, Nickel CH, et al. Patients presenting to the emergency department with non-specific complaints: the Basel non-specific complaints (BANC) study. Acad Emerg Med 2010;17(3):284–92.
8. McQuown C. Weakness and functional decline. In: Mattu A, Grossman SA, Rosen PL, editors. Geriatric emergencies: a discussion-based review. 1st edition. Chichester, UK: John Wiley & Sons, Ltd; 2016. p. 252–63.
9. Bhalla MC, Wilber ST, Stiffler KA, et al. Weakness and fatigue in older ED patients in the United States. Am J Emerg Med 2014;32(11):1395–8.
10. Wachelder JJH, Stassen PM, Hubens LPAM, et al. Elderly emergency patients presenting with non-specific complaints: characteristics and outcomes. PLoS One 2017;12(11):e0188954.
11. Peng A, Rohacek M, Ackerman S, et al. The proportion of correct diagnoses is low in emergency patients with nonspecific complaints presenting to the emergency department. Swiss Med Wkly 2015. https://doi.org/10.4414/smw.2015.14121.
12. Carlson LC, Zachrison KS, Yun BJ, et al. The association of demographic, socioeconomic, and geographic factors with potentially preventable emergency department utilization. West J Emerg Med 2021;22(6):1283–90.
13. Birrenbach T, Geissbühler A, Exadaktylos AK, et al. A dangerously underrated entity? Non-specific complaints at emergency department presentation are associated with utilisation of less diagnostic resources. BMC Emerg Med 2021;21(1):133.
14. Ibsen S, Dam-Huus KB, Nickel CH, et al. Diagnoses and mortality among prehospital emergency patients calling 112 with unclear problems: a population-based cohort study from Denmark. Scand J Trauma Resusc Emerg Med 2022;30(1):70.
15. Conroy S, Carpenter C, Banerjee J Silver Book II Quality Care for Older People With Urgent Care Needs Online. Available at: https://www.bgs.org.uk/silverbook2. Accessed 21 December, 2021.
16. Powell VD, Kumar N, Galecki AT, et al. Bad company: loneliness longitudinally predicts the symptom cluster of pain, fatigue, and depression in older adults. J Am Geriatr Soc 2022;70(8):2225–34.
17. Hashimoto K, Takeuchi T, Murasaki M, et al. Psychosomatic symptoms related to exacerbation of fatigue in patients with medically unexplained symptoms. J Gen Fam Med 2022;24(1):24–9.
18. Hals G, LoVecchio F. Geriatric psychosocial issues in the emergency department. J Emerg Med Case Rep 2010;31(11):125–31.

19. Rosen T, Stern ME, Elman A, et al. Identifying and initiating intervention for elder abuse and neglect in the emergency department. Clin Geriatr Med 2018;34(3): 435–51.
20. Burgdorf J, Mulcahy J, Amjad H, et al. Family caregiver factors associated with emergency department utilization among community-living older adults with disabilities. Journal of Primary Care and Community Health 2019;10:1–9.
21. Ankuda CK, Maust DT, Kabeto MU, et al. The association of spousal caregiver wellbeing with patients healthcare expenditures. Journal of the American Geriatric Society 2017;65(10):2220–6.
22. Deschodt M, Devriendt E, Sabbe M, et al. Characteristics of older adults admitted to the emergency department (ED) and their risk factors for ED readmission based on comprehensive geriatric assessment: a prospective cohort study. BMC Geriatr 2015;15:54.
23. Huang HH, Chang JC, Tseng CC, et al. Comprehensive geriatric assessment in the emergency department for the prediction of readmission among older patients: a 3-month follow-up study. Arch Gerontol Geriatr 2021;92:104255.
24. Gettel CJ, Serina PT, Uzamere I, et al. Emergency department-to-community care transition barriers: a qualitative study of older adults. J Am Geriatr Soc 2022; 70(11):3152–62.
25. Castrén M, Kurland L, Liljegard S, et al. Non-specific complaints in the ambulance; predisposing structural factors. BMC Emerg Med 2015;15:8.
26. Ibsen S, Lindskou TA, Nickel CH, et al. Which symptoms pose the highest risk in patients calling for an ambulance? A population-based cohort study from Denmark. Scand J Trauma Resusc Emerg Med 2021;29(1):59.
27. Ivic R, Kurland L, Vicente V, et al. Serious conditions among patients with non-specific chief complaints in the pre-hospital setting: a retrospective cohort study. Scand J Trauma Resusc Emerg Med 2020;28(1):74.
28. Karakoumis J, Nickel CH, Kirsch M, et al. Emergency presentations with nonspecific complaints-the burden of morbidity and the Spectrum of underlying disease: nonspecific complaints and underlying disease. Medicine (Baltim) 2015;94(26): e840.
29. Patzen A, Simon NR, Jauslin AS, et al. Nonspecific complaints in emergency medicine: contribution of clinical chemistry and diagnostic imaging to final diagnosis. An observational study. Signa Vitae 2021;17(4):49–54.
30. Cortes-Penfield NW, Trautner BW, Jump RLP. Urinary tract infection and asymptomatic bacteriuria in older adults. Infect Dis Clin North Am 2017;31(4):673–88.
31. Rosen T, Elman A, Clark S, et al. Vulnerable Elder Protection Team: Initial experience of an emergency department-based interdisciplinary elder abuse program. J Am Geriatr Soc 2022;70(11):3260–72.
32. Lesser A, Israni J, Kent T, et al. Association between physical therapy in the emergency department and emergency department revisits for older adult fallers: a nationally representative analysis. J Am Geriatr Soc 2018;66(11):2205–12.
33. Nickel CH, Ruedinger JM, Messmer AS, et al. Drug-related emergency department visits by elderly patients presenting with non-specific complaints. Scand J Trauma Resuscitation Emerg Med 2013;21(15). https://doi.org/10.1186/1757-7241-21-15.
34. Birrenbach T, Hoffmann M, Hautz SC, et al. Frequency and predictors of unspecific medical diagnoses in the emergency department: a prospective observational study. BMC Emerg Med 2022;22(1):109.

35. Simpson M, Sergi C, Malsch A, et al. Association of Geriatric Emergency Department post-discharge referral order and follow-up with healthcare utilization. J Am Geriatr Soc 2022. https://doi.org/10.1111/jgs.18137.
36. Huang YL, McGonagle M, Shaw R, et al. Models of care for frail older persons who present to the emergency department: a scoping review of the literature. Int Emerg Nurs 2023;66:101250. https://doi.org/10.1016/j.ienj.2022.101250.
37. Balzaretti PL, Reano A, Canonico S, et al. A geriatric re-evaluation clinic is associated with fewer unplanned returns in the Emergency Department: an observational case-control study. Eur Geriatr Med 2022;1–7. https://doi.org/10.1007/s41999-022-00726-1.
38. Ellis G, Whitehead MA, O'Neill D, et al. Comprehensive geriatric assessment for older adults admitted to hospital. Cochrane Database Systematic Review 2011;7: CD006211.
39. Hwang U, Dresden SM, Rosenberg MS, et al. Geriatric emergency department innovations: transitional care nurses and hospital use. J Am Geriatr Soc 2018; 66(3):459–66.
40. Hwang U, Dresden SM, Vargas-Torres C, et al. Association of a geriatric emergency department innovation program with cost outcomes among Medicare beneficiaries. Journal of American Medical Association 2021;4(3):e2037224.

Older Adult Falls in Emergency Medicine, 2023 Update

Kalpana N. Shankar, MD, MSc, MSHP[a],*, Angel Li, MD, MBA[b]

KEYWORDS

- Emergency medicine • Accidental fall • Geriatric • Trauma • Implementation
- Emergency medical services • Technology • Falls prevention

KEY POINTS

- Low-level falls occur in one-third of adults older than 65 each year and are a leading cause of death in developed nations.
- Prehospital providers should represent the first-line health care professionals to manage falls and initiate innovative approaches to alleviate emergency department crowding.
- Emergency department falls research is limited by uncertainty regarding reliable and feasible approaches to identity and intervene on fallers at increased risk for recurrent falls.
- Systematic reviews have shown that emergency department falls screening is associated with fall reduction when interventions are done through the emergency department.
- Innovative technological approaches are showing promising results to assess dynamic fall risk, at home fall reduction interventions and identification of high risk fall patients.

EPIDEMIOLOGY OF FALLS

Of 4 older adults, 1 will fall each year in the United States. Based on 2020 data from the Centers of Disease Control, about 36 million older adults fall each year, resulting in 32,000 deaths.[1] Emergency departments (ED) see about 3 million older adults for fall-related injuries[1] with falls having the ability to cause serious injury such as catastrophic head injuries and hip fractures.[2] One-third of older fall patients discharged from the ED experience one of these outcomes at 3 months.[3] Between 36% and 50% of patients have an adverse event, such as a recurrent fall, ED revisit, or death within 1 year after a fall.[4,5] Not only do falls lead to adverse health outcomes and disability, but also substantial economic burdens for the family and health system.[2,6]

[a] Department of Emergency Medicine, Brigham and Women's Hospital, 75 Francis Street, Neville House, Boston, MA 02115, USA; [b] Department of Emergency Medicine, The Ohio State University, 376 West 10th Avenue, Columbus, OH 43210, USA
* Corresponding author.
E-mail address: knshankar@mgb.org

Clin Geriatr Med 39 (2023) 503–518
https://doi.org/10.1016/j.cger.2023.05.010
0749-0690/23/© 2023 Elsevier Inc. All rights reserved.

The Prevention of Falls Network Europe (ProFaNE) is the most widely accepted definition for falls, stating that it is "an unexpected event in which the participants come to rest on the ground, floor or lower level."[7] The prevalence of falls is largely derived from single-center retrospective studies or secondary analyses of administrative databases, both of which may simultaneously underestimate the scope of fall injuries and overestimate the observed value of diagnostic and therapeutic interventions.[8] However, algorithmic approaches to improve the value of Medicare data are now under way,[9] as well as chart review methods that augment International Classification of Diseases, Tenth Revision (ICD-10) codes with the patient's chief complaint[10] with newer research suggesting that Natural Language Processing can accurately identify falls based on ED notes compared to using ICD or chief complaint coding.[11]

Frailty is an important predictor of falls, but widely used measures of vulnerability among older adults in ED settings do not exist.[12,13] Similarly, existing constructs of "frailty" fail to accurately identify subsets of nursing home residents at increased risk for falls.[14] However, injurious falls presenting to ED trauma units are more commonly community-dwelling individuals.[15] Geography is another factor in assessing the sequelae of falls. Rural fall victims are less likely to be hospitalized, have a shorter duration of hospital length of stay, and demonstrate higher 1-month readmission rates and mortality.[16]

In the United States, direct medical costs associated with falls totaled $754 million for fatal and $49.6 billion for nonfatal injurious falls in 2015, with significant variability between states.[17,18] As fall-related hospitalizations and associated costs continue to rise, ED identification of older adults at higher risk for fall-related injuries will become increasingly relevant. Nonetheless, ED fall interventions have yet to demonstrate cost-effectiveness, so quantifying the benefits and harms of fall-prevention strategies remains an unmet challenge.[19,20] This review focuses on prehospital and ED fall-risk screening and interventions and real-world barriers to implementation of these concepts, while exploring evolving approaches to management, such as post–ED falls clinics and technological approaches to monitor falls and fall risk factors.

TECHNOLOGICAL ADVANCES WITH PRE-HOSPITAL FALLS DETECTION

Technology-based interventions have been used in a wide range of fall-prevention efforts, including diagnosing and managing fall risk, improving intervention adherence, and fall detection.[21,22] For example, a feasibility study using calcaneal ultrasound as one quantitative predictor of falls was recently published[23] as well as a study looking at sarcopenia as a marker for frailty and falls.[24] Other devices (ie, mobile phone–based systems) have many advantages, namely their popularity, decreasing costs, and portability.[25,26] Most smartphones also integrate all the required elements to develop autonomous and self-sufficient fall-detection applications.

Technology also has been seen as a means to help patients self-assess their risk of falling, which can potentially save money if patients do not need to do initial screening with a clinician.[21] This may be key to reducing costs as well as improving quality of care. The "Aachen Fall Prevention App" (AFPA) is the first reported mobile health application that empowers older patients (>50 years) to self-assess and monitor their fall risk[27]; however, there have been numerous other applications that have also demonstrated feasibility and usability.[28–32] Although technology is an important step in aiding in falls detection, a recent review of the literature on technology-based falls applications underscores a few important points: including older adults in the IT society for application development and ensuring ease of use, designing solutions that fit the older adult physical and cognitive profile, and ensuring that all design principles help practitioners develop proper devices for older adults.[22]

Early detection of falls is also important, as long waiting times on the ground increase the risk of hospitalization and death.[33] Traditionally, fall alert systems depend on the older adult pushing a button and communicating with a central operating system. These systems may be less useful if the range of the device is restricted to the home or if the person cannot push the button (eg, if he or she is unconscious). Hence, using the accelerometer feature in today's smartphones, which older adults can easily carry, represents a promising new technology.[26,34] There is a plethora of work being conducted to develop smartphone-based fall-detection systems.[22] False negatives (fall has occurred but device did not recognize a fall) might be problematic using smartphones and the rate of missed falls will depend on the type of falls (forward vs lateral vs backward falls), type of algorithm used to determine if a fall has occurred, and where the smartphone or associated sensor is placed.[22] The percentage of false negatives ranges from 1.2% to 29.9% depending on the type of fall and the different application algorithms. False-positive (no fall occurred but device alarms as if a fall did happen) rates range from 5.9% to 21.9% depending on the various algorithms. No algorithm had an efficiency higher than 95% or 90% to avoid false positives and false negatives, respectively.[25] Biomedical engineers are now assessing the combined ability of smartphones and smartwatches to detect falls. Vilarinho and colleagues[35] found that together the smartphone/smartwatch could correctly identify 63% of falls. The Apple Watch Series 4 can detect falls and call EMS if a faller does not respond or agrees with the call, a technology currently being investigated by the GapCare II Intervention.[36]

Passive monitoring systems also exist and can be used in assisted living facilities to monitor falls. Patel and Gunnarsson[37] described a passive monitoring system that uses advanced motion sensor technology that learns the daily patterns of community residents in a senior home and sends alerts when abnormal events occur. Monitoring resulted in reduced falls and improved resident retention compared with the control group. However, among immigrant older adults, passive monitoring devices seem less likely to be used and interventions should be mindful of patients' social values in shaping how people and families interact with technology based older adult care interventions.[38]

SYSTEMS-BASED PREHOSPITAL FALLS DETECTION RISK ASSESSMENT AND PREVENTIVE INTERVENTIONS

Emergency medical services (EMS) report a 3-fold increase in fall-related calls between 2007 and 2017.[39] Although pain or altered functional status is associated with transportation to the ED, EMS calls from personal alarm devices are less likely to be associated with the patient being transported as well as falls that occur in public locations or result in no clinical detection of apparent illness or injury.[40,41] The traditional scoop and run paradigm has shifted to a more evaluative, patient-centered process that empowers paramedics and paramedic extenders to assess intrinsic and extrinsic risks for future falls, because a subset of patients are heavy EMS users who infrequently require transportation.[42,43] ED and primary care providers often are not aware of EMS fall evaluations when patients are not transported to the hospital; however, there is evidence that combined effort between EMS providers and ED staff can result in a successful future falls prevention strategy.[44] Reducing recurrent injurious falls among patients in either prehospital or ED settings depends on reliable patient follow-up and often patient adherence to behavioral changes such as physical therapy,[45] as well as identification of the subset of fall victims most likely to benefit from preventive interventions.[41] When fall victims are not transported to the ED, they may be referred to a "Falls Clinic" (discussed later) or provided information about other fall-prevention services.

EMS research thus far has demonstrated inconsistent fall-prevention benefits and no effect on reducing injurious falls.[46] One British EMS protocol trained prehospital providers to use an algorithm assessing fall risk and refer appropriate fallers who were not transported to the ED to a "Fall Clinic." This intervention reduced future emergency calls but did not decrease or increase short-term injury risk and had a mean cost of $23 per patient.[47] There are more recent trials looking at a personalized intervention for older adult falls not transported to the ED, but results are not yet published.[48]

Multiple issues likely underlie the failure of EMS interventions to consistently reduce fall-related injuries. First, each region's EMS system represents a unique domain with variable institutional interest in healthy aging or falls prevention buried within a constellation of competing priorities. Adapting EMS educational priorities with the guidance of a geriatric emergency medicine opinion leader has successfully overcome this inertia in some settings.[49] Second, reliably accurate, widely accepted, and routinely available EMS protocols to risk-stratify and intervene on fall victims do not exist.[46] The disappointing results of prior research may indicate selection of the patients less likely to benefit from specific interventions, because fall victims have a heterogeneous mixture of risk factors and comorbid illness burden. Third, referral to a "Falls Clinic" or to primary care is often dependent on patient compliance and effectiveness of the subsequent fall-reduction interventions, as is discussed later.

EMERGENCY DEPARTMENT AND POST–EMERGENCY DEPARTMENT FALL RISK ASSESSMENT AND INTERVENTIONS

Management of geriatric trauma patients for ground level falls is increasingly being managed primarily by emergency medicine physicians even at designated trauma centers. Studies have even shown EM physicians have a 30% lower rate of admission compared to the trauma team with no difference in associated risk of mortality.[50] In addition to primary management of trauma, the ED is responsible for managing the complexities of caring for an older patient.

Unfortunately, most geriatric fall victims who are transported by EMS (or arrive by other transportation) to the ED do not receive guidelines-directed care.[51,52] Multiple emergency medicine and geriatrics professional societies have endorsed fall management guidelines (**Fig. 1**),[12] yet these recommendations remain largely untested and unavailable for many ED settings. In resource-strained ED settings, it is neither cost-effective nor feasible to label every older adult as high risk for ED or post-discharge falls. Yet relative to the injury burden falls represent, there is a paucity of ED research to develop instruments and predictors to distinguish high-risk from low-risk future fallers.[46] Triage nurses also evaluate fall risk, which can be a useful process for ED providers and inpatient services if effectively communicated between providers.[53]

Fall screening for high-risk individuals in the community setting has proven to be difficult, and multiple studies have shown poor predictive ability of screening for future falls in the outpatient setting, including the most commonly used "Timed Up and Go".[54,55] Pooled analysis from the US Preventive Task Force shows the most beneficial interventions have been recruitment from the ED to reduce the number of falls independent of the screening tools used during the study. This suggests that patients

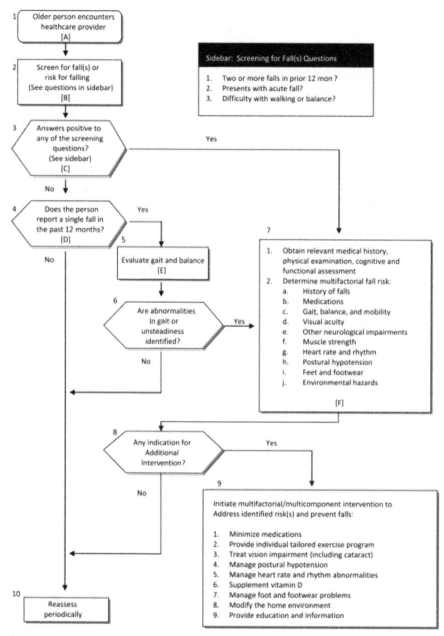

Fig. 1. American Geriatric Society/British Geriatric Society Guidelines to prevent falls in community-residing elderly. (*From* Panel on Prevention of Falls in Older Persons, American Geriatrics Society, British Geriatrics Society. Summary of the updated American Geriatrics Society/British Geriatrics Society clinical practice guideline for prevention of falls in older persons. J Am Geriatr Soc 2011;59(1):150; with permission.)

presenting for a fall to the ED are already by definition high risk.[56] These findings suggest the ED be a larger stakeholder in future falls prevention research and intervention.

Objective functional assessments like "Get Up and Go" have not accurately predicted future fall risk in ED patients.[45,57–59] This inaccuracy may reflect patient selection rather than test properties, because the "Timed Up and Go" test is more accurate in lower functioning older adults than in healthier community-dwelling individuals.[60] Emergency medicine nursing studies focus primarily on falls within the ED, which are not comparable with post–ED fall instruments or interventions. In addition, nursing studies of fall instruments oftentimes do not measure quantitative results for comparison with other screening instruments.[61,62] Ongoing efforts to derive, validate, and evaluate the impact of fall-risk instruments have proven challenging because of the large number of intrinsic and extrinsic factors associated with older adult falls and fall-related injuries.

The most recent Cochrane review of multifactorial interventions to reduce falls in community-dwelling older adults included 62 trials, but only 1 based in the ED.[63,64] The Prevention of Falls in the Elderly Trial (PROFET) randomized cognitively intact patients older than 65 following an ED falls-related visit to either routine care or to a detailed collaborative evaluation by a geriatrician and occupational therapist within 1 week of ED discharge. They determined that exercise and balance training are still the most effective tools in multifactorial interventions for future falls prevention. The comprehensive geriatric evaluation assessed visual acuity, balance, affect, mental status, and postural hypotension in a "day clinic," with appropriate referrals based on these findings.[65] Few EDs have access to a "day clinic," geriatrician, or occupational therapist, and the PROFET results have not been replicated. A telephone-based patient centered program RESPOND reduced falls and fall injuries in older patient populations in a 6-month intervention program from the ED in Australia. In this RCT, the number of falls decreased but not fall-related injuries. The intervention included a home visit, telephone follow-up, and module training.[66]

The Geriatric Acute and Post-acute Fall Prevention (GAPcare) is a recent ED randomized controlled trial of 110 adults over the age of 65 years with a recent fall. The study consisted of an assessment by an ED clinician with the GAPcare intervention involving a pharmacist conducting a bedside evaluation and physical therapy consult performing a fall risk assessment and plan. The intervention patients were half as likely to experience a subsequent ED visit and a third as likely to have fall-related ED visit within 6 months.[67]

Online Emergency Department Fall Resources

ED providers rely on outpatient fall resources for comprehensive risk assessment and definitive prevention interventions. Identifying these resources real time during a clinical shift is challenging because no central repository exists. Web-based resources from "fall clinics" include the CDC STEADI initiative, University of Wisconsin Medicine, and Live Long Walk Strong at Spaulding Rehabilitation Center in Cambridge, Massachusetts. **Table 1** provides a nonexhaustive list of Web addresses for representative "fall clinics." CDC STEADI initiative is the most comprehensive for health care professionals and includes a fall risk checklist, case studies, functional assessments, patient information, and more. The University of North Carolina has an Otago exercise program with resources for finding Otago trained therapists. The American College of Emergency Physicians' (ACEP) Geriatric ED Guidelines outlines an extensive workup for fall patients.[68] ACEP also created the *7 Step Fall Challenge*, a 7-minute video available on YouTube that clinicians can share with ED patients to educate them on fall risk and prevention.[69] In addition, Free Open Access Medical Education (FOAMed)

Table 1 Online fall resources	
Fall Clinics	
CDC STEADI	https://www.cdc.gov/steadi/index.html
University of Wisconsin	http://www.fammed.wisc.edu/northeast-clinic-takes-steps-prevent-elderly-falls/
University of North Carolina	https://www.med.unc.edu/aging/cgwep/courses/exercise-program/
Live Long Walk Strong	http://spauldingrehab.org/conditions-and-treatments/live-long-walk-strong
Emergency Medicine Cases	
ACEP 7 Step Fall Challenge	https://www.youtube.com/watch?v=-ehHhdoJ2k8
ALiEM	https://www.aliem.com/geriatric-em-falls-sentinel-events/
The Skeptics Guide to Emergency Medicine	https://thesgem.com/2021/11/sgem351-how-to-stop-geriatrics-from-free-fallin/
Geri-EM	https://geri-em.com/
GEMCAST	https://gempodcast.com/2017/03/13/ems-preventing-falls/#more-459
CDEM geriatric curriculum	https://www.saem.org/about-saem/academies-interest-groups-affiliates2/cdem/for-students/online-education/m4-curriculum

resources increasingly highlight fall management challenges, including EM Cases and Skeptics Guide to Emergency Medicine. Geri-EM is an interactive e-learning web site focused on geriatric emergencies and including free continuing medical education with topics ranging from falls to end-of-life issues. Finally, the Clerkship Directors in Emergency Medicine in collaboration with the Academy of Geriatric Emergency Medicine for SAEM has created a geriatric curriculum for medical students.

POST–EMERGENCY DEPARTMENT FALLS CLINIC

Access to falls clinics in the United States is inconsistent, but health outcomes researchers continue to explore the key attributes and efficacy of these outpatient resources. In Malaysia, a falls clinic was effectively able to use the STOPP/START criteria in identifying inappropriate prescribing practices that could have led to a fall.[70] Telephone-based phone follow-up with home-based services and education resulted in decreased falls and associated fractures, but no effect on fall injuries.[66] In the Netherlands, there are 23 fall clinics. Screening ED and primary care patients with the CAREFALL Triage Instrument suggests that on average, patients referred to a fall clinic from the ED have more fall risk factors than do those referred by primary care.[71] More importantly, patients referred from an ED have risk factors different from those referred from primary care, which may influence the impact of interventions.

Linking high-risk fall patients in the ED with appropriate outpatient resources is challenging. Simply distributing information about local falls prevention programs is unlikely to reduce fall rates or injuries.[57] In addition, although ED patients may report willingness to follow-up with a falls clinic, actual compliance rates are often quite low.[45] Patients in 2 separate pilot fall-prevention referral study report low compliance secondary to transportation barriers, conflicting social determinants such as caregiving duties, disinterest, unwillingness in seeing someone other than their primary care physician, and lack of sufficient motivation.[45,72] Reducing recurrent falls will also depend on identifying and overcoming barriers to patient follow-up. Shared decision making and fall-specific patient aids may be one approach to improving patient compliance with fall-reduction interventions,[58] while keeping in mind potential barriers to shared decision making that are unique to the ED.[73]

Another approach addressing the barriers to follow up is to use telehealth in hospital at home model.[74] Telehealth in emergency medicine has been increasing due to the Coronavirus disease 2019 (COVID-19) pandemic, and multiple modalities have been adopted across the country.[75] The rapid adoption is due in part to changes in November 25, 2020 where the Center for Medicare & Medicaid services announced a home waiver and reimburse for "home hospital" services.[76] A pilot program for fall prevention from the ED is being performed at Massachusetts General Hospital and involves the use of virtual observation units. The intervention includes a virtual visit with an emergency physician for a safety evaluation and in-home safety evaluation by paramedics. The program also aims to identify patients who are high risk for need of further intervention and creating a treatment plan.

RESOURCE ALLOCATION FOR FALLS MANAGEMENT IN THE EMERGENCY DEPARTMENT

Falls pose a significant financial burden for the healthcare system and only continue to grow with the increasing aging population. The continual shortage of healthcare professionals and services raises concerns on how these resources will be allocated.

The COVID-19 pandemic disproportionately impacted older adults in illness severity and hospitalization rates, and exposed the limitations of inpatient capacity to accommodate surges in hospitalization. In response, the American Geriatric Society (AGS) published a position statement for stakeholders in developing resource allocation strategies.[77] Although the consensus statement focuses primarily on policies in times of crisis, these recommendations extend to management of falls in the ED.

Clear identification and communication of available resources in a hospital or system setting is needed to create a more ethical resource allocation strategy. No consensus exists on fall screening tools for the ED.[19] Future research will need to focus on developing accurate tools for high-risk future fallers for appropriate allocation of fall-related interventions. Multifactorial intervention in the ED is costly and resource intensive; however, studies have shown a positive return on investment for community-based fall intervention that covered both implementation cost and program delivery cost.[78,79]

Unfortunately, determining which patients to screen, when to screen them, and who is best suited to screen them is the first issue. Although all older adults who come to the ED should be evaluated for fall risk, the feasibility of this type of approach is limited with so many other competing priorities. A more tangible approach would focus on recent fallers (within the past 2–4 weeks) because their chief complaint likely is related to their fall; the ED visit as a sentinel event could serve as an opportune teachable moment for high-risk patients.[62] Another option is to use other screens such as nutrition risk and frailty to target high-risk patients,[80] machine learning to categorize high-risk falls for appropriate resource allocation[81] or only intervene on fall patients who are discharged home. Ethical and pragmatic issues with delirium or nursing home patients also exist. These vulnerable subsets are more likely to be at risk of recurrent falls, but also may be the most difficult to prevent recurrent falls secondary to underlying frailty, disease burden, and cognitive impairment. For example, one multifactorial intervention in cognitively impaired ED patients was ineffective,[63] but exercise in and of itself can still be helpful and decreasing falls risk in this population.[82]

An even more challenging issue is what type of interventions are effective, available, and feasible for ED fall patients and their health care providers. Similarly, ED physicians will be hesitant to change sleep, depression, anxiety, and cardiovascular medications that specialists and primary care physicians have prescribed. However, the ongoing opioid epidemic is refocusing attention on analgesic prescribing and falls.[83,84] Practically speaking, ED physicians are likely only to implement interventions that are streamlined and highly effective in reducing recurrent falls. One challenge is the need to create fall programs in the ED that follow implementation science principles and/or quality improvement strategies to maximize successful outcomes.[59,66,85,86]

Another challenge is that it takes a village to be successful at managing an individual's fall risk.[65] Although family members, patients, EMS, and ED providers are often the first clinicians to see someone after a fall, the primary care doctors, physical therapists, case managers, and geriatricians often manage the sequelae. That said, all have a stake in fall management and must work collectively as a team. For example, physical therapy services in the ED are associated with fewer revisits up to 2 months[87] with the GAPcare study showing a 6-month reduction in future ED encounters with a combined physical therapy and pharmacy evaluation.[67] Multidisciplinary hip fracture pathways can reduce ED and hospital length of stay, while also reducing inpatient complications.[88–90] However, rarely are transdisciplinary falls experts and stakeholders at the same national/international meetings or institutional grand rounds to discuss lessons learned or to share stories of success. Though with development of surgical and EDs geriatric accreditation pathways, health systems are slowly beginning to see the benefits of such cross collaboration to stimulate support, innovation, and inspiration.

NEXT STEPS

Knowledge translation begins with definitive research evidence. One immediate challenge for emergency medicine falls intervention is that much of the evidence regarding risk assessment and intervention has been developed for primary care doctors (eg, one guideline from the American Geriatrics Society, one from Stopping Elderly Accidents Death and Injuries, and another from the US Preventive Services Task Force).[56,60,91] No single, well-accepted, simple test or risk factor exists for falls and no single prehospital falls detection system exists that can accurately capture and intervene upon falls, particularly in the ED setting. Fall risk assessments are complex, multifactorial endeavors that can consume 10 to 15 minutes. Furthermore, a qualitative study indicated a number of barriers in implementing comprehensive falls assessment in the ED including lack of knowledge, paucity of evidence, heterogeneous self-perceived skills, perceived increased time, and workload.[92] In addition, ED fall patients often have acute injuries, weakness, dementia, delirium, or other chief complaints that make using commonly cited risk assessment instruments challenging.[59] The following important unanswered questions remain.

1. Which patients should undergo a risk assessment?
2. What functional tests should be conducted, if any?
3. What interventions are feasible in the ED?

Most ED clinicians cannot identify the approximate proportion of community-dwelling elderly patients who fall annually, and two-thirds of ED clinicians are unfamiliar with Geriatric Emergency Department fall-prevention guidelines.[68] Although 80% of respondents in one survey believe it is very important for them to prevent recurrent falls among elderly ED patients, 46% would spend less than 2 minutes to do so. Most (87%) providers believe that there is not enough time to implement geriatric falls prevention in the ED. There is a need to do more training to general ED providers about fall risk factors, but education alone is unlikely to sustainably improve ED falls management.[52,93] Nonetheless, the ED can be an ideal place for a multimodal intervention as an ED fall is often a sentinel event for poor outcomes where patients have the most to gain out of an intervention. Thus, these visits may necessitate prioritizing specific interventions such as exercise or PT regimens and med reconciliations which demonstrated promising results for falls reduction,[67] creative interventions that do not depend on ED providers, such as a mobile falls assessment team, pre-hospital falls assessments/interventions, geriatric/physical therapy consults in the ED, telehealth appointments or home visits for safety evaluations,[94] or outside-the-box interventions such as incentives for ED providers who implement fall-prevention interventions.

CLINICS CARE POINTS

- Emergency departments should develop tangible criteria and solutions when deciding how to initiate falls screening, such as frailty or timing of their most recent fall.
- Education and training for falls risk factors should be performed in conjunction with real time, multi-modal interventions.
- Emergency departments should consider pre-hospital care and resources outside of the emergency setting when trying to initiate both falls screening and falls interventions.

DISCLOSURE

The authors have no commercial or financial conflicts of interest.

REFERENCES

1. Centers for Disease Control, Injury Prevention & Control. Keeping On Your Feet-Preventing Older Adult Falls. Available at: https://www.cdc.gov/injury/features/older-adult-falls/index.html. Accessed January 12, 2023.
2. Gill TM, Murphy TE, Gahbauer EA, et al. Association of injurious falls with disability outcomes and nursing home admissions in community-living older persons. Am J Epidemiol 2013;178(3):418–25.
3. Sirois MJ, Émond M, Ouellet MC, et al. Cumulative incidence of functional decline after minor injuries in previously independent older Canadian individuals in the emergency department. J Am Geriatr Soc 2013;61(10):1661–8.
4. Liu SW, Obermeyer Z, Chang Y, et al. Frequency of ED revisits and death among older adults after a fall. Am J Emerg Med 2015;33(8):1012–8.
5. Sri-On J, Tirrell GP, Bean JF, et al. Revisit, subsequent hospitalization, recurrent fall, and death within 6 Months after a fall among elderly emergency department patients. Ann Emerg Med 2017;70(4):516–21.e2.
6. Spaniolas K, Cheng JD, Gestring ML, et al. Ground level falls are associated with significant mortality in elderly patients. J Trauma Inj Infect Crit Care 2010;69(4):821–5.
7. Lamb SE, Jørstad-Stein EC, Hauer K, et al, Prevention of Falls Network Europe and Outcomes Consensus Group. Development of a common outcome data set for fall injury prevention trials: the Prevention of Falls Network Europe consensus. J Am Geriatr Soc 2005;53(9):1618–22.

8. Hoffman JR, Carpenter CR. Guarding against overtesting, overdiagnosis, and overtreatment of older adults: thinking beyond imaging and injuries to weigh harms and benefits. J Am Geriatr Soc 2017;65(5):903–5.
9. Kim SB, Zingmond DS, Keeler EB, et al. Development of an algorithm to identify fall-related injuries and costs in Medicare data. Inj Epidemiol 2016;3(1):1.
10. Patterson BW, Smith MA, Repplinger MD, et al. Using chief complaint in addition to diagnosis codes to identify falls in the emergency department. J Am Geriatr Soc 2017;65(9):E135–40.
11. Patterson BW, Jacobsohn GC, Maru AP, et al. RESEARCHComparing strategies for identifying falls in older adult emergency department visits using EHR data. J Am Geriatr Soc 2020;68(12):2965–7.
12. Carpenter CR, Shelton E, Fowler S, et al. Risk factors and screening instruments to predict adverse outcomes for undifferentiated older emergency department patients: a systematic review and meta-analysis. Acad Emerg Med 2015; 22(1):1–21.
13. Bandeen-Roche K, Seplaki CL, Huang J, et al. Frailty in older adults: a nationally representative profile in the United States. J Gerontol A Biol Sci Med Sci 2015; 70(11):1427–34.
14. Buckinx F, Croisier JL, Reginster JY, et al. Prediction of the incidence of falls and deaths among elderly nursing home residents: the SENIOR study. J Am Med Dir Assoc 2018;19(1):18–24.
15. Evans D, Pester J, Vera L, et al. Elderly fall patients triaged to the trauma bay: age, injury patterns, and mortality risk. Am J Emerg Med 2015;33(11):1635–8.
16. Sukumar DW, Harvey LA, Mitchell RJ, et al. The impact of geographical location on trends in hospitalisation rates and outcomes for fall-related injuries in older people. Aust N Z J Public Health 2016;40(4):342–8.
17. Florence CS, Bergen G, Atherly A, et al. Medical costs of fatal and nonfatal falls in older adults: medical costs of falls. J Am Geriatr Soc 2018;66(4):693–8.
18. Haddad YK, Bergen G, Florence CS. Estimating the economic burden related to older adult falls by state. J Public Health Manag Pract 2019;25(2):E17–24.
19. Harper KJ, Barton AD, Arendts G, et al. Failure of falls risk screening tools to predict outcome: a prospective cohort study. Emerg Med J 2018;35(1):28–32.
20. Matchar DB, Eom K, Duncan PW, et al. A cost-effectiveness analysis of a randomized control trial of a tailored, multifactorial program to prevent falls among the community-dwelling elderly. Arch Phys Med Rehabil 2019;100(1):1–8.
21. Hamm J, Money AG, Atwal A, et al. Fall prevention intervention technologies: a conceptual framework and survey of the state of the art. J Biomed Inform 2016;59:319–45.
22. Iancu I, Iancu B. Designing mobile technology for elderly. A theoretical overview. Technol Forecast Soc Change 2020;155:119977.
23. Ou LC, Chang YF, Chang CS, et al. Epidemiological survey of the feasibility of broadband ultrasound attenuation measured using calcaneal quantitative ultrasound to predict the incidence of falls in the middle aged and elderly. BMJ Open 2017;7(1):e013420.
24. Benton E, Liteplo AS, Shokoohi H, et al. A pilot study examining the use of ultrasound to measure sarcopenia, frailty and fall in older patients. Am J Emerg Med 2021;46:310–6.
25. Luque R, Casilari E, Morón MJ, et al. Comparison and characterization of Android-based fall detection systems. Sensors 2014;14(10):18543–74.
26. González-Cañete FJ, Casilari E. Consumption analysis of smartphone based fall detection systems with multiple external wireless sensors. Sensors 2020;20(3):622.

27. Rasche P, Mertens A, Bröhl C, et al. The "Aachen fall prevention App" - a Smartphone application app for the self-assessment of elderly patients at risk for ground level falls. Patient Saf Surg 2017;11:14.
28. Hsieh KL, Roach KL, Wajda DA, et al. Smartphone technology can measure postural stability and discriminate fall risk in older adults. Gait Posture 2019;67: 160–5.
29. Hsieh KL, Frechette ML, Fanning J, et al. The developments and iterations of a mobile technology-based fall risk health application. Front Digit Health 2022;4: 828686.
30. Hsieh K, Fanning J, Frechette M, et al. Usability of a fall risk mHealth app for people with multiple sclerosis: mixed methods study. JMIR Hum Factors 2021;8(1): e25604.
31. Hsieh KL, Chen L, Sosnoff JJ. Mobile technology for falls prevention in older adults. J Gerontol A Biol Sci Med Sci 2022. https://doi.org/10.1093/gerona/glac116. glac116.
32. Taheri-Kharameh Z, Malmgren Fänge A, Ekvall Hansson E, et al. Development of a mobile application to screen and manage fall risks in older people. Disabil Rehabil Assist Technol 2022;17(3):362–7.
33. Gurley RJ, Lum N, Sande M, et al. Persons found in their homes helpless or dead. N Engl J Med 1996;334(26):1710–6.
34. González-Cañete FJ, Casilari E. A feasibility study of the use of smartwatches in wearable fall detection systems. Sensors 2021;21(6):2254.
35. Vilarinho T, Farshchian B, Bajer DG, et al. A Combined Smartphone and Smartwatch Fall Detection System. In: 2015 IEEE International Conference on Computer and Information Technology; Ubiquitous Computing and Communications; Dependable, Autonomic and Secure Computing; Pervasive Intelligence and Computing. Meeting held in Liverpool UK, 26-28 October 2015, IEEE; 2015:1443-1448. https://doi.org/10.1109/CIT/IUCC/DASC/PICOM.2015.216.
36. Strauss DH, Davoodi NM, Healy M, et al. The geriatric acute and post-acute fall prevention intervention (GAPcare) II to assess the use of the apple Watch in older emergency department patients with falls: protocol for a mixed methods study. JMIR Res Protoc 2021;10(4):e24455.
37. Patel PA, Gunnarsson C. A passive monitoring system in assisted living facilities: 12-month comparative study. Phys Occup Ther Geriatr 2012;30(1):45–52.
38. Berridge C, Chan KT, Choi Y. Sensor-based passive remote monitoring and discordant values: qualitative study of the experiences of low-income immigrant elders in the United States. JMIR Mhealth Uhealth 2019;7(3):e11516.
39. Quatman CE, Mondor M, Halweg J, et al. Ten years of EMS fall calls in a community: an opportunity for injury prevention strategies. Geriatr Orthop Surg Rehabil 2018;9. 2151459318783453.
40. Jeruzal JN, Boland LL, Jin D, et al. Trends in fall-related encounters and predictors of non-transport at a US emergency medical services agency. Health Soc Care Community 2022;30(5):e1835–43.
41. Simpson PM, Bendall JC, Toson B, et al. Predictors of nontransport of older fallers who receive ambulance care. Prehosp Emerg Care 2014;18(3):342–9.
42. Munjal KG, Shastry S, Loo GT, et al. Patient perspectives on EMS alternate destination models. Prehosp Emerg Care 2016;20(6):705–11.
43. Quatman CE, Anderson JP, Mondor M, et al. Frequent 911 fall calls in older adults: opportunity for injury prevention strategies. J Am Geriatr Soc 2018; 66(9):1737–43.

44. Chiang TL, Hsu CP, Yuan YJ, et al. Can EMS providers and emergency department nurses work together to identify home risk factors for falls in older people? Medicine 2022;101(38):e30752.

45. Shankar KN, Treadway NJ, Taylor AA, et al. Older adult falls prevention behaviors 60 days post-discharge from an urban emergency department after treatment for a fall. Inj Epidemiol 2017;4(1):18.

46. Zozula A, Carpenter CR, Lipsey K, et al. Prehospital emergency services screening and referral to reduce falls in community-dwelling older adults: a systematic review. Emerg Med J 2016;33(5):345–50.

47. Snooks HA, Anthony R, Chatters R, et al. Support and Assessment for Fall Emergency Referrals (SAFER) 2: a cluster randomised trial and systematic review of clinical effectiveness and cost-effectiveness of new protocols for emergency ambulance paramedics to assess older people following a fall with referral to community-based care when appropriate. Health Technol Assess 2017;21(13): 1–218.

48. Bouzid W, Tavassoli N, Berbon C, et al. Impact of a personalised care plan for the elderly calling emergency medical services after a fall at home: the RISING-DOM multi-centre randomised controlled trial protocol. BMC Geriatr 2022;22(1):182.

49. Shah MN, Caprio TV, Swanson P, et al. A novel emergency medical services-based program to identify and assist older adults in a rural community. J Am Geriatr Soc 2010;58(11):2205–11.

50. Skochko S, Grigorian A, Eshraghi C, et al. Emergency medicine (EM) can safely manage geriatric trauma patients sustaining ground level falls: fostering EM autonomy while safely offloading a busy trauma service. Am J Surg 2022;224(5): 1314–8.

51. Tirrell G, Sri-on J, Lipsitz LA, et al. Evaluation of older adult patients with falls in the emergency department: discordance with national guidelines. Shah MN. Acad Emerg Med 2015;22(4):461–7.

52. McEwan H, Baker R, Armstrong N, et al. A qualitative study of the determinants of adherence to NICE falls guideline in managing older fallers attending an emergency department. Int J Emerg Med 2018;11(1):33.

53. Southerland LT, Slattery L, Rosenthal JA, et al. Are triage questions sufficient to assign fall risk precautions in the ED? Am J Emerg Med 2017;35(2):329–32.

54. Lusardi MM, Fritz S, Middleton A, et al. Determining risk of falls in community dwelling older adults: a systematic review and meta-analysis using posttest probability. J Geriatr Phys Ther 2017;40(1):1–36.

55. Gates S, Smith LA, Fisher JD, et al. [No title found]. JRRD (J Rehabil Res Dev) 2008;45(8):1105.

56. Guirguis-Blake JM, Michael YL, Perdue LA, et al. Interventions to prevent falls in older adults: updated evidence report and systematic review for the US preventive services Task Force. JAMA 2018;319(16):1705–16.

57. Baraff LJ, Lee TJ, Kader S, et al. Effect of a practice guideline on the process of emergency department care of falls in elder patients. Acad Emergency Med 1999;6(12):1216–23.

58. Hogan TM, Richmond NL, Carpenter CR, et al. Shared decision making to improve the emergency care of older adults: a research agenda. Acad Emerg Med 2016;23(12):1386–93.

59. Carpenter CR, Lo AX. Falling behind? Understanding implementation science in future emergency department management strategies for geriatric fall prevention. Acad Emerg Med 2015;22(4):478–80.

60. Panel on prevention of falls in older persons, American geriatrics society and British geriatrics society. Summary of the updated American geriatrics society/British geriatrics society clinical practice guideline for prevention of falls in older persons: AGS/BGS clinical practice guideline for prevention of falls. J Am Geriatr Soc 2011;59(1):148–57.

61. Hess EP, Grudzen CR, Thomson R, et al. Shared decision-making in the emergency department: respecting patient autonomy when seconds count. Acad Emerg Med 2015;22(7):856–64.

62. Tinetti ME, Baker DI, McAvay G, et al. A multifactorial intervention to reduce the risk of falling among elderly people living in the community. N Engl J Med 1994; 331(13):821–7.

63. Shaw FE, Bond J, Richardson DA, et al. Multifactorial intervention after a fall in older people with cognitive impairment and dementia presenting to the accident and emergency department: randomised controlled trial. BMJ 2003;326(7380):73.

64. Hopewell S, Adedire O, Copsey BJ, et al. Multifactorial and multiple component interventions for preventing falls in older people living in the community. Cochrane Database Syst Rev 2018;7. https://doi.org/10.1002/14651858.CD012221.pub2.

65. Ganz DA, Alkema GE, Wu S. It takes a village to prevent falls: reconceptualizing fall prevention and management for older adults. Inj Prev 2008;14(4): 266–71.

66. Barker A, Cameron P, Flicker L, et al. Evaluation of RESPOND, a patient-centred program to prevent falls in older people presenting to the emergency department with a fall: a randomised controlled trial. PLoS Med 2019;16(5):e1002807.

67. Goldberg EM, Marks SJ, Resnik LJ, et al. Can an emergency department-initiated intervention prevent subsequent falls and health care use in older adults? A randomized controlled trial. Ann Emerg Med 2020;76(6):739–50.

68. American College of Emergency Physicians. American geriatrics society, emergency nurses association, society for academic emergency medicine, geriatric emergency department guidelines Task Force. Geriatric emergency department guidelines. Ann Emerg Med 2014;63(5):e7–25.

69. 7 Step Fall Challenge.; 2017. Available at: https://www.youtube.com/watch?v=-ehHhdoJ2k8. Accessed February 21, 2023.

70. Chiam R, Saedon N, Khor HM, et al. Potentially inappropriate prescribing in a falls clinic using the STOPP and START criteria. Int J Clin Pharm 2022;44(1):163–71.

71. Schoon Y, Hoogsteen-Ossewaarde ME, Scheffer AC, et al. Comparison of different strategies of referral to a fall clinic: how to achieve an optimal casemix? J Nutr Health Aging 2011;15(2):140–5.

72. van Wijck S FM, Rizzo C, S. Tsegai N, et al. Unexpected challenges to preventing falls in older adults: a mixed methods study of an emergency department-based falls prevention referral pilot project. Health Edu Care 2019;4(2). https://doi.org/10.15761/HEC.1000158.

73. Schoenfeld EM, Goff SL, Elia TR, et al. Physician-identified barriers to and facilitators of shared decision-making in the Emergency Department: an exploratory analysis. Emerg Med J 2019;36(6):346–54.

74. Rosen JM, Adams LV, Geiling J, et al. Telehealth's new horizon: providing smart hospital-level care in the home. Telemedicine and e-Health 2021;27(11): 1215–24.

75. Hayden EM, Davis C, Clark S, et al. Telehealth in emergency medicine: a consensus conference to map the intersection of telehealth and emergency medicine. Acad Emerg Med 2021;28(12):1452–74.

76. Ouchi K, Liu S, Tonellato D, et al. Home hospital as a disposition for older adults from the emergency department: benefits and opportunities. Journal of the American College of Emergency Physicians Open 2021;2(4). https://doi.org/10.1002/emp2.12517.

77. Farrell TW, Francis L, Brown T, et al. Rationing limited healthcare resources in the COVID-19 era and beyond: ethical considerations regarding older adults. J Am Geriatr Soc 2020;68(6):1143–9.

78. Stevens JA, Lee R. The potential to reduce falls and avert costs by clinically managing fall risk. Am J Prev Med 2018;55(3):290–7.

79. Carande-Kulis V, Stevens JA, Florence CS, et al. A cost–benefit analysis of three older adult fall prevention interventions. J Saf Res 2015;52:65–70.

80. Hutchins-Wiese H, Argeros G, Walsh SE. Frailty and nutrition risk predict falls and emergency department visits in home-delivered meal clients. J Nutr Gerontol Geriatr 2023;1–14. https://doi.org/10.1080/21551197.2023.2167030.

81. Wang HH, Huang CC, Talley PC, et al. Using healthcare resources wisely: a predictive support system regarding the severity of patient falls. J Healthc Eng 2022;2022:3100618.

82. Chan WC, Yeung JWF, Wong CSM, et al. Efficacy of physical exercise in preventing falls in older adults with cognitive impairment: a systematic review and meta-analysis. J Am Med Dir Assoc 2015;16(2):149–54.

83. Daoust R, Paquet J, Moore L, et al. Recent opioid use and fall-related injury among older patients with trauma. CMAJ (Can Med Assoc J) 2018;190(16):E500–6.

84. Santosa KB, Lai YL, Brummett CM, et al. Higher amounts of opioids filled after surgery increase risk of serious falls and fall-related injuries among older adults. J Gen Intern Med 2020;35(10):2917–24.

85. Neta G, Glasgow RE, Carpenter CR, et al. A framework for enhancing the value of research for dissemination and implementation. Am J Public Health 2015;105(1):49–57.

86. Stoeckle A, Iseler JI, Havey R, et al. Catching quality before it falls: preventing falls and injuries in the adult emergency department. J Emerg Nurs 2019;45(3):257–64.

87. Lesser A, Israni J, Kent T, et al. Association between physical therapy in the emergency department and emergency department revisits for older adult fallers: a nationally representative analysis. J Am Geriatr Soc 2018;66(11):2205–12.

88. Wallace R, Angus LDG, Munnangi S, et al. Improved outcomes following implementation of a multidisciplinary care pathway for elderly hip fractures. Aging Clin Exp Res 2019;31(2):273–8.

89. Salvador-Marín J, Ferrández-Martínez FJ, Lawton CD, et al. Efficacy of a multidisciplinary care protocol for the treatment of operated hip fracture patients. Sci Rep 2021;11(1):24082.

90. Li Y, Tung KK, Cho YC, et al. Improved outcomes and reduced medical costs through multidisciplinary co-management protocol for geriatric proximal femur fractures: a one-year retrospective study. BMC Geriatr 2022;22(1):318.

91. Stevens JA, Phelan EA. Development of STEADI: a fall prevention resource for health care providers. Health Promot Pract 2013;14(5):706–14.

92. Parks A, Eagles D, Ge Y, et al. Barriers and enablers that influence guideline-based care of geriatric fall patients presenting to the emergency department. Emerg Med J 2019;36(12):741–7.

93. Cameron ID, Dyer SM, Panagoda CE, et al. Interventions for preventing falls in older people in care facilities and hospitals. Cochrane Bone, Joint and Muscle Trauma Group. Cochrane Database Syst Rev 2018;2020(1). https://doi.org/10.1002/14651858.CD005465.pub4.
94. Bernocchi P, Giordano A, Pintavalle G, et al. Feasibility and clinical efficacy of a multidisciplinary home-telehealth program to prevent falls in older adults: a randomized controlled trial. J Am Med Dir Assoc 2019;20(3):340–6.

Trauma (Excluding Falls) in the Older Adult

Kyle R. Burton, MD, MPP[a], Phillip D. Magidson, MD, MPH[b],*

KEYWORDS

- Geriatric trauma • Older patient • Triage • Critical care • Trauma • Geriatrics

INTRODUCTION

Trauma in the geriatric population is a growing concern that will increasingly have significant implications for the United States health care system. By 2030, 69 million Americans are expected to be older than 65 years of age.[1] Although geriatric patients represent 31% of all trauma patients encountered, this proportion is anticipated to grow as the population ages and life expectancy increases.[2] Older adults who experience trauma face worse outcomes compared with their younger counterparts. Increasing age is an independent predictor of poor outcome following trauma, with a 2.4 to 5.6 greater risk of death.[3–6] The traumatic case fatality rate nearly doubles after age 65 years, and geriatric patients with traumatic injuries have an increased 12-month mortality; more than 55,000 individuals in the United States die from unintentional injury each year.[7,8] Although ground-level falls are much more prevalent than other mechanisms of trauma in geriatric patients, other modes typically seen include motor vehicle accidents, pedestrians struck by a vehicle, injuries related to other forms of transport, firearm injuries, and penetrating injuries. This article excludes trauma from falls while outlining the physiologic vulnerabilities, specific injury considerations, and management strategies among older patients.

Undertriage in Geriatric Trauma

Challenges with the management of geriatric trauma patients start before the patient has arrived in the emergency department (ED). Trauma centers often rely on protocolized care structures. Geriatric patient-specific considerations are not always included within such protocols resulting in undertriage of these patients.[9,10] Geriatric trauma patients who have comprehensive trauma evaluations by a trained trauma team ultimately have fewer complications and stay in the ED and hospital for less time.[11] Although undertriage challenges must be addressed, physicians can mitigate the lack of a trauma team with early recognition of traumatic injuries and an expedited,

[a] Department of Emergency Medicine, Johns Hopkins Hospital, 1830 Eas, Monument Street, Suite 6-110, Baltimore, MD 21287, USA; [b] Johns Hopkins Hospital, Johns Hopkins Bayview Medical Center, 4940 Eastern Avenue, Suite A150, Baltimore, MD 21224, USA
* Corresponding author. 4940 Eastern Avenue, Suite A150, Baltimore, MD 21224.
E-mail address: pmagidson@jhmi.edu

Clin Geriatr Med 39 (2023) 519–533
https://doi.org/10.1016/j.cger.2023.05.005
0749-0690/23/© 2023 Elsevier Inc. All rights reserved.

thorough evaluation of geriatric trauma patients. Timely imaging diagnostics and early involvement of consulting services has been shown to improve outcomes and decrease patient length of stay.[12] Some institutions have gone as far as to use age as a qualifier for trauma team activation. One level 1 trauma center found that activating the team for any trauma patient greater than age 70 years resulted in both decreased ED length of stay and overall improvement in mortality.[13] This finding should be considered in institutional protocol that intends to improve outcomes in geriatric trauma management.

Physiologic Changes Associated with Aging

Older patients have a higher incidence of medical comorbidities and lower physiologic reserves, increasing their susceptibility to even minor trauma and their mortality risk fivefold.[3,14] Although some of these comorbidities contribute to trauma, others complicate the trauma examination and injury management.

Neurologic/cognitive considerations

Cognitive impairment affects 25% of older adults who present to EDs.[15] This greatly contributes to the challenges of caring for older adults, delaying presentation, and creates difficulty obtaining a history. Patients may not be able to report critical patient information such as the use of anticoagulants and injury mechanism. If unsupported in their living space, those with cognitive impairment are at risk for trauma through motor vehicle operation. Those with cognitive comorbidities may have a decreased ability to request pain medications, leading to further suffering. Agitation and behavioral disturbance from cognitive impairment may complicate the obtaining a history, examination, and diagnostic tests. Furthermore, these patients have an increased risk of developing delirium from trauma and injury-specific management.

In addition, geriatric patients are more likely to have had prior cerebrovascular accidents, often with residual neurologic deficits, than their younger counterparts.[16] This makes identifying new deficits from a traumatic injury more challenging.

Respiratory considerations

Relatively poor baseline pulmonary function and underlying lung disease makes older patients more vulnerable to traumatic sequelae. Older adults have increased chest wall rigidity, worsened kyphosis, decreased respiratory muscle strength, and decreased elastic recoil of the lung, leading to decreased vital capacity.[17] Geriatric patients often have loss of the protective cough mechanism, decreased mucociliary clearance, decreased diffusion capacity, increased ventilation/perfusion heterogeneity, and dysfunction of the central and peripheral chemoreceptors.[18] These changes can result in reduced respiratory reserve and increased risk of uncompensated hypoxia and hypercarbia, which can cause encephalopathy if inappropriately managed. Pulmonary comorbidities among older patients help explain how the most common post-traumatic hospital complication is pneumonia, which can have delayed resolution in those with poor baseline pulmonary function and have 24% mortality.[19,20]

Cardiovascular considerations

As patients age, there is progressive stiffening of both the arterial vasculature and the myocardium.[17] This leads to higher baseline blood pressure, which can increase the risk for acute coronary syndrome and the traumatic injuries that can result from having myocardial ischemia. Older patients with blunt chest trauma have a higher risk of dissection and higher mortality with existing cardiac conditions.[21] Vascular stiffening and decreased peripheral perfusion from peripheral vascular disease in older adults also leads to a more precipitous drop in blood pressure from stressors such as trauma. The geriatric population is also much more likely to be on medications that alter hemodynamics slowing the heart rate (HR) artificially or blunting a physiologic tachycardic response to stress or hemorrhage.

Renal considerations

The number of glomeruli decreases with age, leading to decreased renal function and decreased ability to retain sodium and water.[22] Glomerular filtration rate lowers by 10% per decade after age 40 years, and this drop worsens in patients with hypertension and chronic heart disease.[23] Given the poor fluid retention ability, this population is at an increased risk of dehydration, especially when combined with a frequently impaired thirst response and poor oral intake from decreased mobility. Dehydration can lead to geriatric trauma.

Musculoskeletal considerations

Higher rates of deconditioning and osteoporosis in geriatric patients make them susceptible to musculoskeletal injuries compared with younger adults.[24] Older patients are more likely to suffer fractures and dislocations from minor trauma. Unfortunately, radiograph imaging has decreased sensitivity for detection of fractures in this age group, such that advanced imaging may be necessary. Orthopedic injuries that may have minimal impact on the lives of younger patients can have a profound impact on functional independence, and even mortality, in geriatric patients. Even a mere ankle sprain can be debilitating enough to limit kitchen, and therefore food, access.

Critical Trauma Stabilization in the Geriatric Patient

The appropriate initial management of geriatric trauma relies on an understanding of several nuances in critical stabilization for older patients. Physicians can perform a systematic trauma assessment that adheres to Advanced Trauma Life Support guidance but should consider the unique vital signs, rapid assessment, and imaging factors that can complicate geriatric trauma care.

Normal vital signs are not as reassuring as they may be in younger patients. Among older patients, mortality is 7% to 13% higher among those with HR greater than 90 beats per minute (bpm) and with systolic blood pressure (SBP) less than 110 mm Hg.[25] Compare this to an HR greater than 130 bpm and an SBP less than 95 mm Hg, which are associated with increased mortality in young patients. The individual HR and SBP are less reliable than the age-adjusted shock index that includes these two measures for accurately predicting mortality in geriatric trauma patients.[26] Vital sign data obtained in the ED should not replace clinical suspicion in determining hemodynamic compromise, as older patients may have delayed vital sign manifestation of shock.

Airway

Unstable geriatric trauma patients, with shock, altered mental status, and/or significant thoracic trauma, warrant early intubation. Goals of care in this population vary, and providers should attempt to establish patient desires before intervention.

Several anatomic changes that occur with aging should be considered in airway management.[17] An increased prevalence of nasal polyps in the older population impairs the passing of nasopharyngeal airways. Atrophy of the orbicularis oris muscle, limited mandibular protrusion, and dental decay, loose teeth, or edentulous anatomy make it difficult to form a proper seal with a bag-valve-mask device. If dentures are securely in place, they should not be removed as they can improve the seal in bag-valve-mask ventilation, but they should be removed before intubation. Temporomandibular joint stiffness can limit mouth opening, making it difficult to place some rescue airway devices. The decreased thyromental distance and submandibular compliance increase difficulty in obtaining an adequate airway view. The increased parapharyngeal fat and a floppy epiglottis due to decreased elastic and collagen fibers increase the likelihood of collapse and obstruction in the older population. Also, degeneration/inflammatory and iatrogenic (ie, radiation, surgery) changes of the cervical spine decrease the neck mobility. Consider using video laryngoscopy for a clear view of the airway if intubation is needed.

Breathing
Lung disease and spinal kyphosis worsen functional lung volumes in the geriatric trauma patient. Ramping up the bed with a reverse Trendelenburg approach can assist with oxygenation and ventilation. Capnography monitoring is recommended in circumstances of underlying lung disease, thoracic injury, and when analgesia or sedatives are provided.

Circulation
In every age group, but especially in older adults, mortality increases dramatically with the presence of shock. Shock is more difficult to identify in older adults, but physicians should diagnose it early and treat it rapidly. Evaluation of the inferior vena cava collapsibility by ultrasound may assist with assessing overall fluid status and guiding resuscitation. The indicators for need of massive transfusion, such as the Assessment of Blood Consumption and the Trauma Associated Severe Hemorrhage scores, are not as sensitive in older adults. Resuscitation with isotonic crystalloid or blood should be initiated rapidly and anticoagulation reversal should be considered in traumatic shock. There are many age-related changes in cardiac output that can impact the critical management of geriatric trauma. There is a significant decrease in the maximum HR that should equate to 220 minus the patient age. Older patients have a decreased response to adrenergic catecholamines due to the reduced responsiveness of membrane receptors. If shock persists beyond fluid resuscitation, pressor support should be available.

Disability
Around 3% of older patients will have intracranial injury without clinical indicators such as loss of consciousness of focal neurologic deficit.[27] Even subtle changes in mental status may be the only sign of traumatic brain injury (TBI), and no combination of findings reliably predicts the absence of intracranial injuries in the older population. It is important to confirm baseline mental status with caregivers.

Exposure
Older patients may not always be able to report or localize their source of pain, so obtaining full exposure is imperative for guiding imaging and management. Even minor wounds can cause serious complications in older patients. Importantly, once exposure has been obtained, it is important to cover the patient with warmed blankets given the thermoregulatory deficits in this population.[28]

Trauma imaging
A low threshold is suggested for liberal use of cross-sectional imaging in older patients involved in high-energy trauma, even in the absence of obvious injuries.[29] By performing an early computed tomography (CT) pan-scan, there is a reduced need for intensive monitoring, which can facilitate early mobilization and shorten periods of fasting, both of which are important for preventing delirium. Similarly, the duration of hospital stay, intensive care unit admission rates, morbidity, and mortality can be decreased

even if the patient has a high acuity trauma.[30] Some may hesitate to obtain contrast imaging of older patients given the higher chance that these patients may have chronic kidney disease. The diagnostic yield of a contrast-enhanced study outweighs the risk of contrast-induced nephropathy which can be managed medically following trauma stabilization.[31] This is especially relevant in view of potential consequences with undertriage.

Injury-Specific Management

Traumatic brain injury

Head trauma among older patients carries a greater risk of intracranial injury irrespective of acuity as well as increased mortality and morbidity when compared with younger trauma patients.[32] TBI can account for up to 58% of deaths from blunt trauma.[33] Increased mortality among older patients with TBI may result from factors such as comorbid illness and higher rates of intracranial hemorrhage (ICH). Increasing vessel fragility, hypertension, and amyloid angiopathy, hematological conditions, alcohol, and anticoagulant use increase the risk of bleeding in all brain compartments.[34]

Although there is an increased risk of hemorrhage in all intracranial sections, this risk is most prevalent in the subdural compartment. As patients age, the incidence of post-traumatic subdural hematoma increases due partly to the inherent changes in vasculature and white matter exacerbated by the increased use of antiplatelet and anticoagulant therapy.[35] As the brain atrophies, the subdural compartment widens, stretching the bridging cortical veins, which are then more susceptible to shearing injury.[3] The early detection and aggressive treatment of traumatic brain abnormalities in the older patient significantly improves overall clinical outcomes and increases the chance of returning to normal independent living.[36] Unfortunately, recovery from serious head injuries often is delayed and results in worse cognitive and psychosocial function in older adults compared with their younger counterparts.[37]

Anticoagulation considerations in traumatic brain injury

The risk of traumatic ICH is greater among patients taking anticoagulants and antiplatelet medications.[38,39] Those on anticoagulation have a four to five times increased risk of mortality from ICH and are more likely to require intervention or experience complications.[40] Those on anticoagulation with confirmed ICH warrant anticoagulant reversal. As with younger patients, those with hemodynamic instability may also benefit from tranexamic acid (TXA) when bleeding is suspected. TXA seems to be as efficient in preventing death in older patients as in the young.[41] Current data suggest that a head CT at the time of presentation is sufficient for older patients with a normal neurologic examination, patients with therapeutic/subtherapeutic international normalized ratio (INR) (if on warfarin), and for those taking novel oral anticoagulants.[42] There remains no consensus on whether serial neurologic examinations are sufficient or if repeat imaging is warranted in patients with a supratherapeutic INR.

Following TBI, it may be challenging to determine whether to continue the anticoagulation that the patient was previously on. It is reasonable to believe, even if the older patient does not suffer ICH that this individual is at increased risk for ICH given the chance of suffering additional trauma. In most cases, the decision of if and when to continue anticoagulation will result from shared decision-making between the primary care physician and patient and/or caretaker. Studies actually suggest that patients with frequent falls do not have an increased risk of major bleeding, thus making it safe to continue anticoagulation if the head CT is unremarkable.[43] Data suggest that patients on warfarin would need to fall 295 times in a year for the risk of fall-related ICH to outweigh the benefit of the warfarin itself.[44] Although data suggest that continuing anticoagulation is safe for patients, in particular those with multiple stroke risk factors, it is prudent for physicians to evaluate each patient individually. One can do this by considering the underlying pathology being addressed with anticoagulation and making a calculated risk–benefit assessment using previously validated clinical decision tools. The CHA2DS2-VASc score assesses the risk of stroke in patients with atrial fibrillation, a common reason for older patients to use anticoagulation.[44] This score provides a stroke risk that can be weighed against the risk of major bleeding while taking anticoagulation calculated by the HAS-BLED score.[45] If the risk of stroke exceeds the risk of major bleeding, then anticoagulation may be favored, even in light of risk for future trauma.

Maxillofacial injury

Patients older than 75 years are most likely to sustain midfacial fractures, particularly orbital wall fractures.[46] There is relative weakness of the bones in the midface compared with the mandible and the calvarium, making the midface particularly vulnerable.[47] With geriatric trauma, there can be serious maxillary sinus pneumatization further weakening the midface if the patients have undergone extraction of the maxillary teeth.[48] Although most maxillofacial fractures are diagnosed by head CT, a dedicated maxillofacial CT should be obtained if clinical findings hint at an injury. The midface is only partially imaged with a head CT, and oral and facial soft tissue injuries may indicate underlying bony injuries that could be missed without focused imaging.[49] Those severely injured patients who do not undergo maxillofacial CT are at risk of increased hospital length of stay because many of these patients will require subsequent scans that could have been completed at initial presentation.

Patients older than 75 years with maxillofacial fractures are at high risk of intracranial injuries, particularly hemorrhage.[50] In addition to an increased risk for intracranial bleeding, these patients often have long bone fractures especially of the forearm. Physicians must perform a thorough examination and consider the injury mechanism when obtaining imaging for these patients.

Neck and spine injury

Although young patients have the highest risk of cervical spine injury at the most mobile portion of the cervical spine (C4–C7), older patients have increased spinal rigidity and are more likely to suffer from injuries to the odontoid process and C2.[51] Spinal fractures are the third most common traumatic injury in older people, of which cervical spine injuries make up around 15%.[52] Conditions such as senescent spondylosis deformans, ankylosing spondylitis, diffuse idiopathic skeletal hyperostosis, and ossification of the posterior longitudinal ligament may result in increased rigidity of the mid and lower cervical spine, with relatively increased mobility of the superior cervical spine (C1 and C2) and craniocervical junction. As a result, up to 60% of spinal fractures in older patients involve the C1 ring and C2 dens.[53] Spondylosis results in an increased incidence of spinal canal stenosis. There is an increased risk of spinal cord injury, with or without bony injury, especially if the paraspinal ligaments and the ligamentum flavum are disrupted.[54] In hyperextension injuries, the bulging ligamentum flavum may compress the spinal cord resulting in a central cord syndrome. Unfortunately, hyperextension injuries may be very subtle or occult on radiography with only slight widening of an intervertebral disc space of a soft tissue hematoma. Patients with an apparently isolated head injury have a 5% risk of additional spinal injury, so cervical spine CT is added to all CT head studies in older patients.[55] Diagnostic value of CT radiographic assessment is limited by reduced bone density and spondylotic changes, so injuries may be missed in up to 40% of adults and 80% of geriatric trauma patients.[53] If a fracture is detected, further assessment for possible contiguous and noncontiguous spinal fractures is required, as 30% to 40% of patients sustain multilevel cervical spinal injuries.[56] MRI is useful in cases of equivocal CT findings, suspected ligamentous injury, spinal cord injury, or occult fractures.[57] A retrospective cohort study of older patients (80–89 years of age) with traumatic odontoid fractures found that operative management had not associated in-hospital mortality and relatively low 30-day mortality (6%).[58] Early interventions in older patients with intense management to prevent complications may be beneficial.

As mentioned earlier, geriatric trauma patients may also have cognitive impairment. Physicians may be challenged with determining whether to obtain MRI studies after CT imaging does not identify abnormalities in a patient with cognitive impairment. The high quality of modern CT scanners likely explains recent data showing the incidence of occult C-spine injuries to be as low as 0.12%, even in obtunded patients.[59] Another systematic review recommends removing the cervical collar after negative high-quality CT scan alone consistent with the Eastern Association for the Surgery of Trauma guidelines.[60] Cervical collars have been shown to cause discomfort, tissue breakdown, increased aspiration risk, and worsened delirium.[61] Some patients may even warrant sedation for MRI, in which case the physician must consider the risks of sedative administration versus the likelihood of advanced imaging changing management. Several factors, including patient wishes, underlying functional status, goals of care, and shared decision-making, should play into the physician's decision in these scenarios.

Osteoporosis is a major risk factor for vertebral compression fractures, particularly in the thoracolumbar spine. This condition is common in postmenopausal women and affects a third of men over 75 years of age, justifying the increased risk in geriatric trauma.[54] Older patients are at greater risk of having a spinal injury, mainly due to poorer osseous mineralization, osteoporosis, and increased spinal rigidity. Spinal injuries tend to occur with seemingly minor trauma and are not infrequently multilevel.[55,56] Because injuries may be clinically unstable and at risk of neurologic decline, the prompt imaging is imperative. The most common site of injury is at the thoracolumbar junction (T12–L2), followed by the mid-thoracic spine.[54] Studies suggest that most of the fractures are nonoperative and that spine immobilization can lead to worse outcomes.[62] Early ambulation with a supportive brace is often indicated for vertebral fractures without neurologic compromise in older patients. Spinal fractures in geriatric trauma are associated with substantial morbidity and mortality (over 40% at 1 year), often because of pneumonia and respiratory failure.[52]

Thoracic injury

Rib fractures are the most common manifestation of blunt thoracic trauma in older patients. Older patients, especially women, are more susceptible to seatbelt-induced thoracic trauma from low or moderate speed crashes than other populations.[63] Thoracic injuries are associated with increased mortality in women 65 years and older, and age is one of the strongest predictors of mortality from rib fractures.[64] Managing rib fractures in older adults are mostly comparable to management in younger adults, with particularly attention for surgical intervention with those having respiratory compromise. Treating flail segments with open reduction and internal fixation has been shown to reduce the need for ventilatory support, shorten the intensive care and overall hospital stay, reduce the incidence of pneumonia and septicemia, reduce the risk of chest deformity, and reduce mortality rate.[65] Although rib fractures without flail segments in geriatric trauma patients historically have been managed conservatively, there has been recent advocacy for operative management, particularly rib plating. Studies on rib plating and fracture fixation have demonstrated lower mortality, decreased post-traumatic complications, and shorter rehabilitation periods than patients managed conservatively.[66]

Geriatric trauma patients with rib fractures have double the mortality rate of young patients with rib fractures, and this number increases proportionately with each additional rib fracture due to secondary pulmonary and cardiac complications.[67] Ninety percent of patients with rib fractures have other traumatic injuries.[68] Rib fractures are often associated with more severe traumatic sequelae, such as cardiac and great vessel injuries, pneumothoraces, pulmonary contusions, and liver and splenic trauma.[5] Patients 60 years and over have a threefold risk of blunt thoracic aortic injury when involved in motor vehicle accidents often due to the deceleration mechanism.[69] Despite this, traumatic vascular injuries are overall uncommon in older patients, occurring in approximately 1% of cases.[70] When present, these vascular injuries have a fourfold increase in adjusted mortality.

Clavicle fractures are associated with a surprisingly high mortality rate in patients over 65 years who have sustained high-impact trauma.[5] These fractures indicate not only severe thoracic but also brain injuries and are associated with a higher mortality rate in older patients.

Abdominal injury
Blunt abdominal trauma is as common in older patients as in younger patients, but associated with a fivefold increase in the mortality rate.[54] For those who suffer from splenic injury, age predicts overall mortality rates.[71] Geriatric trauma patients who suffer from abdominal trauma have a lower likelihood of qualifying for operative management, and those who undergo surgery have worse outcomes than younger patients.[72] Given these findings, physicians should prioritize identifying intra-abdominal injuries early to allow for maximal medical management.

Pelvic and hip injury
The average age of patients with hip fractures is more than 70 years of age, and nearly 80% are women.[73] Older patients tend to sustain hip injuries that result in significant morbidity and mortality from low-energy mechanisms.[74] Lateral compression fractures are five times more common than anteroposterior compression fractures in the geriatric population, a reversal of the normal pattern observed in younger patients.[75] Lateral compression fractures can have associated vascular injury necessitating invasive procedures.[75] Exsanguination is the common cause of death in the first 6 hours following a severe pelvic fracture, and older patients have an eightfold risk of significant pelvic bleeding compared with younger adults.[76] Furthermore, geriatric trauma patients have higher rates of pelvic bleeding requiring blood transfusions and a greater need for angiographic treatment.[77] During the trauma examination, physicians can look for gross hematuria to be an indicator of severe pelvic fractures. Missed pelvic and hip fractures may lead to increased nonunion, avascular necrosis, and morbidity.[78] It is important to maintain a high level of suspicion for pelvic and hip fractures and to have a low threshold of more advanced imaging in those with significant pain or difficulty ambulating in the setting of nondiagnostic radiographs. Older patients who sustain pelvic trauma have a fourfold increase in mortality rate (up to 20%) when compared with younger patients, on par with the mortality of 24% in adults over age 65 years with acute myocardial infarction (MI).[76,79] Surgical intervention is recommended in most geriatric trauma hip fractures, and even those who are minimally ambulatory may have palliative benefits from surgery. Physicians should

maintain urgency in pursuing surgical intervention. In older patients undergoing operative repair of a hip fracture, the pulmonary complications were decreased if the surgery was performed within less than 24 hours and 30-day mortality is decreased with repair within 12 hours.[80,81]

Orthopedic extremity injury

Geriatric trauma patients have higher incidence of osteoporosis and sarcopenia, increasing the likelihood of bony injury after trauma, most commonly forearm fractures.[72,82] Sarcopenia increases the likelihood that older patients need rehabilitation and possible prolonged hospitalization after injuries.[16] The incidence of distal radius fractures increases with age, especially in women, and nearly 10% sustain concurrent median nerve injury.[83,84] Femoral neck fractures are intracapsular injuries in which the 1-year mortality increases with associated medical comorbidities, such as chronic renal failure and congestive heart failure.[85] Intertrochanteric fractures occur between the greater and lesser trochanter and typically occur in an older age group than those with femoral neck fractures. A retrospective chart review of the Ottawa Ankle Rules found comparable sensitivities between the nongeriatric and geriatric cohorts, speaking to the applicability of these guidelines to older adults.[86] It is important to have a low threshold for radiographs.

Polytrauma

Polytrauma carries a mortality rate of 36% for geriatric trauma patients.[72] The most common complications of polytrauma in one study were delirium, pneumonia, and electrolyte abnormalities.[87]

Interdisciplinary Support

Physicians, already tasked with critical stabilization and trauma management, should not be expected to address all geriatric trauma patient needs through their efforts alone. Fortunately, a growing number of institutions are learning the value of the interdisciplinary team in providing complete care. Having a geriatrician available for consulting on trauma patients has been shown to improve outcomes in geriatric trauma patients and decrease hospital length of stay.[88] These providers help perform a comprehensive assessment of geriatric patients to reduce hospital-acquired complications, such as falls, functional decline, and delirium while also evaluating new and existing medical conditions.[89] Because a formal comprehensive geriatric assessment improves outcomes for medical and surgical geriatric patients alike, this service is strongly recommended for trauma patients.

The early involvement of a palliative care team can strongly benefit patients with an increased risk of death while also benefiting their families and the hospital system as a whole.[90,91] Early palliative care consultation, even when initiated from the ED, can decrease patient pain and suffering, decrease family anxiety, improve patient/family understanding of goals of care, decrease hospital length of stay, decrease intensive care unit admissions, and decrease hospital system costs.[92]

Disposition Planning

Geriatric patients with many traumatic injuries may be admitted to a trauma service with a geriatric consult so that specific injuries can be addressed, whereas holistic evaluation of their medical condition is conducted. Literature indicates admitting geriatric trauma patients to internal medicine can unnecessarily and significantly increase length of stay, but each institution may have systems set in place that optimize patient care.[93] It is helpful to draft interdepartmental protocols that allow for expedited intervention.

All ages of trauma patients have been shown to have increased mortality up to 1 year after the initial event compared with non-trauma patients, but this discrepancy is markedly increased in older patients.[94] These findings emphasize the need for longer follow-up periods of geriatric trauma patients. Both patients and family members should be engaged early to establish goals of care after serious injuries. Geriatric trauma patients rely on consideration of injuries sustained and the conditions that precipitated those injuries, complicating their management. Adequate analgesia, early mobilization, and prevention of complications can have a positive impact on morbidity and mortality.

CLINICS CARE POINTS

- Older patients have a higher incidence of comorbidities that increase susceptibility to trauma and complicate the trauma examination and injury management.
- The appropriate critical stabilization of older trauma patients relies on the recognition of the nuances to geriatric physiology.
- Injury-specific management in geriatric trauma can optimize outcomes of this vulnerable population.
- The early involvement of ancillary support providers can address circumstances that may have led to the patient traumatic event and could avoid future events.
- Comprehensive older patient outpatient follow-up coordination can have a positive impact on patient morbidity and mortality.

DISCLOSURES

Nothing to disclose.

REFERENCES

1. Trauma Facts - The American association for the surgery of trauma Available at: https://www.aast.org/trauma-facts. Accessed January 15, 2023.
2. Chang MC. National trauma data bank annual report. Chicago, IL: American College of Surgeons; 2016.
3. Grossman MD, Miller D, Scaff DW, et al. When is an elder old? Effect of pre-existing conditions on mortality in geriatric trauma. J Trauma 2002;52:242–6.
4. Gubler KD, Davis R, Koepsell T, et al. Long-term survival of elderly trauma patients. Arch Surg 1997;132:1010–4.
5. Keller JM, Sciadini MF, Sinclair E, et al. Geriatric trauma: demographics, injuries, and mortality. J Orthop Trauma 2012;26:e161–5.
6. Jacobs DG. Special considerations in geriatric injury. Curr Opin Crit Care 2003;9:535–9.
7. Friesendorff M, von McGuigan FE, Wizert A, et al. Hip fracture, mortality risk, and cause of death over two decades. Osteoporos Int 2016;10(7):2945–53.
8. Available at: https://www.cdc.gov/injury/wisqars/pdf/leading_causes_of_death_by_age_group_2017-508.pdf. Accessed December 27, 2022.
9. Hung KK, Yeung JHH, Cheung CSK, et al. Trauma team activation criteria and outcomes of geriatric trauma: 10 year single centre cohort study. Am J Emerg Med 2019;37(3):450–6.

10. Ryb GE, Dischinger PC. Disparities in trauma center access of older injured motor vehicular crash occupants. J Trauma 2011;71(3):742–7.
11. Wiles LL, Day MD. Delta alert: expanding gerotrauma criteria to improve patient outcomes. J Trauma Nurs 2018;25(3):159–64.
12. Fernandez FB, Ong A, Martin AP, et al. Success of an expedited emergency department triage evaluation system for geriatric trauma patients not meeting trauma activation criteria. Open Access Emerg Med 2019;11:241–7.
13. Hammer PM, Storey AC, Bell T, et al. Improving geriatric trauma outcomes: a small step toward a big problem. J Trauma Acute Care Surg 2016;81(1):162–7.
14. McGwin G Jr, MacLennan PA, Fife JB, et al. Preexisting conditions and mortality in older trauma patients. J Trauma 2004;56(6):1291–6.
15. Wilber S, Han JH. Altered mental status in the elderly. In: Kahn J, Maguaran B, Olshaker J, editors. Geriatric emergency medicine: principles and practice. Cambridge: Cambridge University Press; 2014. p. 102–13.
16. Llompart-Pou JA, Pérez-Bárcena J, Chico-Fernández M, et al. Severe trauma in the geriatric population. World J Crit Care Med 2017;6(2):99–106.
17. Perera T, Cortijo-Brown A. Geriatric resuscitation. Emerg Med Clin North Am 2016;34(3):453–67.
18. Johnson KN, Botros DB, Groban L, et al. Anatomic and physiopathologic changes affecting the airway of the elderly patient: implications for geriatric-focused airway management. Clin Interv Aging 2015;10:1925–34.
19. Bergeron E, Lavoie A, Clas D, et al. Elderly trauma patients with rib fractures are at greater risk of death and pneumonia. J Trauma 2003;54(3):478–85.
20. Wutzler S, Bläsius FM, Störmann P, et al. Pneumonia in severely injured patients with thoracic trauma: results of a retrospective observational multi-centre study. Scand J Trauma Resusc Emerg Med 2019;27:31.
21. Singh S, Angus LD. Blunt cardiac injury. StatPearls, StatPearls Publishing; 2020. Available at: https://www.ncbi.nlm.nih.gov/books/NBK532267/.
22. El-Sharkawy AM, Sahota O, Maughan RJ, et al. The pathophysiology of fluid and electrolyte balance in the older adult surgical patient. Clin Nutr 2014;33(1):6–13.
23. Wiggins J, Patel SR. In: Halter J, Ouslander J, Studenski S, et al, editors. Aging of the kidney. 7th edition. Hazzard's geriatric medicine and gerontology. 7th edition. New York: McGraw-Hill; 2017. p. 1275–82.
24. Reske-Nielsen C, Medzon R. Geriatric trauma. Emerg Med Clin North Am 2016;34(3):483–500.
25. Heffernan DS, Thakkar RK, Monaghan SF, et al. Normal presenting vital signs are unreliable in geriatric blunt trauma victims. J Trauma 2010;69(4):813–20.
26. Pandit V, Rhee P, Hashmi A, et al. Shock index predicts mortality in geriatric trauma patients: an analysis of the National Trauma Data Bank. J Trauma Acute Care Surg 2014;76(4):1111–5.
27. Mack LR, Chan SB, Silva JC, et al. The use of head computed tomography in elderly patients sustaining minor head trauma. J Emerg Med 2003;24:157–62.
28. Rösli D, Schnüriger B, Candinas D, et al. The impact of accidental hypothermia on mortality in trauma patients overall and patients with traumatic brain injury specifically: a systematic review and meta-analysis. World J Surg 2020 Dec;44(12):4106–17.
29. Hruska K, Ruge T. The tragically hip: trauma in elderly patients. Emerg Med Clin North Am 2018 Feb;36(1):219–35.
30. Dwyer CR, Scifres AM, Stahlfeld KR, et al. Radiographic assessment of ground-level falls in elderly patients: is the "PAN-SCAN" overdoing it? Surgery 2013;154:816–22.

31. Atinga A, Shekkeris A, Fertleman M, et al. Trauma in the elderly patient. Br J Radiol 2018;91(1087):20170739.
32. Rathlev NK, Medzon R, Lowery D, et al. Intracranial pathology in elders with blunt head trauma. Acad Emerg Med 2006;13:302–7.
33. Brazinova A, Rehorcikova V, Taylor MS, et al. Epidemiology of traumatic brain injury in Europe: a living systematic review. J Neurotrauma 2016;38(10):1411–40.
34. Samaras N, Chevalley T, Samaras D, et al. Older patients in the emergency department: a review. Ann Emerg Med 2010;56:261–9.
35. O'Neill KM, Jean RA, Savetamal A, et al. When to admit to observation: predicting length of stay for anticoagulated elderly fall victims. J Surg Res 2020;250:156–60.
36. Wutzler S, Lefering R, Wafaisade A, et al. Aggressive operative treatment of isolated blunt traumatic brain injury in the elderly is associated with favourable outcome. Injury 2015;46(9):1706–11.
37. Gardner RC, Dams-O'Connor K, Morrissey MR, et al. Geriatric traumatic brain injury: epidemiology, outcomes, knowledge gaps, and future directions. J Neurotrauma 2018;35(7):889–906.
38. Boltz MM, Podany AB, Hollenbeak CS, et al. Injuries and outcomes associated with traumatic falls in the elderly population on oral anticoagulant therapy. Injury 2015;46(9):1765–71.
39. Smith K, Weeks S. The impact of pre-injury anticoagulation therapy in the older adult patient experiencing a traumatic brain injury: a systematic review. JBI Libr Syst Rev 2012;10(58):4610–21.
40. Mina AA, Knipfer JF, Park DY, et al. Intracranial complications of preinjury anticoagulation in trauma patients with head injury. J Trauma 2002;53:668–72.
41. Roberts I, Edwards P, Prieto D, et al. Tranexamic acid in bleeding trauma patients: an exploration of benefits and harms. Trials 2017;18(1):48.
42. Battle B, Sexton KW, Fitzgerald RT. Understanding the value of repeat head CT in elderly trauma patients on anticoagulant or antiplatelet therapy. J Am Coll Radiol 2018;15(2):319–21.
43. Gage BF, Birman-Deych E, Kerzner R, et al. Incidence of intracranial hemorrhage in patients with atrial fibrillation who are prone to fall. Am J Med 2005;118(6):612–7.
44. Ntaios G, Lip GYH, Makaritsis K, et al. CHADS$_2$, CHA$_2$S$_2$DS$_2$-VASc, and long-term stroke outcome in patients without atrial fibrillation. Neurology 2013;80(11):1009–17.
45. Pisters R, Lane DA, Nieuwlaat R, et al. A novel user-friendly score (HAS-BLED) to assess 1-year risk of major bleeding in patients with atrial fibrillation: the euro heart survey. Chest 2010;138(5):1093–100.
46. Kloss FR, Tuli T, Hächl O, et al. The impact of ageing on cranio-maxillofacial trauma—a comparative investigation. Int J Oral Maxillofac Surg 2007;36:1158.
47. Gassner R, Tuli T, Hächl O, et al. Cranio-maxillofacial trauma: a 10 year review of 9543 cases with 21 067 injuries. J Cranio-Maxillo-Fac Surg 2003;31:51.
48. Sharan A, Extractions Madjar D. A radiographic study. Int J Oral Maxillofac Implants 2008;23:48.
49. Holmgren EP, Dierks EJ, Homer LD, et al. Facial computed tomography use in trauma patients who require a head computed tomogram. J Oral Maxillofac Surg 2004;62:913.
50. Toivari M, Suominen AL, Lindqvist C, et al. Among patients with facial fractures, geriatric patients have an increased risk for associated injuries. J Oral Maxillofac Surg 2016;74:1403.

51. Sadro CT, Sandstrom CK, Verma N, et al. Geriatric trauma: a radiologist's guide to imaging trauma patients aged 65 years and older. Radiographics 2015;35(4): 1263–85.

52. Benchetrit S, Blackham J, Braude P, et al. Emergency management of older people with cervical spine injuries: an expert practice review. Emerg Med J 2022; 39(4):331–6.

53. Ehara S, Shimamura T. Cervical spine injury in the elderly: imaging features. Skeletal Radiol 2001;30:1–7.

54. Sadro CT, Sandstrom CK, Verma N, et al. Geriatric trauma: a radiologist's guide. Radiographics 2015;35:1263–85.

55. Bub LD, Blackmore CC, Mann FA, et al. Cervical spine fractures in patients 65 years and older: a clinical prediction rule for blunt trauma. Radiology 2005;234: 143–9.

56. Lomoschitz FM, Blackmore CC, Mirza SK, et al. Cervical spine injuries in patients 65 years old and older: epidemiologic analysis regarding the effects of age and injury mechanism on distribution, type, and stability of injuries. AJR Am J Roentgenol 2002;178:573–7.

57. Bernstein M. Easily missed thoracolumbar spine fractures. Eur J Radiol 2010; 74:6–15.

58. Ryang YM, Török E, Janssen I, et al. Early morbidity and mortality in 50 very elderly patients after posterior atlantoaxial fusion for traumatic odontoid fractures. World Neurosurg 2016;87:381–91.

59. Malhotra A, Wu X, Kalra VB, et al. Utility of MRI for cervical spine clearance after blunt traumatic injury: a meta-analysis. Eur Radiol 2017;27(3):1148–60.

60. Patel MB, Humble SS, Cullinane DC, et al. Cervical spine collar clearance in the obtunded adult blunt trauma patient: a systematic review and practice management guideline from the Eastern association for the surgery of trauma. J Trauma Acute Care Surg 2015;78(2):430–41.

61. Dehner C, Hartwig E, Strobel P, et al. Comparison of the relative benefits of 2 versus 10 days of soft collar cervical immobilization after acute whiplash injury. Arch Phys Med Rehabil 2006;87(11):1423–7.

62. Weerink LBM, Folbert EC, Kraai M, et al. Thoracolumbar spine fractures in the geriatric fracture center: early ambulation leads to good results on short term and is a successful and safe alternative compared to immobilization in elderly patients with two-column vertebral fractures. Geriatr Orthop Surg Rehabil 2014; 5(2):43–9.

63. Lee WY, Yee WY, Cameron PA, et al. Road traffic injuries in the elderly. Emerg Med J 2006;23(1):42–6.

64. Brasel KJ, Guse CE, Layde P, et al. Rib fractures: relationship with pneumonia and mortality. Crit Care Med 2006;34(6):1642–6.

65. Schulte K, Whitaker D, Attia R. In patients with acute flail chest does surgical rib fixation improve outcomes in terms of morbidity and mortality? Interact Cardiovasc Thorac Surg 2016;23:314–9.

66. Fitzgerald MT, Ashley DW, Abukhdeir H, et al. Rib fracture fixation in the 65 years and older population: a paradigm shift in management strategy at a Level I trauma center. J Trauma Acute Care Surg 2017;82(3):524–7.

67. Bulger EM, Arneson MA, Mock CN, et al. Rib fractures in the elderly. J Trauma 2000;48(6):1040–7.

68. Coary R, Skerritt C, Carey A, et al. New horizons in rib fracture management in the older adult. Age Ageing 2020;49(2):161–7.

69. McGwin G Jr, Metzger J, Moran SG, et al. Occupant- and collision-related risk factors for blunt thoracic aorta injury. J Trauma 2003;54(4):655–60.

70. Konstantinidis A, Inaba K, Dubose J, et al. Vascular trauma in geriatric patients: a national trauma databank review. J Trauma 2011;71:909–16.

71. Da Costa J-P, Laing J, Kong VY, et al. A review of geriatric injuries at a major trauma centre in South Africa. S Afr Med J 2020;110(1):44–8.

72. Clare D, Zink KL. Geriatric trauma. Emerg Med Clin North Am 2021;39(2):257–71.

73. Vaidya R, Scott A, Tonnos F. Patients with pelvic fractures from blunt trauma . What is the cause of mortality and when? Am J Surg 2016;211(3):495–500.

74. Brown JV, Yuan S. Traumatic injuries of the pelvis. Emerg Med Clin North Am 2020;38(1):125–42.

75. Henry SM, Pollak AN, Jones AL, et al. Pelvic fracture in geriatric patients: a distinct clinical entity. J Trauma 2002;53:15–20.

76. Kimbrell BJ, Velmahos GC, Chan LS, et al. Angiographic embolization for pelvic fractures in older patients. Arch Surg 2004;139:728–32.

77. Kanezaki S, Miyazaki M, Notani N, et al. Clinical presentation of geriatric poly-trauma patients with severe pelvic fractures: comparison with younger adult patients. Eur J Orthop Surg Traumatol 2016;26(8):885–90.

78. Parker MJ. Missed hip fractures. Arch·Emerg Med 1992;9(1):23–7.

79. Schnell S, Friedman SM, Mendelson DA, et al. The 1-year mortality of patients treated in a hip fracture program for elders. Geriatr Orthop Surg Rehabil 2010; 1(1):6–14.

80. Fu MC, Boddapati V, Gausden EB, et al. Surgery for a fracture of the hip within 24 hours of admission is independently associated with reduced short-term post-operative complications. Bone Joint Lett J 2017;99-B(9):1216–22.

81. Bretherton CP, Parker MJ. Early surgery for patients with a fracture of the hip decreases 30-day mortality. Bone Joint Lett J 2015;97-B(1):104–8.

82. Siris ES, Adler R, Bilezikian J, et al. The clinical diagnosis of osteoporosis: a position statement from the national bone health alliance working group. Osteoporos Int 2014;25(5):1439–43.

83. Danna NR, Zuckerman JD. Musculoskeletal injuries in the elderly. In: Busby-Whitehead J, Arenson C, Durso SC, et al, editors. Reichel's care of the elderly: clinical aspects of aging. New York: Cambridge University Press; 2016. p. 462–76.

84. Clement ND, Duckworth AD, McQueen MM, et al. The outcome of proximal humeral fractures in the elderly. Bone Joint Lett J 2014;96-B(7):970–7.

85. Brox WT, Roberts KC, Taksali S, et al. The American academy of orthopaedic surgeons evidence-based guideline on management of hip fractures in the elderly. J Bone Joint Surg Am 2015;97:1196.

86. Murphy J, Weiner DA, Kotler J, et al. Utility of Ottawa ankle Rules in an aging population: evidence for addition of an age criterion. J Foot Ankle Surg 2020;59(2): 286–90.

87. de Vries R, Reininga IHF, Pieske O, et al. Injury mechanisms, patterns and outcomes of older polytrauma patients-An analysis of the Dutch trauma registry. PLoS One 2018;13(1):e0190587.

88. Eagles D, Godwin B, Cheng W, et al. A systematic review and meta-analysis evaluating geriatric consultation on older trauma patients. J Trauma Acute Care Surg 2020;88(3):446–53.

89. Fallon WFJ, Rader E, Zyzanski S, et al. Geriatric outcomes are improved by a geriatric trauma consultation service. J Trauma Acute Care Surg 2006;61(5): 1040–6.

90. Bowman J, George N, Barrett N, et al. Acceptability and reliability of a novel palliative care screening tool among emergency department providers. Acad Emerg Med 2016;23(6):694–702.
91. George N, Barrett N, McPeake L, et al. Content validation of a novel screening tool to identify emergency department patients with significant palliative care needs. Acad Emerg Med 2015;22(7):823–37.
92. Wu FM, Newman JM, Lasher A, et al. Effects of initiating palliative care consultation in the emergency department on inpatient length of stay. J Palliat Med 2013; 16(11):1362–7.
93. Greenberg SE, VanHouten JP, Lakomkin N, et al. Does admission to medicine or orthopaedics impact a geriatric hip patient's hospital length of stay? J Orthop Trauma 2016;30(2):95–9.
94. Hwabejire JO, Kaafarani HM, Lee J, et al. Patterns of injury, outcomes, and predictors of in-hospital and 1-year mortality in nonagenarian and centenarian trauma patients. JAMA Surg 2014;149(10):1054–9.

Delirium and Delirium Prevention in the Emergency Department

Sangil Lee, MD, MS[a],*, Matthew A. Howard III, MD[b],
Jin H. Han, MD, MSc[c,d]

KEYWORDS

- Altered mental status • Delirium • Encephalopathy • Subtype • Prevention
- Treatment

KEY POINTS

- Delirium is a common and serious brain dysfunction of which every emergency medicine clinician should be aware.
- Accurate delirium assessment and outcome measurement facilitate the further evaluation of the underlying etiology.
- The prevention and treatment of delirium are still based on expert opinions except for the application of evidence-proven prevention from the hospital and intensive care unit.

INTRODUCTION

Delirium is a common and dangerous form of acute brain dysfunction among older emergency department patients.[1] Delirium is associated with higher mortality, accelerated cognitive and functional decline, and increased hospital length of stay.[2,3] Unfortunately, emergency department providers miss delirium in most cases, because they do not routinely screen for this diagnosis.[4] Using a delirium assessment can improve recognition; several brief and easy-to-use delirium assessments are feasible to use for the emergency department. Once delirium is detected, the emergency physician's primary goal is to find and treat the underlying etiology. A significant proportion of older emergency department patients without delirium will develop delirium during hospitalization.[5] Because preventing delirium is by far the most effective way to maximize older patient outcomes, emergency departments should consider implementing

[a] Department of Emergency Medicine, University of Iowa Carver College of Medicine, 200 Hawkins Drive, Iowa City, IA 52242, USA; [b] Department of Neurosurgery, University of Iowa, 200 Hawkins Drive, Iowa City, IA 52242, USA; [c] Department of Emergency Medicine, Vanderbilt University Medical Center, 312 Oxford House, Nashville, TN 37232-4700, USA; [d] Geriatric Research, Education, and Clinical Center, Tennessee Valley Healthcare System, 1310 24th Avenue South, Nashville, TN 37212-2637, USA
* Corresponding author.
E-mail address: sangil-lee@uiowa.edu

Clin Geriatr Med 39 (2023) 535–551
https://doi.org/10.1016/j.cger.2023.05.006
0749-0690/23/© 2023 Elsevier Inc. All rights reserved.

nonpharmacologic, multicomponent delirium prevention protocols, especially for those at moderate-to-high risk for developing delirium.

The emergency department plays a critical role in the evaluation and management of older patients with delirium. The emergency department is often the initial point of entry for geriatric hospital utilizations[6] and serves the role of rapidly identifying those who are critically ill while efficiently identifying the underlying etiology and promptly initiating life-saving therapies. In the United States alone, the emergency department sees approximately 18 million patients who are 65 years and older each year.[7] Because of the projected exponential growth of the US aging population over the next several decades, the number of elder emergency department patient visits will also grow at a similar pace.[8] Thus, the emergency physician must be adept in evaluating and managing delirium in the emergency department. This article discusses the epidemiology, assessment, treatment, and prevention of delirium in the emergency department setting.

DELIRIUM DEFINITION AND EPIDEMIOLOGY IN THE EMERGENCY DEPARTMENT

According to the Diagnostic and Statistical Manual of Mental Disorders, Fifth Edition, Text Revision (DSM-5-TR), delirium is defined as a disturbance in attention and awareness that is accompanied by an acute (hours to days) loss in cognition that cannot be better accounted for by a pre-existing or evolving neurocognitive disorder such as dementia.[9] Delirium occurs in 6% to 36% of patients of older emergency department patients[2–4,10–18] and is associated with increased in-hospital and long-term death,[2,15,18,19] accelerated functional and cognitive decline,[20] longer hospital length of stays,[19,21] unanticipated intensive care unit (ICU) admissions,[19] discharge to a skilled nursing facility,[19] and increased 30-day rehospitalizations.[19]

DELIRIUM'S HETEROGENEITY

Delirium is a heterogeneous syndrome that can vary by psychomotor activity and may have prognostic implications.[22,23] Subtyping delirium by psychomotor activity is generally the most widely studied nomenclature.[24] Psychomotor subtyping is based on the patient's motor activity, speech, and level of arousal.[25] The 4 psychomotor subtypes of delirium are hypoactive, hyperactive, mixed[26] and no subtype,[27–30] and it is hypothesized that each psychomotor subtype has its own distinct underlying pathophysiology and etiologies.[26,31,32] Hypoactive delirium is described as quiet delirium; patients with this subtype appear drowsy, somnolent, or lethargic. Because its clinical presentation can be subtle, hypoactive delirium is frequently missed by health care providers[33] and may be misinterpreted as depression or fatigue.[34,35] On the other hand, patients with hyperactive delirium have increased psychomotor activity; these patients may seem restless, anxious, agitated, or combative. Hyperactive delirium is more easily recognized by health care providers; yet this is the least common subtype of delirium in older emergency department patients.[3] Mixed-type delirium exhibits fluctuating levels of psychomotor activity; the patient can exhibit hypoactive symptomatology at 1 moment and hyperactive symptomatology several hours or even seconds later. Hypoactive delirium tends to portend the worst prognosis and is associated with higher mortality rates.[30,36–38]

DELIRIUM AND DEMENTIA

Delirium is often confused with dementia, but they are 2 distinct syndromes with different characteristics and prognoses. **Table 1** shows the key differences between these 2 conditions.

Table 1		
Key differences between delirium and dementia		
Characteristic	**Delirium**	**Dementia**
Onset	Acute onset over a period of hours or days	Gradual onset over months or years
Course	Fluctuating	Stable
Inattention	Present	Absent
Impairment of arousal	Usually present	Typically absent
Disorganized thinking	May be present	Typically absent
Disturbed sleep-wake cycle	Present	Typically absent
Perceptual disturbances and hallucinations	May be present	Typically absent
Is cognitive decline reversible?	Usually reversible	Often not reversible
Precipitated by a medical or surgical illness?	Usually	Rarely
Life threatening?	Potentially	Rarely

Classically, delirium is considered reversible and precipitated by an underlying medical or surgical illness. There is a proportion of patients, however, who develop long-term cognitive impairment after delirium.[39,40] Dementia is traditionally characterized as chronic, irreversible, and not secondary to an underlying medical illness. Delirium usually has neurocognitive (inattention, disorganized thinking, and perceptual disturbances) and non-neurocognitive (impaired arousal and sleep-wake disturbance) impairments that are not typically observed in dementia.

Distinguishing delirium from advanced dementia can be challenging, because the clinical features can overlap. Patients with advanced dementia can be inattentive and have impaired arousal, disorganized thinking, sleep-wake cycle disturbances, and perceptual disturbances in the absence of delirium.[41] When patients with advanced dementia develop delirium, an acute change in mental status is still observed, and any pre-existing cognitive and noncognitive abnormalities can worsen.

RISK FACTORS FOR DELIRIUM

When considering the if an older emergency department patient is delirious or is at risk for developing delirium, the emergency physician must consider vulnerability and precipitating factors of delirium (**Table 2**). Dementia is the most consistently reported and powerful vulnerability factor for delirium across multiple clinical settings.[3,19,42–49] Infection is the most common precipitating factor for delirium,[43,46,47,50–53] but is important to note that most patients with delirium will have more than 1 etiology.[51,54] The development of delirium involves complex interplay between patient vulnerability and precipitating factors. For example, patients with high vulnerability to developing delirium, such as a 90-year-old with Alzheimer dementia who requires complete assistance to perform activities of daily living, requires a relatively lower intensity insult like an uncomplicated urinary tract infection (UTI) to develop delirium. Patients with little vulnerability to developing delirium, such as a fully functional 70-year-old who still works as an engineer, will require a more noxious insult, such as severe sepsis, to trigger delirium. In patients with little or no vulnerability to developing delirium, emergency physicians should look for a precipitating life-threatening illness.

Table 2
Vulnerability and precipitous factors

Vulnerability Factors	Precipitating Factors

Demographics
  Advanced age, educational level, male
	Systemic illness
	  Infection, inadequate pain control, trauma, surgery

Medications and drugs
  Polypharmacy, psychoactive medications, alcohol and substance use disorder
	Medications and drugs
	  Medication changes, alcohol and recreation drug use or withdrawal

Comorbidities
  Dementia, comorbidity burden, chronic kidney disease, chronic liver disease, terminal illness, frailty
	Metabolic
	  Vitamin (ie, thiamine) deficiencies, electrolyte disturbances, hypo- or hyperglycemia, thyroid dysfunction

Sensory impairment
  Hearing impairment, visual impairment
	Organ dysfunction
	  Acute kidney injury, acute liver failure, acute heart failure, acute respiratory failure, shock

Decreased oral intake
  Malnutrition (chronic)
	Decreased oral intake
	  Dehydration, malnutrition (acute)

Functional status
  Functional impairment, immobility
	Central nervous system
	  Cerebrovascular accident, intraparenchymal hemorrhage, subdural/epidural hematoma, seizures, meningitis, encephalitis

Psychiatric
  Depression
	Iatrogenic
	  Physical restraints, indwelling catheter use, prolonged emergency department length of stay

MEDICATION RISK FACTORS FOR DELIRIUM

It is important to note that delirium can be precipitated by medication side effects or withdrawals. Thus, it is imperative to obtain medication history, including nonprescription medications, recent changes or altered compliance with medications, and missed medications. Medication lists obtained from the electronic medical record (EMR) may not be accurate and should be clarified. High-risk medications include sedatives, corticosteroids, antihistamines, anticholinergics, tricyclic antidepressants, and muscle relaxants.[54] Opioids have the potential to precipitate delirium, although clinicians need to consider treating pain first.[55,56]

UNDER RECOGNITION OF DELIRIUM IN THE EMERGENCY DEPARTMENT

Despite the high morbidity and mortality associated with delirium, emergency health care providers fail to detect delirium in 57% to 83% of cases,[3,4,10,16,35,57,58] because it is not actively screened for using a validated delirium assessment.[59] The evidence suggests that delirium remains underrecognized in the emergency department.[4,10,12,13,16] When delirium is unrecognized in the emergency department, the inpatient providers will also miss delirium in 95% of cases.[3] Missing delirium has several negative implications for clinical care.[57] Because delirium is frequently misdiagnosed as dementia or psychiatric illnesses, such as depression,[35] some may be inappropriately admitted to a psychiatric ward or discharged, thus delaying the diagnosis of delirium and their underlying medical condition.[58] Studies suggest that 25% of delirious older emergency department patients are actually discharged and sent home[10,21] and may not be able to fully comprehend their diagnosis or discharge instructions[60] leading to noncompliance, return visits, and other adverse outcomes.[61]

ASSESSMENT OF DELIRIUM IN THE EMERGENCY DEPARTMENT

Using a validated delirium assessment is vital to improving recognition (see **Table 2**). There are 3 types of delirium assessments: patient-based, proxy-based, and observational. Patient-based delirium assessments require the rater to interact with the patient and usually incorporate bedside cognitive testing to assess the features of delirium. The advantage of this approach is that it has a potentially high ceiling for diagnostic accuracy (> 95% sensitive and > 95% specific). The disadvantages to this approach, however, are that to achieve high diagnostic accuracy, it may require significant training and a lengthier delirium assessment.[62] It also requires raters to conduct additional cognitive testing on the patient, which may be difficult in a setting with significant time constraints such as the emergency department.

The most widely used patient-based delirium assessment is the Confusion Assessment Method (CAM) algorithm and its derivatives. The short-form CAM algorithm consists of 4 features: (1) altered mental status or fluctuating course, (2) inattention, (3) disorganized thinking, and (4) altered level of consciousness.[63] A patient is considered to meet the criteria for delirium if both features 1 and 2 and either 3 or 4 are present. The CAM's features are evaluated by subjective impression after performing a brief global cognitive assessment. For this reason, the CAM may require substantial training, and its diagnostic accuracy may depend on an operator's level of training and experience. To reduce operator dependence, increase ease of use, and reduce training burden, several delirium assessments have incorporated brief, objective assessments into the CAM algorithm. Examples of these CAM-based assessments are the Brief Confusion Assessment Method (bCAM), Confusion Assessment Method for the Intensive Care Unit (CAM-ICU), and 3D-CAM. The bCAM, among the most commonly used delirium screening tools besides CAM, was specifically tailored for the emergency department and takes less than 2 minutes to perform with high inter-rater reliability.[62,64] **(Table 3)**

The 4AT is another widely used patient-based delirium assessment and has 4 components: (1) alertness, (2) orientation, (3) attention, and (4) acute change or fluctuating course. The 4AT also takes 2 minutes to perform with excellent diagnostic accuracy.[67] Ultrabrief delirium patient-based assessments exist, such as the MOTYB-12 task, but diagnostic accuracy is often sacrificed for brevity. Alternatively, a 2-step approach to delirium assessment has been proposed for the emergency department to increase screening efficiency. A highly sensitive delirium assessment such as the Delirium Triage Screen (DTS) or 2-Item Ultra-Brief (UB-2) delirium assessment can be performed to rapidly rule out delirium. Because DTS or UB-2 have moderate specificity, a positive test requires a confirmatory delirium assessment with a higher specificity such as the bCAM, 3D-CAM, or 4AT.[62]

Proxy-based delirium assessments asks a family member about the presence of delirium features. An example of a proxy-based delirium assessment SQiD,[73,74] where the clinical asks proxy if the patient has been more confused lately. Although this approach has moderately good diagnostic accuracy, a proxy is unavailable in the emergency department for approximately 25% to 75% of patients.[75] Observation-based delirium assessment simply observes the patient for delirium features during routine clinical interaction. Because this requires subjective assessment, extensive training may be needed to maximize diagnostic accuracy. RASS assesses the patients

Table 3
Selected examples of delirium screening tools

Instrument	Synopsis	Sensitivity	Specificity	Time
CAM[65]	A bedside cognitive test is used to determine 1. Altered mental status or fluctuating course 2. Inattention 3. Disorganized thinking 4. Altered level of consciousness using clinical impression	86%	93%	5–10 min
CAM-ICU[66]	CAM modified to include cognitive assessments and test of attention that can be used for ventilated patients in ICU	95%–100%	89%–93%	2–3 min
bCAM[62]	Uses the CAM algorithm but uses the months of the year backwards task from December to July to evaluate inattention and 4 yes/no questions and simple command to evaluate disorganized thinking	84% (95% confidence interval [CI] 72–92)	96% (95% CI 93%-97%)	< 2 min
4AT[67]	Evaluates alertness, orientation, attention, and fluctuation	89.7%	64.9%	< 2 min
Delirium Triage Screen (DTS)[62]	Evaluates inattention using object testing and level of consciousness using DTS followed by more specific test to confirm	98% (95% CI 90%–100%)	55% (95% CI 50%–60%)	< 30 s

Tool	Description			Time
Ultra-Brief 2-item Screener[68] (UB-2)	2 questions, "Tell me the day of the week" and "please tell me the months of the year backwards"	93% (95% CI 81%–99%)	64% (95% CI 56%–70%)	<1 min
Nursing Delirium Screening Scale (Nu-DESC)[69]	5 items- disorientation, inappropriate behavior	86% (95% CI 65%–95%)	87% (95%CI 73%–94%)	1-2 min based on 8 h of observation
Delirium Observation Screening Scale (DOSS)[70]	7 areas (consciousness, attention, thought process, orientation, psychomotor, mood, perception)	90%	91%	5 min based on 8 h of observation
Month of the year backwards – 12 mo (MOTYB-12)[71]	Asks the patient to recite the months of the year backwards from December to July	80.0% (95% CI 60.9%–91.1%)	57.1% (95% CI, 50.4%- 63.7%)	<1 min
Richmond Agitation Sedation Scale (RASS)[72]	A structured evaluation of level of consciousness based on your observation of the patient during routine clinical evaluation	84.0% (95% CI 73.8% to 94.2%)	87.6% (95% CI 84.2% to 91.1%)	<10 s
Single Question in Delirium (SQiD)[73,74]	1 question 'Do you think [name of patient] has been more confused lately?'	80% (95% CI 28.3%–99.5%)	71% (95% CI 41.9%–91.6%)	<10 s

level of arousal and is 82% sensitive and 85% specific for delirium.[72] Observing a change in RASS increases the specificity for delirium to 92%.[76]

THE DIAGNOSTIC EVALUATION ONCE DELIRIUM IS DETECTED IN THE EMERGENCY DEPARTMENT

When delirium is detected, the first and most important priority is to find and treat the underlying etiology. Because older adults with delirium cannot provide an accurate history,[60] emergency physicians should contact family or their caregivers to obtain collateral information. If from a skilled nursing facility, the facility's staff should be contacted. In addition to obtaining a history of why the patient is in the emergency department, the physician should elicit patients' baseline mentation and level of functioning from the collateral historian and how quickly the mental status change occurred.[73] An abrupt (within seconds) change in mental status may indicate a stroke as the cause for the patient's delirium.

Because adverse drug reactions and withdrawal from medications are common delirium etiologies, obtaining an accurate medication history, including over-the-counter (OTC) medications, is vital. Emergency physicians should ask about recent changes in or noncompliance with medications. High-risk medications that may contribute to delirium include: sedative-hypnotic agents, steroids, antihistamines, anticholinergics, tricyclic antidepressants, and muscle relaxants.[77] The use of opioids for pain was considered the risk factor for delirium, yet recent studies did not show a significant association.[55,56] Rather, it is emphasized that painful conditions are treated aggressively to minimize the risk of delirium and avoid certain opioids, such as meperidine. Lastly, ask the patient or collateral historian about substance use disorder (eg, alcohol, opioid, sedative-hypnotics, and illicit drug use).

After history taking, emergency physicians should conduct a comprehensive physical examination, including vital signs. Point-of-care tests for glucose may identify hypo- or hyperglycemia. A full examination of the patient is necessary to inspect the back, sacrum, genitalia, and feet for possible infections or drug patches that may have contributed to delirium. The detailed neurological examination should also be performed. Focal neurological findings may suggest a stroke or intracranial hemorrhage as the cause of delirium. This examination can provide an opportunity to evaluate for trauma: accidental, self-inflicted, or nonaccidental.

Emergency department patients with delirium typically require a broad laboratory evaluation including serum electrolytes, glucose, blood urea nitrogen, creatinine, and transaminases, and a urinalysis. Measuring serum drug concentrations of psychoactive medications such as lithium, anticonvulsants, theophylline, digoxin, and aspirin should be considered if the delirious patient is on these medications. Because acute myocardial infarction can precipitate delirium, and chest pain may be absent from the history,[78,79] a 12-lead electrocardiogram should also be considered. Urinalysis is a routine diagnostic test for older adults because of UTI. Older adults tend to have a higher proportion of abnormal urinalysis without active UTI, which leads to a risk of diagnostic anchoring on abnormal urinalysis and missing another potentially more serious cause of delirium.

Radiographic testing should be guided by the history and physical examination. Because delirious emergency department patients are older, have decreased visceral and peritoneal pain responses, and have difficulty with communication, a lower threshold to perform radiographic imaging may be needed to fully evaluate patients with relatively mild somatic complaints. A chest radiograph should be considered patients who are tachypneic, have abnormal lung auscultation, or have respiratory complaints. There is little evidence-based guidance on when to perform head computed tomography (CT). In a systematic review that included 909 older emergency department patients with altered mental status or confusion, 15.6% had abnormal head CT.[80] However, many of these studies did not use a delirium assessment, and the patients included likely had more severe impairments. Inpatient studies have reported that head CTs have low diagnostic yield in older adults with delirium, but these studies have limited generalizability to the emergency department.[81,82] A head CT should be strongly considered in delirious patients with impaired level consciousness (eg, decreased level of arousal or somnolence), likely to only be relevant when there is a recent history of a fall or head trauma, if the patient is on anticoagulation, or a focal neurological deficit is found on clinical examination.[80–82] Brain MRI should be considered in delirious patients with an abrupt onset of mental status changes or focal neurologic symptoms to rule out a cerebrovascular accident in the setting of a non-diagnostic head CT scan.

NONPHARMACOLOGICAL MANAGEMENT OF DELIRIUM

Aside from finding the underlying etiology delirium, there is no universally accepted intervention for delirium after it has occurred, especially for the emergency department setting.[83] A recent systematic review on delirium prevention and treatment in the emergency department showed limited evidence on 3 nonrandomized controlled trials (non-RCTs) that employed a multifactorial delirium prevention program; 3 non-RCTs evaluated regional anesthesia for hip fractures; and 1 study evaluated the use of Foley catheter, medication exposure, and risk of delirium.[84] One observational cohort study on the use of Foley catheters in the emergency department showed increased duration of delirium (proportional odds ratio [OR] 3.1, 95% CI 1.3–7.4).[85]

If a patient is found to meet the criteria for delirium in the emergency department, the goal is to reduce the risk of agitation if the patient has hypoactive delirium or mitigate the worsening agitation if the patient has mixed-type or hyperactive delirium. Delirious patients often have perceptual disturbances (ie, hallucinations and delusions) and can easily become more agitated in the noisy and overstimulating emergency department environment. Because of the acute loss in cognition, they have difficulty understanding what is going on or have difficulty communicating. To achieve this goal, Flaherty and colleagues recommend the "TADA" approach, which stands for "Tolerate, Anticipate, Don't Agitate:"[86]

- *Tolerate* – The first step is to tolerate seemingly dangerous behaviors. Tolerating behaviors allows patients to respond naturally to their circumstances and may provide them a sense of control while in their delirious state. Because delirious patients are often unable to adequately communicate, these behaviors may also indicate that something is bothering them such as needing to urinate or unaddressed pain.
- *Anticipate* – This step requires the health care provider to anticipate what the patient might do and proactively avoids inciting agents that may cause or exacerbate agitation. This includes avoiding unnatural tethers that are not absolutely needed for clinical care, including oxygen, intravenous lines, urinary catheters, and other monitoring devices. Getting out of bed is also anticipated and encouraged by this approach as long as patient's safety can be ensured.
- *Don't Agitate*– This is the final step and considered the golden rule of this approach. Some agitators are obvious. Reorientation can be unpredictable, as it can occasionally worsen agitation and should only be attempted if the patient is amenable to it.

PHARMACOLOGICAL MANAGEMENT FOR DELIRIUM IN THE EMERGENCY DEPARTMENT

Drug therapy for delirium has been extensively evaluated. Because there are no rigorous mortality or long-term benefits, the goal of pharmacological therapy is to control agitation while avoiding oversedation.[87] The oral route is usually preferred over injections to minimize the discomfort of the injection, subsequent agitation due to injection, and arrhythmia.[88] It is imperative to note that many of these agents were tested for agitated patients, and not all were specific to older adults with delirium.

DISPOSITION OF PATIENTS WITH DELIRIUM

Currently, there are few evidence-based guidelines to whether an emergency department patient with delirium requires a hospitalization or can be discharged home. In general, a significant proportion of those with delirium will require hospitalization because of the severity or acuity of the underlying medical illness that precipitated the delirium. Delirious emergency department patients with severe neurocognitive symptoms, limited home social support, or with poor access to outpatient care will also likely require an admission even for simple clinical conditions that require some form of patient monitoring to continue treatment.

However, there is a potential risk that the symptoms of delirium may worsen during hospitalization, because the patient will be in an unfamiliar environment or be exposed to deliriogenic iatrogenesis. As a result, emergency department discharge should be considered if

The delirium symptoms are mild or have resolved
The etiology is unequivocally obvious and can be managed as an outpatient
The patient can be closely monitored at home by a family member or caregiver
Close outpatient follow-up with transportation can be arranged

For patients who reside in a long-term care facility, depending on cause of delirium and degree of agitation or somnolence, some individuals with delirium may return to their long-term care facility for treatment. If feasible, disposition to skilled nursing facility may also be an option.

NONPHARMACOLOGICAL MANAGEMENT (PREVENTION) IN THE EMERGENCY DEPARTMENT

Up to 30% of older emergency department patients who are nondelirious on hospital admission will develop delirium during a hospital stay leading to significant mortality and morbidity.[89] Because there is no intervention that has been shown to effectively reduce negative sequelae associated with delirium after it occurs,[83] a greater emphasis has been on placed delirium prevention to improve older patient outcomes.

Nonpharmacologic, multicomponent delirium prevention protocols have been shown to be effective in preventing delirium and its resultant outcomes.[90] Some components of these protocols can be considered in the emergency department, especially as boarding is an persistent issue. The most widely used and evidence-based delirium prevention program is the Hospital Elder Life Program (HELP).[91–94] HELP is a multicomponent, nonpharmacologic intervention to reduce delirium risk factors. The HELP program includes reorientation, cognitive stimulation activities, reestablishment of sleep-wake cycles, minimized use of psychoactive medications, maximized mobility, optimal hydration and nutrition, and visual and hearing aids for those with sensory impairment. Although many of the HELP components may be difficult to implement in the emergency department, certain components can be adapted and tailored to the emergency department to decrease the development of delirium in high-risk patients.[95] Observational studies showed that ED length of stays greater than 10 to 12 hours might increase the risk of developing delirium[96,97] especially in patients with pre-existing cognitive impairment.[96] Clinicians should mobilize the resources to prevent any unnecessary emergency department stays for those who have an increased risk of delirium. For example, in times of high boarding in the emergency department, institutions should consider adopting processes that prioritize inpatient bed assignment for persons at high risk of delirium. A recent study showed that higher physical therapy and occupational therapy intensity may be a useful intervention to shorten delirium duration.[98]

ASSESS, DIAGNOSE, EVALUATE, PREVENT, AND TREAT TOOL FOR DELIRIUM CARE

A working group of content experts convened to develop a point-of-care tool to assist physicians in the care of older adults in the emergency department, and it was designed to present and explain the Assess, Diagnose, Evaluate, Prevent, and Treat (ADEPT) tool. Five core principles were identified by the group to ensure adequate and thorough care for older adults with delirium. The ADEPT tool[99] developed by American College of Emergency Physicians gives collective knowledge from an expert panel on delirium evaluation and management.

FUTURE DIRECTIONS

It has been nearly 15 years since recommendations from the American Geriatrics Society and Society for Academic Emergency Medicine to prioritize delirium care, yet emergency medicine still has consensus-based recommendations and tools to formulate delirium treatment protocols.[84] Since 2012, 7 Cochrane reviews have synthesized delirium interventions across various patient populations and clinical settings, but none included studies from the emergency department. The Geriatric Emergency Care Applied Research (GEAR) Network reviewed a similar question and still did not identify any emergency department-based research upon which to base interventions.[96] The authors encourage emergency departments to start implementing processes to minimize delirium risk associated with emergency care.[100,101]

SUMMARY

Delirium has been an elusive condition that did not have an effective screening process in the emergency department until recently. When identified, emergency clinicians must identify the underlying cause, as this is the primary goal of treatment. Further research is needed into processes to improve identification of individuals at risk of delirium and emergency department processes to prevent and mitigate the adverse effects of delirium.

CLINICS CARE POINTS

- Delirium has been an elusive condition that did not have an effective screening process in the emergency department until recently.
- When delirium was identified, emergency clinicians must identify the underlying cause.

DISCLOSURE

Dr S. Lee and Dr M.A. Howard have no disclosure. Dr J.H. Han receives funding from the National Institute on Aging, United States under award number NIA R01 AG065249 and the Geriatric Research Education and Clinical Center, United States.

REFERENCES

1. Han JH, Suyama J. Delirium and dementia. Clin Geriatr Med 2018;34(3):327–54.
2. Han JH, Shintani A, Eden S, et al. Delirium in the emergency department: an independent predictor of death within 6 months. Ann Emerg Med 2010;56(3): 244–52.e1.
3. Han JH, Zimmerman EE, Cutler N, et al. Delirium in older emergency department patients: recognition, risk factors, and psychomotor subtypes. Acad Emerg Med 2009;16(3):193–200.
4. Lewis LM, Miller DK, Morley JE, et al. Unrecognized delirium in ED geriatric patients. Am J Emerg Med 1995;13(2):142–5.
5. Lee S, Harland K, Mohr NM, et al. Evaluation of emergency department derived delirium prediction models using a hospital-wide cohort. J Psychosom Res 2019;127:109850.
6. Schuur JD, Venkatesh AK. The growing role of emergency departments in hospital admissions. N Engl J Med 2012;367(5):391–3.
7. Niska R, Bhuiya F, Xu J. National hospital ambulatory medical care survey: 2007 emergency department summary. Natl Health Stat Report 2010;(26):1–31.
8. He W, Sengupta M, Velkoff V, et al. 65+ in the United States: 2005. Current population reports, P23-209. US Government Printing Office; 2005. Published online December 2005. Available at: https://www.census.gov/content/dam/Census/library/publications/2005/demo/p23-209.pdf. Accessed December 22, 2022.
9. American Psychiatric Association. Diagnostic and statistical manual of mental disorders, 5th edition, text revision (DSM-5-TR). Washington, DC: American Psychiatric Association Publishing; 2022. https://doi.org/10.1176/appi.books.9780890425787.
10. Hustey FM, Meldon SW, Smith MD, et al. The effect of mental status screening on the care of elderly emergency department patients. Ann Emerg Med 2003; 41(5):678–84.
11. Naughton BJ, Moran MB, Kadah H, et al. Delirium and other cognitive impairment in older adults in an emergency department. Ann Emerg Med 1995; 25(6):751–5.
12. Elie M, Rousseau F, Cole M, et al. Prevalence and detection of delirium in elderly emergency department patients. CMAJ (Can Med Assoc J) 2000;163(8): 977–81.
13. Hustey FM, Meldon SW. The prevalence and documentation of impaired mental status in elderly emergency department patients. Ann Emerg Med 2002;39(3): 248–53.
14. Hustey FM, Meldon S, Palmer R. Prevalence and documentation of impaired mental status in elderly emergency department patients. Acad Emerg Med 2000;7(10):1166.
15. Kakuma R, du Fort GG, Arsenault L, et al. Delirium in older emergency department patients discharged home: effect on survival. J Am Geriatr Soc 2003;51(4): 443–50.
16. Suffoletto B, Miller T, Frisch A, et al. Emergency physician recognition of delirium. Postgrad Med J 2013;89(1057):621–5.

17. Hare M, Arendts G, Wynaden D, et al. Nurse screening for delirium in older patients attending the emergency department. Psychosomatics 2014;55(3): 235–42.

18. Hsieh SJ, Madahar P, Hope AA, et al. Clinical deterioration in older adults with delirium during early hospitalisation: a prospective cohort study. BMJ Open 2015;5(9):e007496.

19. Kennedy M, Enander RA, Tadiri SP, et al. Delirium risk prediction, healthcare use and mortality of elderly adults in the emergency department. J Am Geriatr Soc 2014;62(3):462–9.

20. Han JH, Vasilevskis EE, Chandrasekhar R, et al. Delirium in the emergency department and its extension into hospitalization (DELINEATE) study: effect on 6-month function and cognition. J Am Geriatr Soc 2017;65(6):1333–8.

21. Han JH, Eden S, Shintani A, et al. Delirium in older emergency department patients is an independent predictor of hospital length of stay. Acad Emerg Med 2011;18(5):451–7.

22. Girard TD, Thompson JL, Pandharipande PP, et al. Clinical phenotypes of delirium during critical illness and severity of subsequent long-term cognitive impairment: a prospective cohort study. Lancet Respir Med 2018;6(3):213–22.

23. Yang FM, Marcantonio ER, Inouye SK, et al. Phenomenological subtypes of delirium in older persons: patterns, prevalence, and prognosis. Psychosomatics 2009;50(3):248–54.

24. de Rooij SE, Schuurmans MJ, van der Mast RC, et al. Clinical subtypes of delirium and their relevance for daily clinical practice: a systematic review. Int J Geriatr Psychiatry 2005;20(7):609–15.

25. Meagher DJ, Moran M, Raju B, et al. Motor symptoms in 100 patients with delirium versus control subjects: comparison of subtyping methods. Psychosomatics 2008;49(4):300–8.

26. Meagher DJ, Trzepacz PT. Motoric subtypes of delirium. Semin Clin Neuropsychiatry 2000;5(2):75–85.

27. Godfrey A, Leonard M, Donnelly S, et al. Validating a new clinical subtyping scheme for delirium with electronic motion analysis. Psychiatry Res 2010; 178(1):186–90.

28. Meagher D, Adamis D, Leonard M, et al. Development of an abbreviated version of the delirium motor subtyping scale (DMSS-4). Int Psychogeriatr 2014;26(4): 693–702.

29. Meagher DJ, Leonard M, Donnelly S, et al. A longitudinal study of motor subtypes in delirium: frequency and stability during episodes. J Psychosom Res 2012;72(3):236–41.

30. Meagher DJ, Leonard M, Donnelly S, et al. A longitudinal study of motor subtypes in delirium: relationship with other phenomenology, etiology, medication exposure and prognosis. J Psychosom Res 2011;71(6):395–403.

31. Ross CA. CNS arousal systems: possible role in delirium. Int Psychogeriatr 1991;3(2):353–71.

32. Ross CA, Peyser CE, Shapiro I, et al. Delirium: phenomenologic and etiologic subtypes. Int Psychogeriatr 1991;3(2):135–47.

33. Inouye SK, Foreman MD, Mion LC, et al. Nurses' recognition of delirium and its symptoms: comparison of nurse and researcher ratings. Arch Intern Med 2001; 161(20):2467–73.

34. Nicholas LM, Lindsey BA. Delirium presenting with symptoms of depression. Psychosomatics 1995;36(5):471–9.

35. Farrell KR, Ganzini L. Misdiagnosing delirium as depression in medically ill elderly patients. Arch Intern Med 1995;155(22):2459–64.
36. Kiely DK, Jones RN, Bergmann MA, et al. Association between psychomotor activity delirium subtypes and mortality among newly admitted post-acute facility patients. J Gerontol A Biol Sci Med Sci 2007;62(2):174–9.
37. Kim S-Y, Kim S-W, Kim J-M, et al. Differential associations between delirium and mortality according to delirium subtype and age: a prospective cohort study. Psychosom Med 2015;77(8):903–10.
38. Jackson TA, Wilson D, Richardson S, et al. Predicting outcome in older hospital patients with delirium: a systematic literature review. Int J Geriatr Psychiatry 2016;31(4):392–9.
39. Marcantonio ER, Simon SE, Bergmann MA, et al. Delirium symptoms in post-acute care: prevalent, persistent, and associated with poor functional recovery. J Am Geriatr Soc 2003;51(1):4–9.
40. Levkoff SE, Evans DA, Liptzin B, et al. Delirium. The occurrence and persistence of symptoms among elderly hospitalized patients. Arch Intern Med 1992;152(2):334–40.
41. Boller F, Verny M, Hugonot-Diener L, et al. Clinical features and assessment of severe dementia. A review. Eur J Neurol 2002;9(2):125–36.
42. Inouye SK, Viscoli CM, Horwitz RI, et al. A predictive model for delirium in hospitalized elderly medical patients based on admission characteristics. Ann Intern Med 1993;119(6):474–81.
43. Schor JD, Levkoff SE, Lipsitz LA, et al. Risk factors for delirium in hospitalized elderly. JAMA 1992;267(6):827–31.
44. Marcantonio ER, Goldman L, Mangione CM, et al. A clinical prediction rule for delirium after elective noncardiac surgery. JAMA 1994;271(2):134–9.
45. Gustafson Y, Berggren D, Brännström B, et al. Acute confusional states in elderly patients treated for femoral neck fracture. J Am Geriatr Soc 1988;36(6):525–30.
46. Jitapunkul S, Pillay I, Ebrahim S. Delirium in newly admitted elderly patients: a prospective study. Q J Med 1992;83(300):307–14.
47. Kolbeinsson H, Jónsson A. Delirium and dementia in acute medical admissions of elderly patients in Iceland. Acta Psychiatr Scand 1993;87(2):123–7.
48. Pompei P, Foreman M, Rudberg MA, et al. Delirium in hospitalized older persons: outcomes and predictors. J Am Geriatr Soc 1994;42(8):809–15.
49. Margiotta A, Bianchetti A, Ranieri P, et al. Clinical characteristics and risk factors of delirium in demented and not demented elderly medical inpatients. J Nutr Health Aging 2006;10(6):535–9.
50. Rockwood K. Acute confusion in elderly medical patients. J Am Geriatr Soc 1989;37(2):150–4.
51. Cirbus J, MacLullich AMJ, Noel C, et al. Delirium etiology subtypes and their effect on six-month function and cognition in older emergency department patients. Int Psychogeriatr 2019;31(2):267–76.
52. Rahkonen T, Mäkelä H, Paanila S, et al. Delirium in elderly people without severe predisposing disorders: etiology and 1-year prognosis after discharge. Int Psychogeriatr 2000;12(4):473–81.
53. George J, Bleasdale S, Singleton SJ. Causes and prognosis of delirium in elderly patients admitted to a district general hospital. Age Ageing 1997;26(6):423–7.
54. Hanlon JT, Semla TP, Schmader KE. Alternative medications for medications in the use of high-risk medications in the elderly and potentially harmful drug-

disease interactions in the elderly quality measures. J Am Geriatr Soc 2015; 63(12):e8–18.

55. Lee S, Okoro UE, Swanson MB, et al. Opioid and benzodiazepine use in the emergency department and the recognition of delirium within the first 24 hours of hospitalization. J Psychosom Res 2022;153:110704.
56. Daoust R, Paquet J, Boucher V, et al. Relationship between pain, opioid treatment, and delirium in older emergency department patients. Acad Emerg Med 2020;27(8):708–16.
57. Sanders AB. Missed delirium in older emergency department patients: a quality-of-care problem. Ann Emerg Med 2002;39(3):338–41.
58. Reeves RR, Parker JD, Burke RS, et al. Inappropriate psychiatric admission of elderly patients with unrecognized delirium. South Med J 2010;103(2):111–5.
59. Press Y, Margulin T, Grinshpun Y, et al. The diagnosis of delirium among elderly patients presenting to the emergency department of an acute hospital. Arch Gerontol Geriatr 2009;48(2):201–4.
60. Han JH, Bryce SN, Ely EW, et al. The effect of cognitive impairment on the accuracy of the presenting complaint and discharge instruction comprehension in older emergency department patients. Ann Emerg Med 2011;57(6):662–71.e2.
61. Clarke C, Friedman SM, Shi K, et al. Emergency department discharge instructions comprehension and compliance study. CJEM 2005;7(1):5–11.
62. Han JH, Wilson A, Vasilevskis EE, et al. Diagnosing delirium in older emergency department patients: validity and reliability of the delirium triage screen and the brief confusion assessment method. Ann Emerg Med 2013;62(5):457–65.
63. Inouye SK, van Dyck CH, Alessi CA, et al. Clarifying confusion: the confusion assessment method. A new method for detection of delirium. Ann Intern Med 1990;113(12):941–8.
64. Santangelo I, Ahmad S, Liu S, et al. Examination of geriatric care processes implemented in level 1 and level 2 geriatric emergency departments. JGME 2023;3(4).
65. Wong CL, Holroyd-Leduc J, Simel DL, et al. Does this patient have delirium? Value of bedside instruments. JAMA 2010;304(7):779–86.
66. Ely EW, Inouye SK, Bernard GR, et al. Delirium in mechanically ventilated patients: validity and reliability of the confusion assessment method for the intensive care unit (CAM-ICU). JAMA 2001;286(21):2703–10.
67. Bellelli G, Morandi A, Davis DHJ, et al. Validation of the 4AT, a new instrument for rapid delirium screening: a study in 234 hospitalised older people. Age Ageing 2014;43(4):496–502.
68. Fick DM, Inouye SK, Guess J, et al. Preliminary development of an ultrabrief two-item bedside test for delirium. J Hosp Med 2015;10(10):645–50.
69. Gaudreau J-D, Gagnon P, Harel F, et al. Fast, systematic, and continuous delirium assessment in hospitalized patients: the nursing delirium screening scale. J Pain Symptom Manage 2005;29(4):368–75.
70. Gavinski K, Carnahan R, Weckmann M. Validation of the delirium observation screening scale in a hospitalized older population. J Hosp Med 2016;11(7):494–7.
71. Marra A, Jackson JC, Ely EW, et al. Focusing on inattention: the diagnostic accuracy of brief measures of inattention for detecting delirium. J Hosp Med 2018;13(8):551–7.
72. Han JH, Vasilevskis EE, Schnelle JF, et al. The diagnostic performance of the Richmond Agitation Sedation Scale for detecting delirium in older emergency department patients. Acad Emerg Med 2015;22(7):878–82.

73. Sands MB, Dantoc BP, Hartshorn A, et al. Single Question in Delirium (SQiD): testing its efficacy against psychiatrist interview, the confusion assessment method and the memorial delirium assessment scale. Palliat Med 2010;24(6): 561–5.

74. Han JH, Wilson A, Schnelle JF, et al. An evaluation of single question delirium screening tools in older emergency department patients. Am J Emerg Med 2018;36(7):1249–52.

75. Wright DW, Lancaster RT, Ratcliff JJ, et al. Proxy identification: a time-dependent analysis. Acad Emerg Med 2004;11(2):204–7.

76. Chester JG, Beth Harrington M, Rudolph JL, VA Delirium Working Group. Serial administration of a modified Richmond Agitation and Sedation Scale for delirium screening. J Hosp Med 2012;7(5):450–3.

77. Steinman MA, Beizer JL, DuBeau CE, et al. How to use the American Geriatrics Society 2015 beers criteria-a guide for patients, clinicians, health systems, and payors. J Am Geriatr Soc 2015;63(12):e1–7.

78. Bayer AJ, Chadha JS, Farag RR, et al. Changing presentation of myocardial infarction with increasing old age. J Am Geriatr Soc 1986;34(4):263–6.

79. Uguz F, Kayrak M, Cíçek E, et al. Delirium following acute myocardial infarction: incidence, clinical profiles, and predictors. Perspect Psychiatr Care 2010;46(2): 135–42.

80. Liu SW, Lee S, Hayes JM, et al. Head computed tomography findings in geriatric emergency department patients with delirium, altered mental status, and confusion: a systematic review. Acad Emerg Med 2022. https://doi.org/10.1111/acem.14622.

81. Naughton BJ, Moran M, Ghaly Y, et al. Computed tomography scanning and delirium in elder patients. Acad Emerg Med 1997;4(12):1107–10.

82. Hirano LA, Bogardus ST, Saluja S, et al. Clinical yield of computed tomography brain scans in older general medical patients. J Am Geriatr Soc 2006;54(4): 587–92.

83. Abraha I, Trotta F, Rimland JM, et al. Efficacy of non-pharmacological interventions to prevent and treat delirium in older patients: a systematic overview. The SENATOR project ONTOP series. PLoS One 2015;10(6):e0123090.

84. Lee S, Chen H, Hibino S, et al. Can we improve delirium prevention and treatment in the emergency department? A systematic review. J Am Geriatr Soc 2022;70(6):1838–49.

85. Noel CB, Cirbus JR, Han JH. Emergency department interventions and their effect on delirium's natural course: the folly may be in the Foley. J Emerg Trauma Shock 2019;12(4):280–5.

86. Flaherty JH, Little MO. Matching the environment to patients with delirium: lessons learned from the delirium room, a restraint-free environment for older hospitalized adults with delirium. J Am Geriatr Soc 2011;59(Suppl 2):S295–300.

87. Zun L, Wilson MP, Nordstrom K. Treatment goal for agitation: sedation or calming. Ann Emerg Med 2017;70(5):751–2.

88. Gault TI, Gray SM, Vilke GM, et al. Are oral medications effective in the management of acute agitation? J Emerg Med 2012;43(5):854–9.

89. Siddiqi N, House AO, Holmes JD. Occurrence and outcome of delirium in medical in-patients: a systematic literature review. Age Ageing 2006;35(4):350–64.

90. Hshieh TT, Yue J, Oh E, et al. Effectiveness of multicomponent nonpharmacological delirium interventions: a meta-analysis. JAMA Intern Med 2015;175(4): 512–20.

91. Inouye SK, Bogardus ST, Charpentier PA, et al. A multicomponent intervention to prevent delirium in hospitalized older patients. N Engl J Med 1999;340(9): 669–76.

92. Inouye SK, Bogardus ST, Baker DI, et al. The Hospital Elder Life Program: a model of care to prevent cognitive and functional decline in older hospitalized patients. Hospital Elder Life Program. J Am Geriatr Soc 2000;48(12):1697–706.

93. Inouye SK, Baker DI, Fugal P, et al, HELP Dissemination Project. Dissemination of the hospital elder life program: implementation, adaptation, and successes. J Am Geriatr Soc 2006;54(10):1492–9.

94. Inouye SK. Prevention of delirium in hospitalized older patients: risk factors and targeted intervention strategies. Ann Med 2000;32(4):257–63.

95. Inouye SK, Westendorp RGJ, Saczynski JS. Delirium in elderly people. Lancet 2014;383(9920):911–22.

96. Bo M, Bonetto M, Bottignole G, et al. Length of stay in the emergency department and occurrence of delirium in older medical patients. J Am Geriatr Soc 2016;64(5):1114–9.

97. Émond M, Grenier D, Morin J, et al. Emergency department stay associated delirium in older patients. Can Geriatr J 2017;20(1):10–4.

98. Jordano JO, Vasilevskis EE, Duggan MC, et al. Effect of physical and occupational therapy on delirium duration in older emergency department patients who are hospitalized. Journal of the American College of Emergency Physicians Open 2023;4(1):e12857.

99. Shenvi C, Kennedy M, Austin CA, et al. Managing delirium and agitation in the older emergency department patient: the ADEPT tool. Ann Emerg Med 2020; 75(2):136–45.

100. Lo AX, Kennedy M. It's time to mobilize: moving mobility interventions for delirium from inpatient units to the emergency department. Journal of the American College of Emergency Physicians Open 2023;4(1):e12900.

101. Kennedy M, Hwang U, Han JH. Delirium in the emergency department: moving from tool-based research to system-wide change. J Am Geriatr Soc 2020;68(5): 956–8.

Elder Mistreatment
Emergency Department Recognition and Management

Elaine Gottesman, MSW, Alyssa Elman, MSW,
Tony Rosen, MD, MPH*

KEYWORDS

- Elder mistreatment • Elder abuse • Caregiver neglect • Emergency department
- Identification • Intervention

KEY POINTS

- Elder mistreatment is experienced by 5% to 15% of community-dwelling older adults each year.
- An emergency department (ED) encounter offers an important opportunity to identify elder mistreatment and initiate intervention.
- Strategies to improve detection of elder mistreatment include identifying high-risk patients; recognizing suggestive findings from the history, physical examination, imaging, and laboratory tests; and/or using screening tools.
- ED management of elder mistreatment includes addressing acute issues, maximizing the patient's safety, and reporting to the authorities when appropriate.

Elder mistreatment is a common phenomenon that can have a significant impact on the health and quality of life of affected older adults. This mistreatment is defined as an intentional act or failure to act that causes or creates a risk of harm to an older adult committed by a trusted person. This mistreatment may include physical abuse, sexual abuse, neglect, verbal/psychological/emotional abuse, and financial exploitation (**Table 1**). Many older adults experience multiple types.[1–5] Self-neglect, defined as a behavior in which an older adult threatens their own health or safety by not performing or refusing assistance with essential self-care, is also common and can be associated with significant negative outcomes but is not the focus of this chapter.

Elder mistreatment is experienced by 5% to 15% of community-dwelling older adults each year,[1–6] with older adults residing in facilities at even higher risk.[7–11] Most of these older adults suffer in silence, with as few as 1 in 24 cases of elder mistreatment identified

Department of Emergency Medicine, Weill Cornell Medical College/NewYork-Presbyterian Hospital, New York, NY, USA
* Corresponding author. 525 East 68th Street, Room 130, New York, NY.
E-mail address: aer2006@med.cornell.edu

Clin Geriatr Med 39 (2023) 553–573
https://doi.org/10.1016/j.cger.2023.05.007
0749-0690/23/© 2023 Elsevier Inc. All rights reserved.

Table 1
Types of elder abuse and neglect

Type	Definition	Examples
Physical abuse	Intentional use of physical force that may result in bodily injury, physical pain, or impairment	• Slapping, hitting, kicking, pushing, pulling hair • Use of physical restraints, force-feeding • Burning, use of household objects as weapons, use of firearms and knives
Sexual abuse	Any type of sexual contact with an elderly person that is nonconsensual or sexual contact with any person incapable of giving consent	• Sexual assault or battery, such as rape, sodomy, coerced nudity, and sexually explicit photographing • Unwanted touching, verbal sexual advances • Indecent exposure
Neglect	Refusal or failure to fulfill any part of a person's obligations or duties to an elder, which may result in harm—may be intentional or unintentional	• Withholding of food, water, clothing, shelter, medications • Failure to ensure elder's personal hygiene or to provide physical aids, including walker, cane, glasses, hearing aids, dentures • Failure to ensure elder's personal safety and/or appropriate medical follow-up
Emotional/psychological abuse	Intentional infliction of anguish, pain, or distress through verbal or nonverbal acts	• Verbal berating, harassment, or intimidation • Threats of punishment or deprivation • Treating the older person like an infant • Isolating the older person from others
Financial/material exploitation	Illegal or improper use of an older adult's money, property, or assets	• Stealing money or belongings • Cashing an older adult's checks without permission and/or forging his or her signature • Coercing an older adult into signing contracts, changing a will, or assigning durable power of attorney against his or her wishes or when the older adult does not possess the mental capacity to do so

Adapted from National Center on Elder Abuse. Types of abuse. Available at: https://ncea.acl.gov/faq/abusetypes.html. Accessed November 21, 2017.

and reported to the authorities.[2] Experiencing elder mistreatment is associated with increases in depression,[12] dementia,[12] and exacerbations of chronic illness. Exposed older adults are more likely than others to present to the emergency department (ED),[13,14] be hospitalized,[15] and be placed in a nursing home.[16,17] As the older adult population grows, elder mistreatment will become an even greater public health concern.[18–27]

In facility settings, mistreatment may be perpetrated by facility staff or other residents.[28] Resident-to-resident elder mistreatment occurs more frequently,[29] as dementia and associated behavioral disturbance is common among residents.

THE EMERGENCY DEPARTMENT ENCOUNTER: A MISSED OPPORTUNITY

An ED encounter is an important opportunity to identify elder mistreatment and initiate intervention. However, this opportunity is often missed. An interaction with a health care clinician may be the only time that an isolated older adult leaves their home, and these older adults more likely present to the ED than an outpatient provider.[13,14,30] An ED visit is typically prolonged, which provides an opportunity for multiple disciplines to observe an older adult and others at the bedside. Opportunities exist to separate the older adult from the potential perpetrator to facilitate disclosure. An ED encounter may directly result from elder mistreatment, increasing the potential for detection.[13] In addition, seeking assistance from an ED may indicate readiness to disclose and change their relationship with the perpetrator.[31] Also resources to initiate intervention for elder mistreatment are available, particularly in well-resourced EDs.[32]

Despite this, ED clinicians almost never diagnose elder mistreatment or report their concerns to the authorities[33,34]; this may be due to limited time and physical space to complete an assessment and proper follow-up, difficulty in distinguishing intentional and unintentional injuries, and hesitation to involve authorities in patients' lives.[34,35] Reasons that an older adult patient may not disclose to an ED clinician include fear of retribution or harming a relationship, particularly when the perpetrator is someone on whom they rely for physical or emotional needs, guilt or self-blame for the mistreatment, hopelessness, and not trusting health care clinicians.[36,37]

IMPROVING DETECTION

To improve detection of elder mistreatment, ED clinicians may consider identifying high-risk patients; performing a comprehensive history; and recognizing suggestive findings from the physical examination, imaging, and laboratory tests. Routine universal or targeted screening may also be helpful.

Identifying Older Adults at High Risk

Research has described characteristics of older adults and potential perpetrators that increase risk for elder mistreatment, as highlighted in **Box 1**.[4,38–40] Notably, older adults who have cognitive or functional impairment or are dependent on others for basic activities of daily living and instrumental activities of daily living are much more susceptible to elder mistreatment.[41–43] Isolation is also an important risk factor. Still, even in the absence of these risk factors, ED clinicians should maintain a high index of suspicion for mistreatment for all older adult patients.

Performing Comprehensive History

For patients presenting with injuries, it is important to get a detailed understanding of the history, including the mechanism, who was present, what led up to the injury, how

---

Box 1
Potential risk factors for elder abuse

For becoming a victim
  Functional dependence or disability
  Poor physical health
  Cognitive impairment/dementia
  Poor mental health
  Low income/socioeconomic status
  Social isolation/low social support
  Previous history of family violence
  Previous traumatic event exposure
  Substance abuse

For becoming a perpetrator
  Mental illness
  Substance abuse
  Caregiver stress
  Previous history of family violence
  Financial dependence on older adult

Data from Refs.[4,38,39]

---

it was handled, and how soon after the injury care was sought. When evaluating a patient with trauma or injuries, ED clinicians should consider whether the physical findings are consistent with the reported mechanism.

Ideally, ED clinicians obtain a comprehensive medical and social history from all older adult patients if concern exists for elder mistreatment; this includes both immediate factors that led to the hospitalization as well as an understanding of the patient's baseline functioning compared with how they are presenting. Clinicians may also obtain an understanding of how the patient is managing their activities at home, including cognition, taking medications, and general care needs.[44] A review of the medical chart may be helpful as well. **Box 2** indicates red flags for elder mistreatment that may be identified when taking a history.

Although it may be tempting to obtain history from a caregiver at bedside if the patient has cognitive impairment or a language barrier, when considering elder mistreatment, it is important to interview the patient alone to ensure privacy and confidentiality. Research indicates that even people with dementia can often accurately describe how an injury occurred.[45,46] If the patient speaks a foreign language, using professional

---

Box 2
Indicators from the medical history of possible elder abuse or neglect[104]

Unexplained injuries

Past history of frequent injuries

Elderly patient referred to as "accident prone"

Delay between onset of medical illness or injury and seeking of medical attention

Recurrent visits to the ED for similar injuries

Using multiple physicians and EDs for care rather than one primary care physician ("doctor hopping or shopping")

Noncompliance with medications, appointments, or physician directions

interpretation services is better than relying on family. The clinician may explore whether the patient feels isolated or helpless, and if concerns exist, the clinician may follow-up with questions about specific types of elder mistreatment.[47] **Figs. 1** and **2** offer specific questions about mistreatment that can be asked to the patient privately. One study suggests that 7% of cognitively intact older adult ED patients report mistreatment when asked directly about it, so it is important to ensure that the patient is given an opportunity to share concerns.[48] Notably, if the patient is unable to provide a full history, the ED clinician and other members of the team may consider obtaining collateral from sources including a patient's outpatient providers, other family, or homecare agencies.[44]

Obtaining a comprehensive social history is essential when assessing for elder mistreatment. In addition to identifying any risk factors (see **Box 1**), a social history should also include an understanding of the risks within the home environment and any barriers to accessing needed resources.[49] The ED clinician should look for any social or functional needs that are not being met.[25,49] In many large EDs, this social assessment for unmet needs may be conducted by a social worker or care coordinator, who takes the lead when an ED clinician has concerns about elder mistreatment.[50–52]

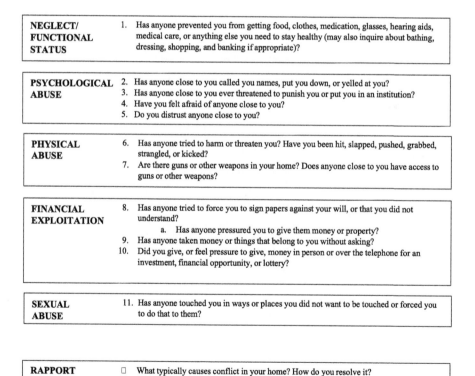

NEGLECT/ FUNCTIONAL STATUS	1. Has anyone prevented you from getting food, clothes, medication, glasses, hearing aids, medical care, or anything else you need to stay healthy (may also inquire about bathing, dressing, shopping, and banking if appropriate)?
PSYCHOLOGICAL ABUSE	2. Has anyone close to you called you names, put you down, or yelled at you? 3. Has anyone close to you ever threatened to punish you or put you in an institution? 4. Have you felt afraid of anyone close to you? 5. Do you distrust anyone close to you?
PHYSICAL ABUSE	6. Has anyone tried to harm or threaten you? Have you been hit, slapped, pushed, grabbed, strangled, or kicked? 7. Are there guns or other weapons in your home? Does anyone close to you have access to guns or other weapons?
FINANCIAL EXPLOITATION	8. Has anyone tried to force you to sign papers against your will, or that you did not understand? a. Has anyone pressured you to give them money or property? 9. Has anyone taken money or things that belong to you without asking? 10. Did you give, or feel pressure to give, money in person or over the telephone for an investment, financial opportunity, or lottery?
SEXUAL ABUSE	11. Has anyone touched you in ways or places you did not want to be touched or forced you to do that to them?

| RAPPORT BUILDING QUESTIONS | ☐ What typically causes conflict in your home? How do you resolve it?
☐ Describe a typical day. Who do you see? What do you do?
☐ Are you aware of supportive community services and crisis services? Have you ever used them?
☐ Are you, your caregiver, or someone close to you interested in receiving additional services or resources? |

Fig. 1. Emergency Department Elder Mistreatment Assessment Tool for Social Workers (ED-EMATS)—Initial Assessment. Please explore any positive responses in detail and strongly consider performing comprehensive social assessment. In the last 6 months.

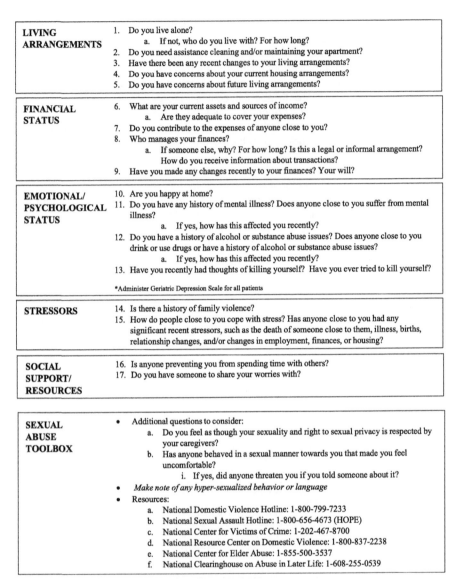

LIVING ARRANGEMENTS	1. Do you live alone? a. If not, who do you live with? For how long? 2. Do you need assistance cleaning and/or maintaining your apartment? 3. Have there been any recent changes to your living arrangements? 4. Do you have concerns about your current housing arrangements? 5. Do you have concerns about future living arrangements?

FINANCIAL STATUS	6. What are your current assets and sources of income?
	    a. Are they adequate to cover your expenses?
	7. Do you contribute to the expenses of anyone close to you?
	8. Who manages your finances?
	    a. If someone else, why? For how long? Is this a legal or informal arrangement? How do you receive information about transactions?
	9. Have you made any changes recently to your finances? Your will?

EMOTIONAL/ PSYCHOLOGICAL STATUS	10. Are you happy at home?
	11. Do you have any history of mental illness? Does anyone close to you suffer from mental illness?
	    a. If yes, how has this affected you recently?
	12. Do you have a history of alcohol or substance abuse issues? Does anyone close to you drink or use drugs or have a history of alcohol or substance abuse issues?
	    a. If yes, how has this affected you recently?
	13. Have you recently had thoughts of killing yourself? Have you ever tried to kill yourself?
	
	*Administer Geriatric Depression Scale for all patients

STRESSORS	14. Is there a history of family violence? 15. How do people close to you cope with stress? Has anyone close to you had any significant recent stressors, such as the death of someone close to them, illness, births, relationship changes, and/or changes in employment, finances, or housing?
SOCIAL SUPPORT/ RESOURCES	16. Is anyone preventing you from spending time with others? 17. Do you have someone to share your worries with?

SEXUAL ABUSE TOOLBOX	• Additional questions to consider:
	    a. Do you feel as though your sexuality and right to sexual privacy is respected by your caregivers?
	    b. Has anyone behaved in a sexual manner towards you that made you feel uncomfortable?
	        i. If yes, did anyone threaten you if you told someone about it?
	• *Make note of any hyper-sexualized behavior or language*
	• Resources:
	    a. National Domestic Violence Hotline: 1-800-799-7233
	    b. National Sexual Assault Hotline: 1-800-656-4673 (HOPE)
	    c. National Center for Victims of Crime: 1-202-467-8700
	    d. National Resource Center on Domestic Violence: 1-800-837-2238
	    e. National Center for Elder Abuse: 1-855-500-3537
	    f. National Clearinghouse on Abuse in Later Life: 1-608-255-0539

Fig. 2. Emergency Department Elder Mistreatment Assessment Tool for Social Workers (ED-EMATS)—Comprehensive Evaluation (if concern remains after initial assessment).

To assist those who may be less comfortable with this, a tool has been developed called the Emergency Department Elder Mistreatment Assessment Tool for Social Workers (ED-EMATS).[50] The preliminary step of this 2-step tool provides questions that all ED clinicians may use to ask directly about types of mistreatment (see **Fig. 1**). The tool also includes a comprehensive social assessment.

When possible, it may be helpful to talk with an older adult's outpatient health care providers. These clinicians may have important insights about their baseline functioning and recent trajectory. They also may be familiar with the dynamics of their relationships with caregivers and other family members.

Recognizing Suggestive Findings from Physical Examination

Although research is still ongoing into injury patterns that may be indicative of elder mistreatment rather than an accidental injury, such as a fall, researchers have found clinically useful findings to assist with elder mistreatment identification. A study comparing physical elder mistreatment victims with older adults presenting with a fall found that the former often had bruises that were large (>5 cm) and found on the face, lateral right arm, or posterior torso.[46] Research has also suggested that physical abuse–related injuries often occur on the head, neck, and upper extremities.[53–55] Older adults experiencing physical abuse are more likely than older adults presenting to the ED with a fall to have injuries to the left cheek/zygoma, with neck and ear injuries occurring commonly in abuse but not due to a fall.[56] In addition, physical elder abuse victims are more likely to have maxillofacial/dental/neck injuries combined with no upper and lower extremity injuries, suggesting that the simultaneous presence and absence of injuries may be helpful in differentiating intentional from unintentional injuries in older adults.[56]

In addition to examining areas of reported injuries, it is important to fully expose an older adult and conduct a head-to-toe examination to ensure a comprehensive assessment of EM; this includes a full skin examination, paying particular attention to any decubitus ulcerations, and fingernail and toenail hygiene. An intraoral examination is also often helpful. **Box 3** provides a comprehensive list of physical findings suggestive of elder mistreatment. No physical finding is diagnostic in isolation. ED clinicians should pay attention to the presence of multiple signs in a single patient, which may raise the index of suspicion.[57–60]

If there is concern for sexual abuse, including evidence of genitourinary trauma or vaginal bleeding, an ED clinician may offer a complete sexual assault examination,

---

Box 3
Physical signs suspicious for potential elder abuse or neglect

Physical Abuse
   Bruising in atypical locations (not over bony prominences/on lateral arms, back, face, ears, or neck)
   Patterned injuries (bite marks or injury consistent with the shape of a belt buckle, fingertip, or other object)
   Wrist or ankle lesions or scars (suggesting inappropriate restraint)
   Burns (particularly stocking/glove pattern suggesting forced immersion or cigarette pattern)
   Multiple fractures or bruises of different ages
   Traumatic alopecia or scalp hematomas
   Subconjunctival, vitreous, or retinal ophthalmic hemorrhages
   Intraoral soft tissue injuries

Sexual Abuse
   Genital, rectal, or oral trauma (including erythema, bruising, lacerations)
   Evidence of sexually transmitted disease

Neglect
   Cachexia/malnutrition
   Dehydration
   Pressure sores/decubitus ulcers
   Poor body hygiene, unchanged diaper
   Dirty, severely worn clothing
   Elongated toenails
   Poor oral hygiene

Data from Refs.[57–61]

including evidence collection by a trained sexual assault forensic examiner if available.[61] If the patient does not have the capacity to consent, the clinician may consider asking for consent from a guardian, if no concerns about mistreatment by this individual exist. Depending on hospital protocols, it is possible the patient may also assent to passive evidence collection.

Considering Evidence from Imaging and Laboratory Testing

Given that findings from diagnostic imaging play a critical role in detecting child abuse, the potential exists for imaging to have a similar role in elder mistreatment.[62–64] Unfortunately, diagnostic radiologists, who receive extensive training in child abuse detection, do not typically receive any education around identifying elder mistreatment.[53,65] Also, there is currently only limited literature describing imaging findings suggestive of elder mistreatment.[53,65,66] Preliminary findings from promising ongoing research have identified potential imaging correlates, including cooccurring old and new fractures, high-energy fractures in the case of a low-energy mechanism, distal ulnar diaphyseal fractures, and small bowel hematomas.[65,66]

If an ED clinician has suspicion for elder mistreatment, they may want to consider communicating concerns to the radiologist and ask the radiologist to comment on whether the imaging findings are consistent with the purported mechanism. In addition, ED clinicians can consider adding imaging tests that screen for elder mistreatment, including maxillofacial computed tomography scan and chest radiograph, to evaluate for acute and chronic fractures; this is analogous to the skeletal survey routinely performed in potential victims of child abuse.[62–64]

Analysis of an older adult's laboratory results can give insight into how they are functioning at home and may be helpful in increasing or decreasing the level of suspicion of elder mistreatment. These tests can help clinicians detect anemia as well as potential dehydration (an elevated BUN/creatinine ratio) or malnutrition (low albumin).[67] Multiple abnormal results may raise the level of suspicion more than a single one. Unusual bruising may be more concerning if platelet levels and coagulation studies are within normal limits. Clinicians can consider checking prescription medication levels (eg, serum levels of antiepileptic drugs, international normalized ratio for patients on warfarin, thyroid-stimulation hormone for patients on levothyroxine) when assessing for mistreatment. Low levels in a patient who is dependent on a caregiver for medication administration may indicate intentional or unintentional withholding, whereas high levels may indicate an intentional or unintentional overdose.[67] The presence of drugs that have not been prescribed or illicit drugs could suggest poisoning.[67] As a result, ED clinicians may also want to use the urine toxicology screen in these cases.[67]

Observing and Working with Caregivers and Others at Bedside

If there is a caregiver or other person present at bedside, the ED clinician and other team members may observe their interactions with the patient for anything concerning for elder mistreatment (shown in **Box 4**). If the patient provides permission, the ED clinician may also interview the caregiver alone to understand the patient's functional status at home.[44] If the caregiver reveals discrepancies from the patient's history or is unfamiliar with the patient's medical history and medications, further assessment may be warranted. The provider might want to explore changes or stressors in the patient's household or direct the caregiver to resources that may ameliorate the care responsibilities. Given the association of caregiving with mistreatment, ED clinician may strive to build trust and rapport, express empathy, and avoid being critical.

Box 4
Observations from older adult/caregiver interaction that should raise concern for elder abuse or neglect[104]

Older adult and caregiver provide conflicting accounts of events

Caregiver interrupts/answers for the older adult

Older adult seems fearful of or hostile toward caregiver

Caregiver seems unengaged/inattentive in caring for the older adult

Caregiver seems frustrated, tired, angry, or burdened by the older adult

Caregiver seems overwhelmed by the older adult

Caregiver seems to lack knowledge of the patient's care needs

Evidence that the caregiver and/or older adult may be abusing alcohol or illicit drugs

---

A Key Role for Emergency Medical Services

Emergency medical services (EMS) providers play a critical role in acute, unscheduled care of older adults, including in elder mistreatment identification.[32,68,69] The observations that EMS providers make inside a home can inform the ED evaluation and identify concerns for potential elder mistreatment. **Box 5** lists concerns about the home environment that may indicate that the older adult is at risk.[70,71] They may also observe the interaction between the caregiver and the patient.[70] A promising tool for EMS providers, Detection of Elder abuse Through Emergency Care Technicians (DETECT), has been developed to ensure that they consider elder mistreatment during their evaluations.[72] In addition, incorporating elder mistreatment into EMS training and specific prompts into their electronic health record may encourage more recognition and documentation of concerns. ED clinicians should attempt to review EMS documentation when caring for older adults. When possible, ED clinicians should try to speak to EMS personnel directly to hear their accounts firsthand, as written reports do not consistently provide important details about the home environment and social situation.[70] Ideally, EMS providers should also feel empowered to express their concerns to the ED team.

Box 5
Concerns about the home environment

Utilities not working correctly (heating or cooling, water, electricity)

Fecal/urine odor

Empty refrigerator/no evidence of available food

Vermin infestation

Extreme clutter/hoarding

Absence of smoke detector

Presence of fire hazard

Expired or unmarked medication bottles or multiple bottles of a single medication

Broken window

Data from Ref.[70,71]

Empowering All Emergency Department Team Members to Contribute

Elder mistreatment may be hard to identify during an ED encounter, particularly given that the perpetrator and even the older adult may be actively trying to conceal it. Given that, it is important to empower all members of the ED team to be observant and contribute.[32] Many team members, including nurses and patient care technologists, typically spend more time at a patient's bedside than other clinicians. They may observe subtle but concerning physical findings when providing personal care[32] or witness troubling interactions between a patient and a caregiver.[32,73] Radiologic technicians have a unique opportunity to assess a patient alone, given that a caregiver may be unwilling to leave a patient's bedside but would not accompany them to the radiology suite.[32] Patients may feel more comfortable disclosing elder mistreatment to nonprovider team members, given that they may perceive fewer consequences from those conversations.[32]

In larger EDs, social workers and care coordinators typically lead sociomedical assessments for older adults, identifying unmet needs and connecting patients, caregivers, and families to resources and supports. The importance of this role as part of geriatric ED care has been increasingly recognized.[51,52] Whenever feasible, it is important to consult social work and/or case management when an older ED patient with suspected or known elder mistreatment is being discharged home, as patients and families may only disclose risk factors or concerns about mistreatment when returning home.

Documenting Completely and Accurately

Any information around elder mistreatment should be completely and accurately documented in the patient's chart. It is important to remember that the medical chart may become part of a legal proceeding, so information included may have significant repercussions on whether the older adult receives justice.[74] ED providers should describe all physical examination findings in detail, including each injury's size, location, stage of healing, and whether the injury is consistent with the reported mechanism. When possible, ED providers should obtain patient permission to take and upload to medical record photos of any significant physical findings. A protocol for photographing injuries in the acute care setting has been published to assist ED providers.[75] Details regarding concern for neglect should be included, such as description of poor hygiene, abnormal laboratory findings, and concerning behavior by the patient's caregiver.[76] Patient responses to direct questions should be documented using the patient's own words. ED providers should also include in their documentation relevant social information, such as the patient's functional status, relationship with the caregiver, and living situation.

Routine Universal or Targeted Structured Screening for Elder Mistreatment

EDs may consider formal universal or targeted structured screening for elder mistreatment in the ED given that the phenomenon is common, serious, and hidden. The American Medical Association, the American College of Emergency Physicians, and the Joint Commission have advocated for assessment for all types of family violence, including elder mistreatment, but have stopped short of recommending universal screening.[77] Notably, the US Preventative Services Taskforce has not recommended screening for elder mistreatment in health care settings given that no evidence yet exists demonstrating that screening results in improved outcomes and lack of data on potential unintended consequences.[78]

Current screening practices in EDs often involve asking a single question, typically some version of "Do you feel safe at home?" Although the efficacy of this approach has not been studied for elder mistreatment, it has been shown to be insensitive for other types of family violence.[77] Several more substantial screening tools have been developed. The Elder Abuse Suspicion Index (EASI) is a short tool validated for cognitively intact patients in ambulatory care.[79] The ED Senior AID (Abuse Identification) tool was designed for EDs and has been shown to be highly sensitive and specific.[80] Because of concern that the ED Senior AID tool may be too lengthy to administer routinely in a busy ED, the Elder Mistreatment Screening and Response Tool (EM-SART) was created.[77] EM-SART involves a multistep process with a brief initial screen for all patients and a more comprehensive assessment with the ED Senior AID tool if concern is identified.[77] The Veteran's Health Administration has successfully integrated EM-SART as part of their geriatric ED initiative.[81] Another screening tool has been developed using tablet technology, Virtual cOaching in making Informed Choices on Elder Mistreatment Self-Disclosure (VOICES). By allowing a patient to interact with a tablet, VOICES minimizes the burden of assessment on ED providers, has the potential to streamline the screening process, and motivates patients to self-report mistreatment while also providing them education around elder mistreatment.[82,83] There are several challenges to developing screening tools in the ED, and development of these instruments is ongoing.[77]

Targeted screening of only high-risk patients would reduce burden on EDs and increase the proportion of patients who screen positive. Risk and protective factors have not yet been completely described, though, and this approach is likely to miss cases.[77] Future strategies may use information from the electronic health record as well as other health care utilization data combined with machine learning approaches to perform automated prescreening to identify high-risk patients who require elder mistreatment assessment.[84]

IMPROVING INTERVENTION AND MANAGEMENT

When elder mistreatment is suspected or confirmed, best practices for management include (1) treating acute issues, (2) maximizing the patient's safety, and (3) reporting to the authorities when appropriate. As with any other patient, ED providers must first assess, stabilize, and treat any acute medical, traumatic, and psychiatric problems, such as bleeding, fractures, dehydration, metabolic abnormalities, infections, delirium, and behavioral symptoms of dementia. The assessment may reveal that the exacerbations of the patient's chronic medical conditions were due to a caregiver failing to give the patient their medications or to provide appropriate care. Hospitalization may be necessary if a patient needs extended treatment.[15,85,86]

A cornerstone of ED management of potential elder mistreatment is trauma-informed care, described in **Box 6**.

Maximizing Patient Safety

It is critical to ensure the patient's immediate safety while they are in the ED. If there are concerns about the perpetrator coming to bedside and interfering with the patient's care or psychological safety, it would be important to include other teams such as security or nursing management to restrict visitation, communication, or provide a security watch. ED and hospital administration and legal may also be helpful in navigating challenging cases, such as when the suspected perpetrator is also the patient's health care decision-maker. If the concerns are high enough, providers may want to identify an alternate living situation for the patient or to consider admitting them for safety.

For patients who will be discharged, it is also important to consider how to address postdischarge unmet needs, safety, and well-being. Team members may want to make

---

Box 6
Trauma-informed care

A cornerstone of ED management of potential elder mistreatment is trauma-informed care. ED providers should try to be sensitive to the potentially deep impact of stressful and traumatic experiences on an older adult's mental and physical health.[105] Also, many patients may have a history of being victimized by medical systems and figures of authority, and these patients may be difficult to engage. In providing trauma-informed care, ED providers should try to maximize victim choice and control while minimizing retraumatization through treatment.
Recommended bedside strategies[106] include the following:
- Using easily understood language and grammar
- Limiting the number of times a victim has to talk about mistreatment
- Avoiding words such as abuse, neglect, or mistreatment if the victim does not perceive their interactions with the perpetrator in this way
- Requesting permission before touching a potential victim
- Maintaining privacy and confidentiality
- Offering an advocate to come to the bedside to support victim if available
- Keeping in mind culturally specific expectations regarding interactions between older adult patients and younger care providers and with male versus female providers

These strategies should also be used for cognitively impaired patients.[106]

---

referrals to providers and services that can increase ongoing supervision of the patient and minimize isolation; this can include a follow-up appointment with a primary care provider or setting up medication delivery. The social worker or case manager should also consider making referrals (options listed in **Box 7**) to help reduce the potential for intentional or unintentional harm. Assistance may look very different depending on the circumstances and the needs of the older adult and perpetrator.[87] Notably, many ED providers may not be familiar with local resources and organizations to which older

---

Box 7
Referrals for assistance in the community

For the Victim
   Homecare agencies
   Crisis hotlines (National Domestic Violence Hotline)
   Meals on Wheels
   Medical transportation services
   Case management (found at local Area Agencies on Aging)
   Senior centers and adult day care
   Geriatric care managers
   Elder attorneys
   Shelter
   Mental health counseling and support groups
   Police reports and victim assistance
   Mobile crisis
   Findhelp.org

For the Caregiver
   Caregiver support groups
   Substance abuse treatment
   Dementia caregiver hotlines
   Respite care options
   Mental health counseling and support groups

Data from Ref.[87]

---

adults can be connected. Online tools such as www.findhelp.org can be used to find available social services by zip code. This tool is particularly relevant in smaller EDs where social workers and care coordinators may not be available to assist and also during nights and weekends. In addition to providing resources and referrals, the ED provider can discuss safety planning to prevent future incidents. The provider may remind the older adult that they can return to the ED whenever they have any future safety concerns.

If an older adult patient refuses intervention, the ED provider may assess if they have the capacity to make this decision. A psychiatric consultation may be helpful. The wishes of an older adult with decision-making capacity who desires to return to an unsafe home situation must be respected, similar to cases of intimate partner violence among younger adults. For older adults who do not have capacity to refuse, an ED clinician may proceed with treatments in the patient's best interest, including hospitalization if appropriate. A summary of guidelines for best practices in elder abuse detection and intervention has been put together by the American College of Surgeons for Trauma Quality Programs.[88]

Reporting Mistreatment

ED providers should report concerns about elder mistreatment to the authorities as well. Only reasonable suspicion is needed to make a report. Adult Protective Services (APS) is the primary agency in most communities that investigates elder mistreatment and protects and supports vulnerable adults. Health care providers are mandated reporters for elder mistreatment in most but not all US states. In many states, elder mistreatment must be reported even if an older adult does not want a report made. ED providers should be aware of requirements in a state in which they practice. Requirements vary by state, and providers should be familiar with the state's guidelines (summary is available at: https://ncEM.acl.gov/NCEM/media/Publication/NCEM_NAPSA_MandatedReportBriefFull.pdf).

In most states, APS only investigates cases of older adults with cognitive or functional impairment and will not act on reports if they find that the older adult does not meet these criteria. In addition, it is important to note that APS works differently than Child Protective Services. APS will not initiate an investigation while a patient is in an ED or hospital, given that this is considered a safe environment. They will only open an investigation after discharge, usually within 72 hours. Given this, ED clinicians may also report to local law enforcement if concerned that a crime has been committed or that an older adult is immediately unsafe. ED clinicians should also make patients aware of a patient's right to report their concerns to local police. When abuse or neglect is suspected or identified in patients from nursing homes, ED providers should report to the state's Department of Health or the long-term care Ombudsman (https://theconsumervoice.org/get_help).

EDs should consider increasing communication and collaboration with APS and other community-based services.[89] In many communities, multidisciplinary teams, which include APS case workers, prosecutors, civil attorneys, law enforcement professionals, financial services professionals, and health care providers, have come together to discuss management of complex elder mistreatment cases. EDs should consider helping launch or joining these teams in their community.[89]

Multidisciplinary Emergency Department–Based Response Team: a Promising Model

Effectively managing complex elder mistreatment cases may be time- and resource-intensive for busy ED providers. To ensure optimal care for potential child abuse victims, ED-based child protection teams were developed more than 50 years ago.[90,91] These on-call multidisciplinary teams with expertise have been shown to increase child abuse identification by ED providers[92] by decreasing disincentives to raising concerns. They also may improve care by providing strategies for next steps in addressing abuse and for allowing frontline ED providers to focus on other critically ill patients. Similar programs for elder mistreatment have only recently been established.[93,94] This new care model is a consultation service including medical providers with forensics expertise and social workers that may assess older adult patients and provide recommendations about appropriate management from an elder mistreatment perspective. Initial experience from these teams has been promising.[95] In one ED, the ED-based response team was activated multiple times each week. Among the patients determined by the response team to have high or moderate suspicion for elder abuse, 75% had a change in living/housing situation or were discharged with new or additional home services (14% discharged to an elder abuse shelter, 39% to a different living/housing situation, and 22% with new or additional home services).[95] ED providers reported that the response team made them more likely to consider/assess for elder abuse and recognized the value of the expertise and guidance the response team provided, with 94% believing that there is merit in establishing similar programs in other EDs.[95]

THE FUTURE

Research is ongoing to inform ED detection and management for elder mistreatment. Similar to extensive research describing findings specific to child abuse, such as metaphyseal fractures and bruising not over bony prominences, elder mistreatment researchers are trying to assist ED clinicians in more accurately and readily detecting elder mistreatment.[96–99] Using these results, clinical prediction rules are being developed to assist ED providers in identifying injuries sustained from physical abuse rather than an accident. In contrast to child abuse detection, it is more difficult to differentiate intentional and unintentional injuries in older adults due to the physiologic changes that occur with normal aging, such as more easily bruising from thin skin and fractures due to osteopenia.[53,57,100–102] Also, older adults commonly use medications such as blood thinners that can affect physical findings.

Box 8
Resources

The Geriatric Emergency Department Collaborative (GEDC), a nationwide collaborative dedicated to improving the quality of ED care for older adults with the goal of reducing harm and improving health care outcomes, has extensive resources for elder mistreatment. Free online continuing education modules for ED providers are available through a collaboration between GEDC and the American Geriatrics Society (https://gedcollaborative.com/course/elder-mistreatment/). The National Collaboratory to Address Elder Mistreatment (NCAEM), a group of US national leaders who have been conducting research and developing innovative elder mistreatment programming, has sought to focus on combating elder mistreatment in EDs. NCAEM has developed and is piloting pragmatic screening, assessment, and management strategies for EDs with varied levels of resources. Working closely with the GEDC, NCAEM has created a toolkit for EDs interested in improving elder mistreatment screening and management (https://gedcollaborative.com/toolkit/elder-mistreatment-emergency-department-toolkit/). In addition, http://www.elderabuseemergency.org provides access to tools, information, and resources that may be useful to ED providers for reference and when working clinically. Comprehensive information about elder mistreatment is available at the National Center on Elder Abuse Web site (https://ncea.acl.gov).

Another area of focus is exploring outcomes for older adults, including unintended consequences, from implementing universal ED elder mistreatment screening. Researchers are also exploring the longer-term impact of multidisciplinary team–based interventions for elder mistreatment.

Improving strategies for identification and intervention is closely linked.[103] Robust screening in many EDs may highlight the need for response strategies and effective interventions. In addition, development of effective and impactful responses may lead to an increased interest in screening.

RESOURCES

Box 8 includes resources available for ED clinicians to improve identification and intervention for elder mistreatment.

SUMMARY

ED providers are in a unique position to identify and initiate intervention for elder mistreatment, which is common, serious, and underrecognized. Providers should maintain a high index of suspicion when providing care to older adults, recognize risk factors, and collaboratively empower all ED team members to contribute. ED management of elder abuse should include treating acute medical and psychological issues, ensuring patient safety, and proper reporting to the authorities. Trauma-informed care should be provided, collaboration with the community should be strengthened, and multidisciplinary interventions including ED-based response teams may be considered.

CLINICS CARE POINTS

- Elder mistreatment is common and may have serious medical and social consequences but is underrecognized. An ED encounter offers an important opportunity to identify elder mistreatment and initiate intervention.

- All ED team members should be empowered to identify elder mistreatment. Emergency Medical Services may play a critical role as well. Formal screening tools may also be useful.

- ED assessment of older adults should include a comprehensive medical and social history, interview of the patient alone, observation of the patient and caregiver interaction, and a head-to-toe physical examination. Imaging and laboratory tests may be useful, as well.

- ED clinicians, including physicians and advanced practice providers, should document any concerns about elder mistreatment and descriptions of their findings in the medical record.

- ED interventions for suspected or confirmed elder mistreatment include treatment of acute medical, traumatic, and psychological conditions; maximizing patient safety; and reporting concerns to the authorities and/or community-based services.

- Health care clinicians are mandated reporters for elder mistreatment in most but not all US states and should consider becoming familiar with the state's guidelines.

REFERENCES

1. Elder Mistreatment: Abuse, Neglect, and Exploitation in an Aging America. Washington D.C: National Academy of Sciences Press; 2003. Available at: https://scholar.google.com/scholar_lookup?title=Elder+Mistreatment:

+Abuse,+Neglect,+and+Exploitation+in+an+Aging+America&publication_
year=2003&.

2. Lifespan of Greater Rochester I, Weill Cornell Medical College, New York City Department for the Aging. Under the Radar: New York State Elder Abuse Prevalence Study. Accessed January 11, 2023. http://www.ocfs.state.ny.us/main/reports/Under%20the%20Radar%2005%2012%2011%20final%20report.pdf.

3. Brandl B, Breckman R, Connolly MT. The Elder Justice Roadmap: A Stakeholder Initiative to Respond to an Emerging Health, Justice, Financial, and Social Crisis. Accessed March 1, 2023. https://www.justice.gov/elderjustice/file/829266/download.

4. Acierno R, Hernandez MA, Amstadter AB, et al. Prevalence and correlates of emotional, physical, sexual, and financial abuse and potential neglect in the United States: the National Elder Mistreatment Study. Am J Public Health 2010;100(2):292–7.

5. Lachs MS, Pillemer K. Elder abuse. Lancet 2004;364(9441):1263–72.

6. Lachs MS, Pillemer KA. Elder abuse. N Engl J Med 2015;373(20):1947–56.

7. Ortmann C, Fechner G, Bajanowski T, et al. Fatal neglect of the elderly. Int J Legal Med 2001;114:191–3.

8. Schiamberg LB, Oehmke J, Zhang Z, et al. Physical abuse of older adults in nursing homes: a random sample survey of adults with an elderly family member in a nursing home. J Elder Abuse Negl 2012;24(1):65–83.

9. Rosen T, Pillemer K, Lachs M. Resident-to-Resident aggression in long-term care facilities: an understudied problem. Aggress Violent Behav 2008;13(2):77–87.

10. Shinoda-Tagawa T, Leonard R, Pontikas J, et al. Resident-to-resident violent incidents in nursing homes. JAMA 2004;291(5):591–8.

11. Rosen T, Lachs MS, Bharucha AJ, et al. Resident-to-resident aggression in long-term care facilities: insights from focus groups of nursing home residents and staff. J Am Geriatr Soc 2008;56(8):1398–408.

12. Dyer CB, Pavlik VN, Murphy KP, et al. The high prevalence of depression and dementia in elder abuse or neglect. J Am Geriatr Soc 2000;48(2):205–8.

13. Dong X, Simon MA. Association between elder abuse and use of ED: findings from the Chicago health and aging project. Research support, N.I.H., Extramural Research Support, Non-U.S. Gov't. Am J Emerg Med 2013;31(4):693–8.

14. Use by older victims of family violence. In: Lachs MS, Williams CS, O'Brien S, et al, editors. Ann Emerg Med 1997;30(4):448–54.

15. Dong X, Simon MA. Elder abuse as a risk factor for hospitalization in older persons. JAMA Intern Med 2013;173(10):911–7.

16. Lachs MS, Williams CS, O'Brien S, et al. Adult protective service use and nursing home placement. Gerontol 2002;42(6):734–9.

17. Dong X, Simon MA. Association between reported elder abuse and rates of admission to skilled nursing facilities: findings from a longitudinal population-based cohort study. Gerontology 2013;59(5):464–72.

18. Roskos, ER and Wilber, ST, 210. The effect of future demographic changes on emergency medicine. Ann Emerg Med, 48 (4), 2006, 65.

19. Wilber ST, Gerson LW, Terrell KM, et al. Geriatric emergency medicine and the 2006 Institute of medicine reports from the committee on the future of emergency care in the U.S. Health system. Acad Emerg Med 2006;13(12):1345–51.

20. Adams JM, U.S. Surgeon General VADM , Robertson L, ACL Administrator and Assistant Secretary for Aging. Elder Abuse: A public health issue that affects all

of us. 2018. Accessed March 30, 2023. https://acl.gov/news-and-events/acl-blog/elder-abuse-public-health-issue-affects-all-us-0.

21. Anetzberger GJ. Caregiving, Primary cause of elder abuse? Generations 2000; 24(2):46–51.

22. Wiehe VR. Understanding Family Violence: Treating and Preventing Partner, Child, Sibling, and Elder Abuse. Thousand Oaks, CA: Sage Publications; 1998.

23. Greenberg J, Mssw M, Ms J. Dependent adult children and elder abuse. J Elder Abuse Negl 1990;2:73–86.

24. Anetzberger GJ, Korbin JE, Austin C. Alcoholism and elder abuse. J Interpers Violence 1994;9(2):184–93.

25. Pillemer K. The dangers of dependency: new findings on domestic violence against the elderly. Soc Probl 1985;33(2):146–58.

26. Anetzberger GJ. The Etiology of Elder Abuse by Adult Offspring. Springfield, IL: C.C. Thomas; 1987.

27. Rosen T, Bloemen EM, LoFaso VM, et al. Acute Precipitants of physical elder abuse: qualitative analysis of legal records from highly Adjudicated cases. J Interpers Violence 2019;34(12):2599–623.

28. Cimino-Fiallos N, Rosen T. Elder abuse-A Guide to Diagnosis and management in the emergency department. Emerg Med Clin North Am 2021;39(2):405–17.

29. Lachs MS, Teresi JA, Ramirez M, et al. The prevalence of resident-to-resident elder mistreatment in nursing homes. Ann Intern Med 2016;165(4):229–36.

30. Platts-Mills TF, Barrio K, Isenberg EE, et al. Emergency physician identification of a cluster of elder abuse in nursing home residents. Ann Emerg Med 2014; 64(1):99–100.

31. Barnett OW. Why battered Women do not leave, Part 1:External Inhibiting factors within society. Trauma Violence Abuse 2000;1(4):343–72.

32. Rosen T, Hargarten S, Flomenbaum NE, et al. Identifying elder abuse in the emergency department: toward a multidisciplinary team-based approach. Ann Emerg Med 2016;68(3):378–82.

33. Blakely BE, Dolon R. Another look at the Helpfulness of Occupational groups in the Discovery of elder abuse and neglect. J Elder Abuse Negl 2003;13(3):1–23.

34. Evans CS, Hunold KM, Rosen T, et al. Diagnosis of elder abuse in U.S. Emergency departments. J Am Geriatr Soc 2017;65(1):91–7.

35. Jones JS, Veenstra TR, Seamon JP, et al. Elder mistreatment: national survey of emergency physicians. Ann Emerg Med 1997;30(4):473–9.

36. Fraga Dominguez S, Storey JE, Glorney E. Help-seeking behavior in victims of elder abuse: a systematic review. Trauma Violence Abuse 2021;22(3):466–80.

37. Smith JR, Difficult. Mothering Challenging Adult Children through Conflict and Commitment. Lanham, MD: Rowman & Littlefield; 2022.

38. Amstadter AB, Zajac K, Strachan M, et al. Prevalence and correlates of elder mistreatment in South Carolina: the South Carolina elder mistreatment study. Research Support, N.I.H., Extramural. J Interpers Violence 2011;26(15):2947–72.

39. Laumann EO, Leitsch SA, Waite LJ. Elder mistreatment in the United States: prevalence estimates from a nationally representative study. Comparative Study Research Support, N.I.H., Extramural. J Gerontol B Psychol Sci Soc Sci 2008; 63(4):S248–54.

40. Friedman LS, Avila S, Tanouye K, et al. A case-control study of severe physical abuse of older adults. J Am Geriatr Soc 2011;59(3):417–22.

41. Cooney C, Howard R, Lawlor B. Abuse of vulnerable people with dementia by their carers: can we identify those most at risk? Int J Geriatr Psychiatry 2006; 21(6):564–71.

42. Lachs MS, Williams C, O'Brien S, et al. Risk factors for reported elder abuse and neglect: a nine-year observational cohort study. Gerontol 1997;37(4):469–74.
43. Wiglesworth A, Mosqueda L, Mulnard R, et al. Screening for abuse and neglect of people with dementia. J Am Geriatr Soc 2010;58(3):493–500.
44. Lachs MS, Fulmer T. Recognizing elder abuse and neglect. Clin Geriatr Med 1993;9(3):665–81.
45. Ziminski CE, Wiglesworth A, Austin R, et al. Injury patterns and causal mechanisms of bruising in physical elder abuse. J Forensic Nurs 2013;9(2):84–91 [quiz: E1-2].
46. Wiglesworth A, Austin R, Corona M, et al. Bruising as a marker of physical elder abuse. J Am Geriatr Soc 2009;57(7):1191–6.
47. Fulmer T, Rodgers RF, Pelger A. Verbal mistreatment of the elderly. J Elder Abuse Negl 2014;26(4):351–64.
48. Stevens TB, Richmond NL, Pereira GF, et al. Prevalence of nonmedical problems among older adults presenting to the emergency department. Acad Emerg Med 2014;21(6):651–8.
49. Elman A, Baek D, Gottesman E, et al. Unmet needs and social challenges for older adults during and after the COVID-19 Pandemic: an opportunity to improve care. J Geriatr Emerg Med 2021;2(11):1.
50. Elman A, Rosselli S, Burnes D, et al. Developing the emergency department elder mistreatment assessment tool for social workers using a modified delphi technique. Health Soc Work 2020;45(2):110–21.
51. Auerbach C, Mason SE. The value of the presence of social work in emergency departments. Soc Work Health Care 2010;49(4):314–26.
52. Hamilton C, Ronda L, Hwang U, et al. The evolving role of geriatric emergency department social work in the era of health care reform. Soc Work Health Care 2015;54(9):849–68.
53. Murphy K, Waa S, Jaffer H, et al. A literature review of findings in physical elder abuse. Can Assoc Radiol J 2013;64(1):10–4.
54. Rosen T, Bloemen EM, LoFaso VM, et al. Emergency department presentations for injuries in older adults independently known to be victims of elder abuse. J Emerg Med 2016;50(3):518–26.
55. Rosen T, Clark S, Bloemen EM, et al. Geriatric assault victims treated at U.S. trauma centers: five-year analysis of the national trauma data bank. Injury 2016;47(12):2671–8.
56. Rosen T, LoFaso VM, Bloemen EM, et al. Identifying injury patterns associated with physical elder abuse: analysis of legally adjudicated cases. Ann Emerg Med 2020;76(3):266–76.
57. Collins KA. Elder maltreatment: a review. Arch Pathol Lab Med 2006;130(9):1290–6.
58. Gibbs LM. Understanding the medical markers of elder abuse and neglect: physical examination findings. Clin Geriatr Med 2014;30(4):687–712.
59. Palmer M, Brodell RT, Mostow EN. Elder abuse: dermatologic clues and critical solutions. J Am Acad Dermatol 2013;68(2):e37–42.
60. Chang ALS, Wong JW, Endo JO, et al. Geriatric dermatology: Part II. Risk factors and cutaneous signs of elder mistreatment for the dermatologist. J Am Acad Dermatol 2013;68(4):533 e1–e533, e10.
61. Speck PM, Hartig MT, Likes W, et al. Case series of sexual assault in older persons. Clin Geriatr Med 2014;30(4):779–806.
62. Kempe CH, Silverman FN, Steele BF, et al. The battered-child syndrome. JAMA 1962;181:17–24.

63. Kleinman PK. Diagnostic imaging in infant abuse. AJR Am J Roentgenol 1990; 155(4):703–12.
64. Nimkin K, Kleinman PK. Imaging of child abuse. Pediatr Clin North Am 1997; 44(3):615–35.
65. Rosen T, Bloemen EM, Harpe J, et al. Radiologists' training, experience, and Attitudes about elder abuse detection. AJR Am J Roentgenol 2016;207(6):1210–4.
66. Wong NZ, Rosen T, Sanchez AM, et al. Imaging findings in elder abuse: a role for radiologists in detection. Can Assoc Radiol J 2017;68(1):16–20.
67. LoFaso VM, Rosen T. Medical and laboratory indicators of elder abuse and neglect. Clin Geriatr Med 2014;30(4):713–28.
68. Shah MN, Bazarian JJ, Lerner EB, et al. The epidemiology of emergency medical services use by older adults: an analysis of the National Hospital Ambulatory Medical Care Survey. Acad Emerg Med 2007;14(5):441–7.
69. Gerson LW, Schelble DT, Wilson JE. Using paramedics to identify at-risk elderly. Ann Emerg Med 1992;21(6):688–91.
70. Rosen T, Lien C, Stern ME, et al. Emergency medical services perspectives on identifying and reporting victims of elder abuse, neglect, and self-neglect. J Emerg Med 2017;53(4):573–82.
71. Cannell MB, Jetelina KK, Zavadsky M, et al. Towards the development of a screening tool to enhance the detection of elder abuse and neglect by emergency medical technicians (EMTs): a qualitative study. BMC Emerg Med 2016;16(1):19.
72. Cannell B, Gonzalez JMR, Livingston M, et al. Pilot testing the detection of elder abuse through emergency care technicians (DETECT) screening tool: results from the DETECT pilot project. J Elder Abuse Negl 2019;31(2):129–45.
73. Sidley CSL. When a "fall" isn't a fall: screening for elder mistreatment. Emergency Physicians Monthly 2015.
74. Coulourides Kogan A, Rosen T, Homeier D, Chennapan K, Mosqueda LJJAGS. Paper abstract-developing a tool to improve documentation of physical findings in injured older adults by health care providers: insights from experts in muliple disciplines. 2017;65:S1-S289.
75. Bloemen EM, Rosen T, Cline Schiroo JA, et al. Photographing injuries in the acute care setting: development and evaluation of a standardized protocol for research, forensics, and clinical practice. Acad Emerg Med 2016;23(5):653–9.
76. Kogan AC, Rosen T, Navarro A, et al. Developing the geriatric injury documentation tool (Geri-IDT) to improve documentation of physical findings in injured older adults. J Gen Intern Med 2019;34(4):567–74.
77. Rosen T, Platts-Mills TF, Fulmer T. Screening for elder mistreatment in emergency departments: current progress and recommendations for next steps. J Elder Abuse Negl 2020;32(3):295–315.
78. USPST Force, Curry SJ, Krist AH, et al. Screening for intimate partner violence, elder abuse, and abuse of vulnerable adults: US preventive services Task Force final recommendation statement. JAMA 2018;320(16):1678–87.
79. Yaffe MJ, Wolfson C, Lithwick M, et al. Development and validation of a tool to improve physician identification of elder abuse: the Elder Abuse Suspicion Index (EASI). J Elder Abuse Negl 2008;20(3):276–300.
80. Platts-Mills TF, Dayaa JA, Reeve BB, et al. Development of the emergency department Senior abuse identification (ED Senior AID) tool. J Elder Abuse Negl 2018;30(4):247–70.
81. Makaroun LK, Halaszynski JJ, Rosen T, et al. Leveraging VA geriatric emergency department accreditation to improve elder abuse detection in older

Veterans using a standardized tool. Acad Emerg Med 2022. https://doi.org/10.1111/acem.14646.

82. Abujarad F, Edwards C, Choo E, et al. Digital health screening tool for identification of elder mistreatment. Gerontechnology : international journal on the fundamental aspects of technology to serve the ageing society. Gerontechnology 2020;19(Suppl 1).

83. Abujarad F, Ulrich D, Edwards C, et al. Development and usability evaluation of VOICES: a digital health tool to identify elder mistreatment. J Am Geriatr Soc 2021;69(6):1469–78.

84. Rosen T, Zhang Y, Bao Y, et al. Can artificial intelligence help identify elder abuse and neglect? J Elder Abuse Negl 2020;32(1):97–103.

85. Hoover RM, Polson M. Detecting elder abuse and neglect: assessment and intervention. Am Fam Physician 2014;89(6):453–60.

86. Ziminski CE, Phillips LR, Woods DL. Raising the index of suspicion for elder abuse: cognitive impairment, falls, and injury patterns in the emergency department. Geriatr Nurs 2012;33(2):105–12.

87. Burnes D, MacNeil A, Nowaczynski A, et al. A scoping review of outcomes in elder abuse intervention research: the current landscape and where to go next. Aggression and Violent Behav 2021;57:101476.

88. Surgeons ACo. ACS Trauma Quality Programs Best Practices Guidelines For Trauma Center Recognition Of Child Abuse, Elder Abuse, and Intimate Partner Violence. Accessed April 3, 2023, https://www.facs.org/media/smbgws45/abuse_guidelines.pdf.

89. Rosen T, Elman A, Dion S, et al. Review of programs to Combat elder mistreatment: focus on hospitals and level of resources needed. J Am Geriatr Soc 2019;67(6):1286–94.

90. Kistin CJ, Tien I, Bauchner H, et al. Factors that influence the effectiveness of child protection teams. Pediatrics 2010;126(1):94–100.

91. Hochstadt NJ, Harwicke NJ. How effective is the multidisciplinary approach? A follow-up study. Child Abuse Negl 1985;9(3):365–72.

92. Powers E, Tiyyagura G, Asnes AG, et al. Early involvement of the child protection team in the care of injured infants in a pediatric emergency department. J Emerg Med 2019;56(6):592–600.

93. Rosen T, Mehta-Naik N, Elman A, et al. Improving quality of care in hospitals for victims of elder mistreatment: development of the vulnerable elder protection team. Jt Comm J Qual Patient Saf 2018;44(3):164–71.

94. Rosen T, Stern ME, Mulcare MR, et al. Emergency department provider perspectives on elder abuse and development of a novel ED-based multidisciplinary intervention team. Emerg Med J 2018;35(10):600–7.

95. Rosen T, Elman A, Clark S, et al. Vulnerable Elder Protection Team: initial experience of an emergency department-based interdisciplinary elder abuse program. J Am Geriatr Soc 2022;70(11):3260–72.

96. Maguire S, Moynihan S, Mann M, et al. A systematic review of the features that indicate intentional scalds in children. Burns 2008;34(8):1072–81.

97. Maguire S, Pickerd N, Farewell D, et al. Which clinical features distinguish inflicted from non-inflicted brain injury? A systematic review. Arch Dis Child 2009;94(11):860–7.

98. Pierce MC, Kaczor K, Aldridge S, et al. Bruising characteristics discriminating physical child abuse from accidental trauma. Pediatrics 2010;125(1):67–74.

99. Sugar NF, Taylor JA, Feldman KW. Bruises in infants and toddlers: those who don't cruise rarely bruise. Puget Sound Pediatric Research Network. Arch Pediatr Adolesc Med 1999;153(4):399–403.
100. Collins KA, Presnell SE. Elder neglect and the pathophysiology of aging. Am J Forensic Med Pathol 2007;28(2):157–62.
101. Collins KA, Sellars K. Vertebral artery laceration mimicking elder abuse. Am J Forensic Med Pathol 2005;26(2):150–4.
102. Rosenblatt DE, Cho KH, Durance PW. Reporting mistreatment of older adults: the role of physicians. J Am Geriatr Soc 1996;44(1):65–70.
103. Kayser J, Morrow-Howell N, Rosen TE, et al. Research priorities for elder abuse screening and intervention: a Geriatric Emergency Care Applied Research (GEAR) network scoping review and consensus statement. J Elder Abuse Negl 2021;33(2):123–44.
104. Rosen T, Stern ME, Elman A, et al. Identifying and initiating intervention for elder abuse and neglect in the emergency department. Clin Geriatr Med 2018;34(3):435–51.
105. Ernst JS, Maschi T. Trauma-informed care and elder abuse: a synergistic alliance. J Elder Abuse Negl 2018;30(5):354–67.
106. Ramsey-Klawsnik H, Miller E. Polyvictimization in later life: trauma-informed best practices. J Elder Abuse Negl 2017;29(5):339–50.

Best Practices in End of Life and Palliative Care in the Emergency Department

Thidathit Prachanukool, MD[a,b,*], Naomi George, MD, MPH[c],
Jason Bowman, MD[b,d], Kaori Ito, MD, PhD, FCCM[e],
Kei Ouchi, MD, MPH[b,d]

KEYWORDS

- Palliative care • Emergency medicine • End-of-life care • Emergency department

KEY POINTS

- Early integration of palliative care at the time of emergency department (ED) visits is important in establishing the comprehensive goals of the entire treatment.
- Primary palliative care is the term for the basic palliative care skills that can be provided in any setting of care, including emergency care, thereby improving the quality of care for overall patients.
- "Serious illness communication skills" are patient-centered communication skills that foster mutual understanding between seriously ill patients and their clinicians.

INTRODUCTION

Three-quarters of patients over the age of 65 visit the ED in the last six months of life.[1,2] Approximately 20% of hospice residents have emergency department (ED) visits.[3] These patients must decide whether to receive emergency care that prioritizes life support, which may not achieve their desired outcomes and might even be futile.[1] The patients in these end-of-life stages could benefit from early palliative care or

[a] Department of Emergency Medicine, Faculty of Medicine, Ramathibodi Hospital, Mahidol University, 270 Rama VI Road, Ratchathewi, Bangkok, 10400, Thailand; [b] Department of Emergency Medicine, Harvard Medical School, Brigham and Women's Hospital, 75 Francis Street, Neville House, Boston, MA 02115, USA; [c] Division of Critical Care Medicine, Department of Emergency Medicine, University of New Mexico School of Medicine, 700 Camino de Salud, Albuquerque, NM 87131, USA; [d] Department of Psychosocial Oncology and Palliative Medicine, Dana Farber Cancer Institute, 75 Francis Street, Neville House, Boston, MA 02115, USA; [e] Department of Emergency Medicine, Division of Acute Care Surgery, Teikyo University School of Medicine, 2-11-1, Kaga, Itabashi-ku, Tokyo 173-8606, Japan
* Corresponding author.
E-mail address: thidathit.pra@mahidol.ac.th

Clin Geriatr Med 39 (2023) 575–597
https://doi.org/10.1016/j.cger.2023.05.011
0749-0690/23/© 2023 Elsevier Inc. All rights reserved.

geriatric.theclinics.com

hospice consultation before they present to the ED. Early integration of palliative care at the time of ED visits is important in determining the goals of treatment.[4–6] In this article, we summarize the current evidence and knowledge about palliative care that is useful in actual clinical practice in the ED, including assessing of palliative care needs in the ED, communicating difficult news, suffering in the last days of life, palliating pain and dyspnea management, caring for hospice patients, and quality metrics for palliative care in the ED.

Palliative care is an interdisciplinary approach encompassing physical, emotional, spiritual, and socioeconomic aspects focused on minimizing suffering for those with serious illness and their loved ones, while simultaneously promoting the best possible quality of life.[7] Two forms of palliative care delivery are commonly recognized: primary palliative care and specialty palliative care.[8] Primary palliative care is the term for the basic palliative care skills that can be provided in any setting of care, including emergency care, thereby improving the quality of care for overall patients. Primary palliative care, which addresses suffering or distress as well as providing support and shared medical decision-making, helps patients establish their goals and values for treatment and outcomes. [8–12]

ASSESSING OF PALLIATIVE CARE NEEDS IN THE EMERGENCY DEPARTMENT

In the ED, assessing for unmet palliative care needs and addressing those needs with either primary palliative care interventions or referral to specialty palliative care can positively impact the lives of patients with serious illness.[13–18] In terms of screening for palliative care needs, 3 ED palliative care screening tools have undergone more rigorous study and focused on identifying ED patients at high risk of poor outcomes: The "Surprise Question," "The Palliative Care and Rapid Emergency Screening (P-CaRES) Tool," and "The Screening for Palliative Needs in the Emergency Department (SPEED) Instrument."[14,19–21] The latter 2 also assess for unaddressed palliative symptoms, such as spiritual distress.[19–21] Most ED-palliative care screening tools are modestly good at predicting mortality, a proxy outcome for unmet palliative care needs,[14] and improve accurate and prompt referral to palliative care consultation.[22–24] Ultimately, the ideal screening tool for palliative care needs will require additional investigation and may depend on hospital-specific factors, such as the patient mix and availability of palliative care consultation. In-depth palliative symptom assessment is less specifically developed or tested in the ED.[21] Comprehensive palliative symptom assessments require time and are not well suited to ED practice.[25] Even though patients with serious illnesses are often dealing with more than one burdensome symptom, using some sort of symptom assessment tool is preferable.[26] One reasonable strategy for symptom assessment is to include questions about each symptom's dimensions (eg, timing, triggers, severity) as well as their meaning (eg, "how does this symptom affect your life?"). Developing an assessment strategy that incorporates psychosocial, spiritual/existential, and caregiver symptom questions is also critical.[27]

Finally, the prognosis for serious illness varies by disease and person, yet the dominant patterns of trajectories have been recognized (**Fig. 1**). Commonly used palliative care assessments focus on "performance status" and can be a helpful tool in developing a global sense of prognosis and trajectory in a patient with terminal disease.[28] In the ED, prognostication is useful to estimate life expectancy, anticipate health deterioration, and prepare for anticipatory symptoms. The prognostication is also helpful in navigating treatment decisions by weighing the risks and benefits.[29] Sharing prognostic information hastily and then shared decision-making requires key steps in high-quality communication.[30,31]

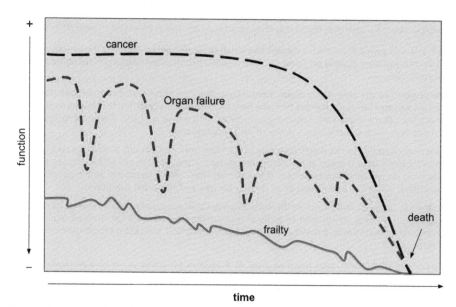

Fig. 1. Common trajectories in serious illness. (*Adapted from* Lunney JR, Lynn J, Foley DJ, Lipson S, Guralnik JM. Patterns of Functional Decline at the End of Life. *JAMA*.2003;289(18):2387–2392. https://doi.org/10.1001/jama.289.18.2387.)

COMMUNICATING DIFFICULT NEWS

The patient-centered communication skills to foster mutual understanding between seriously ill patients and their clinicians are known as "serious illness communication skills." Thoughtful incorporation of serious illness communication skills will allow emergency clinicians to provide acute care most consistent with patients' values and preferences.

Breaking Bad News

As in **Box 1**, an example of a case highlights the importance of serious illness communication skills. These disclosures of unanticipated, bad news are difficult for seriously ill patients and emergency clinicians for the following reasons.[6]

1. Patients are not expecting to hear bad news
2. No existing long-term relationships exist between the patient and emergency clinicians
3. Prognostic uncertainty exists in the new diagnosis or new changes in illness trajectories presenting in the ED (eg, patients may require additional tests).

To overcome these barriers, best practices exist to deliver this bad news.[31,32] The essential elements of delivering bad news for emergency clinicians and why they are essential are shown in **Table 1**. These steps would allow emergency clinicians to deliver the bad news in a patient-centered approach to facilitate patients' understanding of the situation. More importantly, these steps allow emergency clinicians to build a therapeutic alliance with the patients (eg, explicitly let patients know that emergency clinicians are committed to delivering the best care possible along with the patients).

Discussing Treatment Goals Based on the Patient's Values and Preferences

As in **Box 2**, an example of a case continues. Emergency clinicians inherently understand the importance of exploring patients' values and preferences for end-of-life

Box 1
An example of a case that highlights the importance of serious illness communication skills

Mr. B is a 65 year old man with stage 3 non-small cell lung cancer, Chronic Obstructive Pulmonary Disease (COPD) on home O2, and recently hospitalized/discharged home for COPD exacerbation.

He presents to the emergency department (ED) with a new chest and abdominal pain for the last 3 days after being discharged from the hospital. The patient describes the insidious onset of sharp pain that's worse with breathing, associated with a mild cough and worsening dyspnea on exertion, with radiation pain down to his epigastric area.

Oncology history: Per the most recent oncology team note, the patient is on a clinical trial for immunomodulator therapy and is doing well so far for the last 8 months. The oncologist is planning on the third-line treatment if he ever fails the current treatment as the patient's functional status has been quite good despite his age and comorbid conditions.

In the ED, patient's vitals were stable with unremarkable examination other than mild end-expiratory wheezes, which seemed to be at his baseline. The ED work-up revealed segmental pulmonary embolisms and new hepatic mass likely metastatic indicating progression of his cancer.

Data from [Kei Ouchi, MD] [Prachanukool T, Aaronson EL, Lakin JR, et al. Communication Training and Code Status Conversation Patterns Reported by Emergency Clinicians. *J Pain Symptom Manage.* 2023;65(1):58-65. https://doi.org/10.1016/j.jpainsymman.2022.10.006].

Table 1
The essential elements of delivering bad news for emergency physicians

Steps	Examples	Why Important?
Set up	Sit down, private settings, avoid interruptions, involve loved ones	Small steps can maximize the delivery of the bad news in the most patient-centered approach.
Perception	Ask what they heard already: "What have you heard about todays' test?"	Understanding patient's perceptions and expectations can allow emergency physicians to anticipate the prognostic awareness.
Invitation	Obtain permission to talk about the news: "Would it be ok if I share bad news?"	When patients are asked for permission, they perceive a sense of control in uncontrollable situations in the ED.
Knowledge	Disclose the news clearly: "The CT scan showed blood clots and a new cancer in the liver – I am worried that the cancer is getting worse."	Avoid jargon like pulmonary embolism, metastatic disease, etc. Clear headlines: short messages and their overall implications for the patient
Emotion	Respond to patient's emotional response: "This is disappointing and overwhelming."	Without acknowledging and empathizing with patients' emotions, patients cannot process the information being communicated.
Summary	Summarize and discuss next steps: "The key things that I want you to know are"	Next steps after

Data from Kei Ouchi, MD.

Box 2
An example of a continuing case that highlights the discussing treatment goals based on patient's value and preferences for emergency clinicians

Case continue
  After delivering the bad news, the emergency physician placed the inpatient bed request. When handing off the patient care to the inpatient team, the inpatient clinician asked, "What the goals of care for this patient?" Knowing that no emergent decisions are necessary for this patient, the emergency physician decided to start exploring this patient's goals of care while he is clinically stable.

Data from Kei Ouchi, MD.

---

care. The key time window to ask about these values and preferences is while patients are relatively clinically stable.[33] However, when the patients are critically ill, it is often difficult to take the time to explore patients' values and preferences due to a lack of time.[34] Therefore, we have explained exactly how to do this in clinically unstable patients.[35] The highlight of how to ask about patients' values and preferences and how these values and preferences should be applied to our clinical recommendations for care, as shown in **Table 2**. Experts in palliative care recommend asking patients with serious illnesses about their baseline function and their values/preferences for end-of-life care. Many of these questions have been tested rigorously in patients and validation during clinical trials.

Applying Patients' Stated Values/Preferences for End-of-Life Care to Make Clinical Recommendations

To make an empathic and goal-concordant recommendation for end-of-life care, it is critically important to integrate patients' values and preferences, clinical information, and baseline physical function. Ask yourself, "In the best-case scenario, would this patient be able to achieve the minimal quality of life worth living for [him] after intubation/ICU stay?" If this answer is a clear "no" or likely outcome would be considered "worse than death" for the patient, emergency clinicians can confidently make a

---

Table 2
The clinical recommendations on applied approaches to asking patients' values and preferences for emergency clinicians

Step	How to Ask
Baseline function	To decide which treatments might help [his] the most, I need to know more about [his]: What type of activities was [he] doing day to day before this illness?
Values *Use question(s) as appropriate*	• Has [he] expressed wishes about the type of medical care [he] would or wouldn't want? • How might [he] feel if treatments today led to: Inability to return to [his] favorite activities? Inability to care for [himself] as much as [he] does? • What abilities are so crucial that [he] wouldn't consider life worth living if [he] lost them? • How much would [he] be willing to go through for the possibility of more time? • Are there states [he] would consider worse than dying?

Data from Kei Ouchi, MD.

recommendation to focus the treatment on the patient's comfort. If the answer is unclear (eg, the surrogate may not know the minimal quality of life that the patient would consider acceptable to live) or likely outcome would be an acceptable quality of life worth living for, emergency clinicians can make a recommendation to focus the treatment on recovering from the illness (**Fig. 2**). Emphasize what you will do (eg, focus on ensuring the patient's comfort). Consider explaining why you would not recommend certain therapies in the context of the baseline function and values. The introduction of a time-limited trial may also be helpful.[36,37]

SUFFERING IN THE LAST DAYS OF LIFE

Patients at the end of life often experience new or worsen physical and/or psychosocial suffering that may result in their presenting to the ED. The emergency clinicians are able to rapidly assess for suffering, simultaneously work up potential reversible etiologies, initiate evidence-based treatment, and, when indicated, seek expert support from subspecialty teams like palliative care. The 2 most common symptoms are pain and dyspnea, which have more detailed guidance in the subsequent sections. The additional symptoms that frequently cause suffering at the end of life (nausea/vomiting, constipation, depression, anxiety, and delirium) are included in **Table 3** for brief guidance on assessment and management.

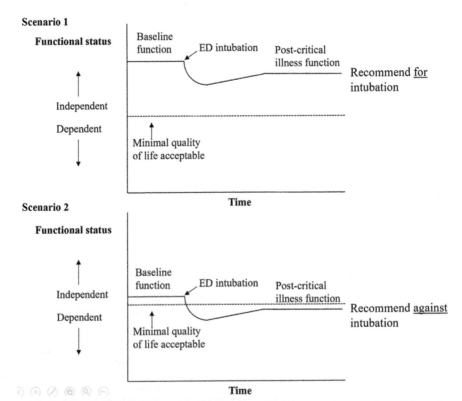

Fig. 2. Recommendation based on quality of life acceptable to patients. (*Adapted from* Ouchi K, Lawton AJ, Bowman J, Bernacki R, George N. Managing Code Status Conversations for Seriously Ill Older Adults in Respiratory Failure. Ann Emerg Med. 2020 12; 76(6):751-756. PMID: 32747084; PMCID: PMC8219473.)

Table 3
Initial pharmacologic management for symptoms in end-of-life emergency department patients

Medication	Detail
Nausea and vomiting	
Ondansetron (serotonin-receptor antagonist)	4–8 mg PO/IV every 8 h. Common "first-line" antiemetic that is generally well tolerated. Also preferred in patients with Parkinson's, Lewy body dementia, or restless leg syndrome as it does not affect dopamine. Constipation is a common side effect.
Metoclopramide and prochlorperazine (dopamine-2-receptor antagonists)	5–10 mg PO/IV every 8 h. Older antiemetics that are still often used for nausea as well as headache. Metoclopramide has a promotility component, so it can be helpful in gastric emptying disorders or constipation, but should be avoided in bowel obstructions. Avoid in patients with Parkinson's, Lewy body dementia, or restless leg syndrome. Acute motor symptoms like dystonic reactions are possible.
Olanzapine (dopamine-2-receptor antagonist)	2.5–5 mg PO/IV every 6–8 h. A newer dopamine antagonist. Generally, well tolerated. Also useful in treating delirium, anxiety, insomnia, and cachexia.
Steroids, anti-histamines, antihistamines and anticholinergics, cannabinoids, etc.	Generally, avoid in the ED unless recommended by a specialist.
Nonpharmacologic	Ginger and mint products can be helpful, as can sniffing isopropyl alcohol swabs.
Constipation	
Sennosides	1–2 tabs (8.6–17.2 mg) once or twice daily. Intestinal stimulant.
Polyethylene glycol	1–2 tablespoons (17–34 g) once or twice daily. Intestinal stimulant.
Docusate	Generally, not helpful as monotherapy. Stool softener. Sometimes used in conjunction with a promotility agent like sennosides.
Bisacodyl enema	Generally dosed once daily. Intestinal stimulant.
Warm tap water and milk of molasses enemas	Can be given up to every 2 h. Work by causing rectal distention and reflex defecation.
Depression and anxiety	
SSRIs, SNRIs, TCAs	Traditional mainstay of depression pharmacotherapy. Generally peak effect takes weeks. Not typically started in the ED. However, may be recommended by palliative and/or psychiatry specialists who see your patients.

(continued on next page)

Table 3
(continued)

Medication	Detail
Mirtazapine	Sometimes used for depression, and also can be helpful for insomnia, nausea, or anorexia. Peak effect shorter than SSRIs, SNRIs, and TCAs, but still not typically started in ED.
Methylphenidate or dextroamphetamine	Stimulants are used to treat depression in patients at the end of life with short (<4 wk) prognosis. Rapid onset. Talk to your palliative and/or psychiatry specialists for guidance.
Olanzapine (dopamine-2-receptor antagonist)	2.5–5 mg PO/IV every 6–8 h. Newer dopamine antagonist. Generally, well tolerated. Also useful in treating delirium, nausea/vomiting, insomnia, and cachexia.
Lorazepam (GABA receptor antagonist)	0.5–1 mg PO/IV every 6–8 h. Rapid onset for relief of anxiety in the ED, but can be deliriogenic. Would generally not prescribe for use at home unless recommended by a palliative care or psychiatry specialist. Higher doses are often needed at end of life.

Delirium
Remember that the first step in treating delirium should be identifying and treating reversible causes. The following are medications that can help improve patients' symptoms and safety.

Medication	Detail
Haloperidol	0.5–1 mg PO/IV/IM, titrating by 2–5 mg every 1 h until effective dose is found. Recommended daily max 100 mg.
Olanzapine	2.5–5 mg PO/IV every 6–8 h. A newer dopamine antagonist. Generally, well tolerated. Also useful in treating, nausea/vomiting, anxiety, insomnia, and cachexia.
Quetiapine	25–50 mg PO once or twice daily. Agent of choice in delirious patients with Parkinson's disease or Lewy body dementia who can take PO.
Thorazine	25–50 mg PO/IV, titration by 25–50 mg every 1 h until effective dose is found. Recommended daily max 2000 mg.
Lorazepam	Generally avoided as they can worsen delirium, though in delirious patients with Parkinson's disease or Lewy body dementia who can't take PO they're sometimes used. Patients with "terminal delirium" can consider combining them with another medication like haloperidol. In this case, start with 0.5–1 mg IV/IM, titrating by 1–2 mg every 1 h until effective dose is found.

Abbreviations: ED, emergency department; IV, intravenous; IM, intramuscular; PO, per oral; SNRIs, serotonin and norepinephrine reuptake inhibitors; SQ, subcutaneous; SSRIs, selective serotonin reuptake inhibitors; TCAs, tricyclic antidepressants.
Data from Jason Bowman, MD.

Nausea and/or vomiting occur in many patients nearing or at the end of life, with reported prevalence ranging from 16% to 68% depending on disease process.[38] Some common reasons for nausea and vomiting include advanced disease, medication effect, infection, bowel obstruction, constipation, intracranial processes, metabolic derangements, or psychosocial distress.[39] In addition to the direct suffering, unmitigated nausea/vomiting can also impact patients' ability to take other oral medications and intake for hydration, sustenance, or pleasure.

Constipation is reported by up to 90% of seriously ill patients and can significantly impact their quality of life.[40] The cause is often multifactorial. When assessing constipation, it is important to inquire about patients' baseline bowel function. Although textbooks suggest a "normal" bowel movement every 1 to 2 days, the reality is that many patients have their own comfortable baseline prior to or earlier in their serious illness. The patients produce stool even if they have little or no oral intake, as an estimated 50% of stool is made up of bowel shedding and other body waste.

Seriously ill patients frequently report depression and/or anxiety as they near the end of life, with published rates for each around 25% to 50%.[41] Although emergency clinicians likely are not initiating or adjusting long-acting medications for these symptoms or providing nonpharmacologic treatment, they can still be the first to explore what the patients are actually experiencing as well as the potential exacerbating triggers (eg, unmitigated physical symptoms, caregivers/social/spiritual distress).

Emergency clinicians frequently encounter patients with delirium, but rates of both hyper- and hypoactive delirium are up to 88% in patients nearing the end of life.[42] Screening can be done using a standardized tool such as the Confusion Assessment Method (CAM). As in all cases of delirium, emergency clinicians should first attempt to identify reversible causes such as pain or other unmitigated symptoms, sleep–wake disruption, and infection.

PALLIATING PAIN MANAGEMENT

Pain is the most common reason for adult patients to present to an ED and is particularly common in patients presenting near or at the end of life. Pain is a complex phenomenon, experienced differently by each patient, and made up of physical, psychological, social, and spiritual components. Commonly used classifications of mechanical/physical pain are (1) nociceptive (such as pressure from a growing tumor), (2) inflammatory (such as from a burn or other traumatic injury), (3) neuropathic (such as in diabetic neuropathy or nerve impingement from tumor or trauma), (4) visceral (such as in Gastrointestinal malignancies, infectious colitis). Psychological, social, and/or spiritual suffering can exacerbate physical pain, or directly cause the perception of pain themselves.[43]

Emergency clinicians can begin a focused assessment of pain in the ED using a tool like OPQRST (**Table 4**) and also ask patients exactly how they have been taking those medications and what effects or adverse effects they have noticed.[44] The emergency clinician should rapidly conduct any indicated work-up for the pain while simultaneously initiating multimodal treatment. Some common options for ED management of pain are described in **Table 5**.[45,46] In addition to traditional options such as oral, topical, intravenous, intramuscular medications, local injections, and nerve blocks are now increasingly performed in the ED. Emergency clinicians can also find support in managing challenging pain from a variety of subspecialty colleagues, including palliative care, acute or chronic pain teams, physical therapy, psychiatry/social work, and

Table 4	
The focused emergency department assessment of pain can begin using a tool like OPQRST	
OPQRST Tool	Detail
1. Onset	What were they doing when it started and how did it start
2. Provocation/palliation	What makes it better or worse
3. Quality	How would they describe (eg, cramping, stabbing, burning, electric shock, pressure)
4. Region/radiation	Where do they feel it and does it move elsewhere
5. Severity	On a scale of 1–10, or mild/moderate/severe
6. Time	When did the pain start and is it constant or intermittent. If the patient has chronic pain, it is also important to assess if their current pain is similar or different to their chronic pain and, if the latter then how it is different.

Data from [Friese G. How to use OPQRST as an effective patient assessment tool. EMS1 Online. 2020. Available at: https://www.ems1.com/ems-products/education/articles/how-to-use-opqrst-as-an-effective-patient-assessment-tool-yd2KWgJIBdtd7D5T/. Accessed Jan 2023.]

even potential surgical options to improve comfort and quality of life, if they are within the patient's goals of care.[46]

PALLIATING DYSPNEA MANAGEMENT

Dyspnea is defined as a subjective sensation of an inability to breathe comfortably, which becomes more prevalent and intense in the last weeks of the patient's life.[47–49] Dyspnea crises can occur and require visits to the ED when acute worsening of dyspnea is experienced with heightened psychosocial-spiritual needs and unprepared caregivers who are overwhelmed to respond.[50] Dyspnea response requires comprehensive, patient-centered assessment and treatment involving coordinating interdisciplinary care teams.[50,51] The step-by-step list describes how emergency clinicians are able to provide quality palliative care for seriously ill patient with dyspnea in the ED (**Table 6**).[47–52] A recommended stepwise approach to dyspnea begins with determining potentially reversible causes, followed by using nonpharmacologic (**Table 7**), and then pharmacologic interventions (**Table 8**) to palliate the suffering of dyspnea. The key to care coordination is communication skills in anticipatory planning, not only with the family regarding goals, concerns, and expected outcomes but also with the health care team. Additionally, a checklist and important step approaches for care could be helpful for ED providers. However, dyspnea can be successfully treated by incorporating an interdisciplinary, multimodal plan, including preparation to anticipate dyspnea before its onset, which can assist in early management and avoid a crisis event.

CARING FOR HOSPICE PATIENTS

Hospice provides palliative care to patients at the end of life with an estimated life expectancy of 6 months or less.[53] When a patient presents with worsening symptoms in the ED, emergency clinicians can prognosticate their life expectancy and offer hospice care suggestions to these patients and their caregivers. On the other hand, the patients receiving hospice care were also reported to have visited the ED. The reasons are primarily related to patient or caregiver factors or hospice care service factors, including inadequate symptom relief,[4,54,55] malfunctioning

Table 5
Initial pharmacologic management of pain in seriously ill or end-of-life emergency department patients

Medication	Details
First-line agents to consider	
Acetaminophen/Tylenol	Excellent, often underutilized and underdosed agent, especially in combination with an NSAID. Consider 650–975 mg PO or IV every 6–8 h. Daily max ranges from 4 g (young and healthy) to 2 g (elderly with underlying liver disease).
Motrin/Advin/ibuprofen, Aleeve/naproxen, Toradol/ketorolac, etc.	Particularly helpful for inflammatory pain. Available in IV/IM/PO forms. Generally, well tolerated at evidence-based doses (example of Ibuprofen 400–600 mg every 6 h, rather than 800 mg as it is not any more effective but has more side effects). Must weigh risk/benefit in each patient (advanced age, systemic anticoagulation, renal disease, etc.), though one-time dosing in ED is generally lower risk than chronic use.
Topical Voltaren/diclofenac (NSAID) gel, lidocaine patches/cream, and other topical agents	Generally, well tolerated and easy to use. Topical NSAID gel can be very helpful for inflammatory pain (musculoskeletal, superficial tumor like posterior spinal metastases, etc.) and systemic absorption is minimal.
Local injections and nerve blocks	Increasingly used in ED patients for a variety of indications with great effect. When done properly, generally very safe and well tolerated. Some examples include trigger point injections for muscle spasm, local injection for dental pain, fascia iliaca blocks for hip fracture, intercostal nerve blocks for rib fracture, etc.
Opioids	
Short-acting	Numerous PO/IV/SQ agents including morphine, hydromorphone, oxycodone, hydrocodone, oxycodone, fentanyl, etc. Can convert between them using an opiate equianalgesic dosing chart or calculator.
	Typically start with the patient's home dose (or equivalent), or in opioid naive patients a dose based on their age/weight/hepato-renal function. Oral medications' peak effect is ~ 45 min, IV morphine and hydromorphone have peaks ~ 20 min, and IV fentanyl is ~ 2 min.
	If effective relief of pain can continue current dose every 2–3 h, adjust as needed. If partial response, repeat initial dose. If no response to initial dose, increase by 50%–100% and give immediately (eg, morphine 4 mg IV → 6 or 8 mg).
Long-acting	Numerous PO and SQ options including long-acting morphine, hydromorphone, oxycodone, fentanyl, methadone, suboxone, etc. An IV opioid infusion ("drip") is another form of "long-acting" or "basal" analgesia.
	ED clinicians should not start these agents without guidance from a subspecialist (palliative care, etc.) but for patients already on one of them it is important to continue basal opioid analgesia while they are in the ED (either their home agent and dose or something equivalent) in addition to using short-acting medications.

(continued on next page)

Table 5 *(continued)*	
Medication	**Details**
	Of note, it can be helpful to think of opioid-dependent patients like patients who are insulin-dependent. In both cases, the long-acting agent (opioid or insulin) can be reduced if indicated (hypoglycemia or delirium respectively, for example) but generally should NOT be stopped entirely. Involve subspecialty consultants early-on in both cases if concerned.
Opioid infusions ("drips")	Historically usually initiated in the ED for patients at the end of life. However, in many cases an opioid infusion is not necessary and intermittent boluses of short-acting opioids can adequately manage the patient's symptoms. In patients no longer able to take their PO long-acting opioids, an equivalently dosed opioid infusion can be started in their place. For patients nearing or at the end of life who require frequent boluses of short-acting opioids over a span of several hours, adding on an opioid infusion can be helpful. A typical starting dose would be the total bolus/PRN needs, divided by the number of hours gone by, multiplied by ½ (eg, if morphine 16 mg IV (4 mg x 4) was needed in PRNs over 4 h, start the infusion at 16 mg/4 h x ½ = 2 mg/h). Worsening pain should be treated with boluses of short-acting opioids (not reflexively increasing the infusion), and the infusion rate adjusted every few hours based on the patient's needs. (Any changes to the infusion rate require several half-lives to take effect.)
Other adjuvants	
Ketamine	Typical ED starting dose for pain is 0.1–0.3 mg/kg IV. Infusing over 10–15 min instead of rapid push can reduce side effects. Continuous infusions of 0.15–0.2 mg/kg/h can also be used for analgesia, though this is less common in the ED. Ketamine be used independently or as an opioid adjuvant.
Other neuropathic agents	Gabapentin, pregabalin, SSRIs, SNRIs, etc. Not started in the ED but, if able, important to continue in patients already on them.
Medications to avoid	
Codeine and Tramadol	Older opioids, previously marketed as "gentle opioids" or [falsely] as "opioid alternatives". They both have variable and unpredictable metabolism as well as high risk of side effects and potentially life-threatening complications. Tramadol in particular has been linked to increased risk of delirium, seizures, refractory hypoglycemia, and death.
Combination drugs (such as Percocet or Vicodin)	Typically, an opioid combined with low (below recommended) dose acetaminophen. However, patients can combine this with OTC acetaminophen and inadvertently overdose. Better to prescribe optimally dose acetaminophen and (if needed) also an opioid.

Abbreviations: ED, emergency department; IM, intramuscular; IV, intravenous; NSAID, nonsteroidal anti-inflammatory drugs; PO, per oral; PRN, pro re nata; SNRIs, serotonin and norepinephrine reuptake inhibitors; SQ, subcutaneous; SSRIs, selective serotonin reuptake inhibitors.
   Data from Jason Bowman, MD.

Table 6
The step-by-step list describes how emergency clinicians are able to provide quality care for palliative dyspnea management

	Detail
1. The systematic screening can	Facilitated early detection and timely intervention.
2. The measurement for patients' distress and discomfort related to dyspnea	• The 0–10 numeric rating scale to the intensity of dyspnea is the most valid, reliable, and widely used measurement for patients' subjective distress and discomfort. • The behavioral approach observed for respiratory distress signs is an option for such a crisis, terminal dyspnea, or patients unable to communicate. The Respiratory Distress Observation Scale (RDOS) consists of 8 variables that are possible to use in the ED but require more studies. • Whenever possible, a comprehensive assessment should be done to determine the severity of dyspnea, potential causes, concomitant symptoms, functional and emotional impacts. • An assessment of family caregiver coping, needs, care participation, and home resources will support and incorporate them into the health care team. Psychoeducational interventions should be provided to caregivers.
3. The treatment for reversible causes and disease-modifying treatments (eg, diuretics, corticosteroids)	Optimized and aligned with patient preferences, goals of care, prognosis, and overall health status. The time-limited trial interventions might be particularly helpful for patients who have uncertain goals of care prior to intubation.
4. A recommended stepwise approach to palliate the suffering of dyspnea	1. Begins with determining potentially reversible causes 2. Using nonpharmacologic (see **Table 7**) 3. Pharmacologic interventions (see **Table 8**)
5. The referral of patients with refractory dyspnea, despite receiving appropriate treatments, to a palliative care specialist	Along with treating the patient's suffering, the goals of care discussion can be facilitated to the patient and their families.
6. Reassessment and adjustment of interventions	Used the same assessment tool for adjustment of dyspnea palliation until the patient's suffering from dyspnea was relieved.

Data from [Weissman DE. Dyspnea at End-of-Life. Palliative Care Network of Wisconsin. 2015. Available at: www.mypcnow.org/fast-fact/dyspnea-at-end-of-life/. Accessed March 2023.] [Ahmed A, Graber MA. Approach to the adult with dyspnea in the emergency department. UpToDate 2022. Available at: https://www.uptodate.com/contents/approach-to-the-adult-with-dyspnea-in-the-emergency-department. Accessed March 2023.] [Hui D, Bohlke K, Bao T, et al. Management of Dyspnea in Advanced Cancer: ASCO Guideline. *J Clin Oncol.* 2021;39(12):1389-1411. https://doi.org/10.1200/JCO.20.03465] [Mularski RA, Reinke LF, Carrieri-Kohlman V, et al. An official American Thoracic Society workshop report: assessment and palliative management of dyspnea crisis. *Ann Am Thorac Soc.* 2013;10(5):S98-S106. https://doi.org/10.1513/AnnalsATS.201306-169ST] [Quest TE, Lamba S. Palliative for adults in the ED: Concepts, presenting complaints, and symptom management. UpToDate 2022. Available at: https://www.uptodate.com/contents/palliative-care-for-adults-in-the-ed-concepts-presenting-complaints-and-symptom-management. Accessed March 2023.]

Table 7
Nonpharmacologic intervention for palliative dyspnea management in the emergency department

Nonpharmacologic Intervention	Detail
Airflow interventions	A fan blowing air toward the patient's face (trigeminal nerve distribution).
Supplemental oxygen	Standard therapy for patients with symptomatic acute hypoxemia on room air (SpO$_2$ ≤ 90%). In other scenarios, a therapeutic trial may be based on symptom relief, which could be helpful in terms of airflow.
Nasal cannula	Patients generally prefer nasal cannula administration to a mask, as is commonly seen in the agitation of imminently dying patients due to the mask. Standard supplemental oxygen is typically delivered through a nasal cannula at 2–6 LPM.
High-flow nasal cannula (HFNC)	• Alleviating dyspnea by increasing oxygenation, improving ventilation with nasopharyngeal washout, stimulation of the trigeminal nerves, augmentation of positive airway pressure, reduction of work of breathing, and heating and humidifying of the inhaled gas • Offered when the patient has severe hypoxemia and the goal is concordant. HFNC could also be used as a time-limited therapeutic trial intervention. • Set the temperature 34°C to 37°C. The flow rate usually starts at 45–50 LPM but may decrease to 20 LPM or increase gradually up to 80 LPM of heated and humidified oxygen, depending on the patient's comfort.
Noninvasive ventilation (NIV)	• Alleviating dyspnea by increased oxygenation, improved ventilation by providing positive end-expiratory pressure, and augmenting respiratory muscles. • More likely to be beneficial for patients with hypercapnic respiratory failure and concordant goals. NIV could also be used as a time-limited therapeutic trial intervention. • The contraindications include facial trauma, a reduced level of consciousness, severe vomiting, the inability to clear secretions, and severe claustrophobia. • The potential adverse events include skin breakdown, muffled communication, claustrophobia, and the inability to eat. Approximately 7% of patients have discontinued due to intolerance.
Positioning	• The head and chest are elevated while in the sitting position, possibly with arms elevated on pillows or a bedside table. • A side-lying position with the "good" lung up or down is helpful for increasing perfusion and/or ventilation.

(continued on next page)

Table 7 (continued)	
Nonpharmacologic Intervention	**Detail**
Bedside breathing exercises	• Abdominal breathing: when inhaling, focus on filling the lungs completely and feel the stomach move outward away. While exhaling, feel the stomach fall slowly and the lungs empty. • Pursed-lip breathing: exhale from the mouth as twice long as inhale. Breathe in through the nose (eg, count 1–2). Pucker the lips and breathe out slowly through the mouth (eg, count 1-2-3-4).
Bedside relaxation techniques	Mindfulness, meditation, guided imagery, and distraction strategies (eg, music, pictures, reading by oneself or a caregiver)
Discontinuing parenteral fluids	In the imminently dying patients

Abbreviations: ED, emergency department; LPM, liter per minutes; SpO_2, peripheral capillary oxygen saturation.

Data from [Weissman DE. Dyspnea at End-of-Life. Palliative Care Network of Wisconsin. 2015. Available at: www.mypcnow.org/fast-fact/dyspnea-at-end-of-life/. Accessed March 2023.] [Ahmed A, Graber MA. Approach to the adult with dyspnea in the emergency department. UpToDate 2022. Available at: https://www.uptodate.com/contents/approach-to-the-adult-with-dyspnea-in-the-emergency-department. Accessed March 2023.] [Hui D, Bohlke K, Bao T, et al. Management of Dyspnea in Advanced Cancer: ASCO Guideline. *J Clin Oncol.* 2021;39(12):1389-1411. https://doi.org/10.1200/JCO.20.03465] [Mularski RA, Reinke LF, Carrieri-Kohlman V, et al. An official American Thoracic Society workshop report: assessment and palliative management of dyspnea crisis. *Ann Am Thorac Soc.* 2013;10(5):S98-S106. https://doi.org/10.1513/AnnalsATS.201306-169ST] [Quest TE, Lamba S. Palliative for adults in the ED: Concepts, presenting complaints, and symptom management. UpToDate 2022. Available at: https://www.uptodate.com/contents/palliative-care-for-adults-in-the-ed-concepts-presenting-complaints-and-symptom-management. Accessed March 2023.]

medical equipment, stress, fear, and difficulty coping with a dying loved one, conflicts regarding the continuation and termination of life-sustaining treatment, conflicts of wills and ideas between the caregiver and patient, caregiver fatigue, and past painful experiences.[56] The important concerns to be addressed in the ED visits are described in **Box 3**.

QUALITY METRICS FOR PALLIATIVE CARE IN THE EMERGENCY DEPARTMENT

The World Health Organization (WHO) defines quality palliative care as quality-of-life care, that is effective, safe, person-centered, timely, equitable, integrated, and efficient.[57] The WHO action keys at the point-of-care level, including the ED, are (1) maintaining and improving the quality of palliative care, (2) collecting and using data to drive improvement efforts, and (3) integrating quality improvement methods into usual practice in the ED.

In 2017, the Palliative Medicine Section of the American College of Emergency Physicians (ACEP) developed a committee to establish consensus on the best practices for providing palliative care in the ED, including metrics and quality measurement in 3 main domains (**Table 9**).[58]

1. Clinical outcome measures focus on assessing the quality of clinical care services provided in the ED for patients with palliative care needs

Table 8
Pharmacologic intervention for palliative dyspnea management in the emergency department

Medication	Detail
The recommended medication for dyspnea palliation	
Systemic opioid	• The primary medication for palliating refractory dyspnea and dyspnea at the end of life, offered when nonpharmacologic interventions are insufficient to relieve the dyspnea • Administered orally, intravenously (IV), subcutaneously, transmurally, and rectally • Monitoring for sedation and confusion. • The doses for acute dyspnea exacerbations are 50% lower than those treating acute pain. • The opioid titration protocol is "low and slow" IV titration of an immediate-release opioid, until the patient reports or displays relief. • The widely studies and recommendations demonstrate significant reductions in dyspnea with the opioid titration protocol administration without evidence of decreased oxygen saturation or respiratory depression.
Opioid for naïve patient	Initial parenteral morphine is 2–5 mg or equivalent, 15–30 min for redosing intervals. Initial oral morphine is 5–15 mg and 60 min for redosing intervals.
Opioid for opioid tolerant patient	A breakthrough dose equivalent to 10%–20% of the previous 24-h opioid dose use (morphine equivalent daily dose: MEDD).
Hydromorphone	Initial IV/subcutaneous dose of 0.2 mg every 5–10 min
Oxycodone	Initial 5 mg orally every 1 h
Benzodiazepine	• The adjunctive addition to the opioid regimen, offered to the patients with anxiety or distress related to dyspnea despite intervention trials • Short-acting benzodiazepines such as midazolam, 2–5 mg every 4 h, may be helpful. In other scenarios, the risk of respiratory depression may further increase due to the benzodiazepines' adverse effects.
Anticholinergic therapy to dry the death rattle (secretions at the end of life)	
Glycopyrrolate	Initial 0.2 mg intravenous bolus every 4–6 h or continuous intravenous/subcutaneous 0.6–1.2 mg/d
Hyoscine BUTYLbromide	Initial 20 mg intravenous bolus every 4–6 h or continuous intravenous/subcutaneous 20–60 mg/d
Hyoscine HYDRObromide	Initial 0.4 mg IV bolus every 4–8 h or continuous intravenous/subcutaneous 1.2–1.6 mg/d. Risk for delirium and agitation

Abbreviations: ED, emergency department; MEDD, morphine equivalent daily dose.

Data from [Weissman DE. Dyspnea at End-of-Life. Palliative Care Network of Wisconsin. 2015. Available at: www.mypcnow.org/fast-fact/dyspnea-at-end-of-life/. Accessed March 2023.] [Ahmed A, Graber MA. Approach to the adult with dyspnea in the emergency department. UpToDate 2022. Available at: https://www.uptodate.com/contents/approach-to-the-adult-with-dyspnea-in-the-emergency-department. Accessed March 2023.] [Hui D, Bohlke K, Bao T, et al. Management of Dyspnea in Advanced Cancer: ASCO Guideline. *J Clin Oncol.* 2021;39(12):1389-1411. https://doi.org/10.1200/JCO.20.03465] [Mularski RA, Reinke LF, Carrieri-Kohlman V, et al. An official American Thoracic Society workshop report: assessment and palliative management of dyspnea crisis. *Ann Am Thorac Soc.* 2013;10(5):S98-S106. https://doi.org/10.1513/AnnalsATS.201306-169ST] [Quest TE, Lamba S. Palliative for adults in the ED: Concepts, presenting complaints, and symptom management. UpToDate 2022. Available at: https://www.uptodate.com/contents/palliative-care-for-adults-in-the-ed-concepts-presenting-complaints-and-symptom-management. Accessed March 2023.]

Box 3

The important information to be addressed in emergency department visits of the patients from the hospice care

The information to be addressed in ED visits of the patients from the hospice care

1. Identify hospice care staff.

2. Identify the trigger for the ED visit.

3. Relieve symptoms of distress.

4. When a medical condition is critical, quick decisions need to be made while providing life-sustaining treatment.
   - Identify the legal decision-maker and confirm the contents of the advance directive.
   - Discuss goals of a care promptly.
   - Provide recommendations.
   - If the patient is already dying, consider cultural/spiritual requests.
   - Diagnostic testing
   - Should be somewhat limited and withheld until discussed with hospice care personnel.
   - Testing should be based on goals of care tailored to the patient's situation.
   - Generally, the first step is to perform a less painful and less invasive procedure for the purpose of clarifying a reversible condition or prognosis.
   - Treatment
   - Engage in treatment based on goals of care tailored to the patient's situation.

5. Determine the disposition.
   - Discuss with hospice care services personnel to develop a plan that meets the patient's goals of care.
   - It may be better to return them home or admit them to an inpatient hospice facility rather than admit them to a hospital.
   - If the patient wants to stay home and is having difficulty relieving symptoms, assistance from 24 hour hospice care services may be coordinated.
   - If hospitalization is required, referral for inpatient hospice care services.

Data from [DeSandra PL, Quest, TE. Palliative Aspects of Emergency Care, First Edition. Oxford University Press; 2013.]

---

2. Operational sustainability measures focus on processes, including patient flow, consultation, disposition, readmissions, and resource utilization
3. Patient satisfaction measures assess the patients, family members, and caregivers' perceptions of the quality of care provided in the ED.

A combination of process indicators and outcome indicators is frequently used to measure the quality of palliative care.[57] One successful strategy for measures in the ED is to make them actionable, easy to collect, and compatible with existing ED processes and staff roles.[58,59] Therefore, **Table 9** is a brief list of widely applied and time-based categories that were ranged along the continuum of the patient's flow in the ED, extending to 72 hours after admission.[16,58] The specific patient measurements specified as a target population in **Table 9** are valuable to the ED for identifying the population of interest, allocating appropriate institutional resources (eg, the number of palliative care consultations or hospice referrals from the ED), and also providing insightful feedback for an organization's strategic investment, including financial impact and outcomes (eg, the elderly patients in the ED transferring from long-term care facilities, the number of ventilators used after the palliative care consultation in the ED).[58] Moreover, the palliative care educational initiatives for ED providers (eg, the providers' attitudes or practices after the trainings) are beneficial in improving the quality of ED palliative care.[58] Entirely, the metrics should be adjustable for each

Table 9
The quality metrics that can be widely applied at the emergency department

Patient Identification and Assessment for Palliative Care Needs	Management of Palliative Care in ED	Transitions of Care
Clinical outcomes		

• Percentage of ED patients screened positive for palliative care eligibility (total and by using each screening tool)
  1. Surprise question: not surprised if the patient died during this admission
  2. Clinical indicators for example, frequent admission with the same problem
  3. Specific disease indicators
• Percentage of patients with X diagnosis who were screened positive for palliative care eligibility
• Percentage of documented screening for palliative care eligibility in the target population (eg, X diagnosis, transfer from the long-term care facility)
• Percentage of patients measured for psychospiritual social needs
• Percentage of family members screened for caregiver strain
	• Percentage of patients with overall/each distressing symptom assessment documented
	• Time from symptom assessment to delivery of medication for symptom relief
	• Percentage of patients prescribed distressing symptom control medications in ED
	• Percentage of documented health proxy or decision maker in medical records in target population
	• Percentage of patients with do not attempt resuscitation status in target population
	• Percentage with documentation of advance directives/POLST/MOLST in target population
	• Percentage of patients who died within 24/48/72 h of ED admission with documented health proxy or decision maker in medical record
		• Percentage of X intervention after ED palliative care consultation
		• Percentage of deaths in the ICU and/or ED after ED palliative care consultation
		• Percentage of repeat ED visits (and/or readmission to the hospital) within 30 d
		• Percentage discharged to home after ED palliative care consultation
		• Percentage discharged to hospice care after ED palliative care consultation

Operational process		
• Time from ED arrival to completion of palliative care screening • Percentage of personnel who completing the screening tool • Percentage of patients transfer from the long-term care facility	• Percentage of X order sets placed by an ED clinician in target population • Percentage of palliative care order sets used in target population • Percentage of order sets used in ED patients with X condition	• Percentage of ED referrals for palliative care consultation/hospice care • Percentage of patients admitted (total, ICU, non-ICU, palliative care unit) after palliative care consultation

(continued on next page)

Table 9
(continued)

Patient Identification and Assessment for Palliative Care Needs	Management of Palliative Care in ED	Transitions of Care
• Percentage of patients who screened positive for palliative care eligibility and multiple ED visits (or hospitalizations) in X time	• Percentage of intensive care in ED (and/or in this admission) in target population (eg, ventilator use, pressor support)	• Time from consult to response by palliative care team or hospice staff • ED length of stay for patients with palliative care consult (and/or in target population) vs ED length of stay for all patients, all discharged patients, all admitted patients • Hospital length of stay for patients with ED palliative care consultations (and/or in target population) • Percentage of canceled palliative care consultations by admitting clinician • Time from ED request for palliative care/hospice consultation to final disposition
Patient and/or family member satisfaction		
• Satisfaction scores on patients who screened positive for palliative care eligibility	• Percentage of patients and/or family members reporting a high level of shared decision making with ED clinicians (eg, ED clinicians listen carefully, explain things in a way that was easy to understand) • Percentage of patients and/or family members reporting high level of satisfaction in end-of-life care for an ED patient death • Percentage of patients and/or family members highly satisfied with pain or symptom management in the ED	• Percentage of patients and/or family members reporting high level of satisfaction with health care team communication • Percentage of patients and/or family members reporting high level of satisfaction in end-of-life care after palliative care consultation in the ED and a patient's hospital death • Percentage of patients and/or family members reporting excellent coordination of care to the next health care setting from the ED

Abbreviations: ED, emergency department; ICU, intensive care unit; MOLST/POLST, medical/physician's/practitioner's orders for life-sustaining treatment.

Data from [Goett R, Isaacs ED, Chan GK, et al. Quality measures for palliative care in the emergency department. *Acad Emerg Med.* 2022;10.1111/acem.14592. https://doi.org/10.1111/acem.14592] [George N, Phillips E, Zaurova M, Song C, Lamba S, Grudzen C. Palliative Care Screening and Assessment in the Emergency Department: A Systematic Review. *J Pain Symptom Manage.* 2016;51(1):108-19.e2. https://doi.org/10.1016/j.jpainsymman.2015.07.017].

ED setting depending on local capacity, resources, experience, and the availability of relevant tools.[57]

SUMMARY

From triage to ED disposition, best practices in end-of-life and palliative care for seriously ill patients have existed. However, some areas require more exploration and study. The continuous and sustainable enhancement of care for seriously ill patients has impacted the entire patient care process within the ED.

CLINICS CARE POINTS

- The ED is crucial for identifying unmet palliative care needs and timely providing palliative care for seriously ill patients who are rapidly declining. Emergency clinicians should not interpret that seriously ill patients, even those in hospice care, visit the ED requesting aggressive life-prolonging treatment.
- Although clinicians attempt a frank appraisal of the prognosis, special consideration must be given to how and when this information is communicated to patients.
- The patient-centered communication skills that foster mutual understanding between seriously ill patients and their clinicians are known as "serious illness communication skills," which include "best practices to deliver bad news" and "discussing treatment goals based on the patient's values and preferences."
- We provided the brief existing guidance on the assessment and management of several suffering symptoms at the end of life that frequently present in the ED.
- Moving palliative care screening "upstream" to the ED rather than after hospital admission would reduce medical utilization and cost.

DISCLOSURE

Dr Kei Ouchi receives consulting fees from Jolly Good, Inc. (a virtual reality company), which has no relation to this manuscript. Other authors have no conflicts of interest to declare.

REFERENCES

1. George N, Bowman J, Aaronson E, et al. Past, present, and future of palliative care in emergency medicine in the USA. Acute Med Surg 2020;7(1):e497.
2. Smith AK, McCarthy E, Weber E, et al. Half of older Americans seen in emergency department in last month of life; most admitted to hospital, and many die there. Health Aff 2012;31(6):1277–85.
3. Aldridge MD, Epstein AJ, Brody AA, et al. The impact of reported hospice preferred practices on hospital utilization at the end of life. Med Care 2016; 54(7):657–63.
4. Grudzen CR, Richardson LD, Morrison M, et al. Palliative care needs of seriously ill, older adults presenting to the emergency department. Acad Emerg Med 2010; 17(11):1253–7.
5. Samaras N, Chevalley T, Samaras D, et al. Older patients in the emergency department: a review. Ann Emerg Med 2010;56(3):261–9.
6. Smith AK, Fisher J, Schonberg MA, et al. Am I doing the right thing? Provider perspectives on improving palliative care in the emergency department. Ann Emerg Med 2009;54(1):86–93, 93 e81.

7. Sepulveda C, Marlin A, Yoshida T, et al. Palliative care: the World health organization's global perspective. J Pain Symptom Manage 2002;24(2):91–6.

8. Quill TE, Abernethy AP. Generalist plus specialist palliative care–creating a more sustainable model. N Engl J Med 2013;368(13):1173–5.

9. Cherny NI, Fallon MT, Kaasa S, et al, editors. Oxford textbook of palliative medicine. 6th edition. Oxford: Oxford University Press; 2021. https://doi.org/10.1093/med/9780198821328.001.0001. Accessed January 12, 2023.

10. Weissman DE, Meier DE. Identifying patients in need of a palliative care assessment in the hospital setting: a consensus report from the Center to Advance Palliative Care. J Palliat Med 2011;14(1):17–23.

11. Carson SS, Cox CE, Wallenstein S, et al. Effect of palliative care-led meetings for families of patients with chronic critical illness: a Randomized clinical trial. JAMA 2016;316(1):51–62.

12. Schenker Y, Arnold R. The Next Era of palliative care. JAMA 2015;314(15): 1565–6.

13. Glajchen M, Lawson R, Homel P, et al. A rapid two-stage screening protocol for palliative care in the emergency department: a quality improvement initiative. J Pain Symptom Manage 2011;42(5):657–62.

14. Kirkland SW, Yang EH, Garrido Clua M, et al. Screening tools to identify patients with unmet palliative care needs in the emergency department: a systematic review. Acad Emerg Med 2022;29(10):1229–46.

15. George N, Phillips E, Zaurova M, et al. Palliative care screening and assessment in the emergency department: a systematic review. J Pain Symptom Manage 2016;51(1):108–119 e102.

16. Wang DH, Heidt R. Emergency department admission triggers for palliative consultation may Decrease length of stay and costs. J Palliat Med 2021;24(4): 554–60.

17. da Silva Soares D, Nunes CM, Gomes B. Effectiveness of emergency department based palliative care for adults with advanced disease: a systematic review. J Palliat Med 2016;19(6):601–9.

18. Wang DH, Heidt R. Emergency department Embedded palliative care service creates value for health systems. J Palliat Med 2023;26(5):646–52.

19. Ouchi K, Jambaulikar G, George NR, et al. The "surprise question" asked of emergency physicians may predict 12-month mortality among older emergency department patients. J Palliat Med 2018;21(2):236–40.

20. George N, Barrett N, McPeake L, et al. Content validation of a Novel screening tool to identify emergency department patients with significant palliative care needs. Acad Emerg Med 2015;22(7):823–37.

21. Richards CT, Gisondi MA, Chang CH, et al. Palliative care symptom assessment for patients with cancer in the emergency department: validation of the Screen for Palliative and End-of-life care needs in the Emergency Department instrument. J Palliat Med 2011;14(6):757–64.

22. Tripp D, Janis J, Jarrett B, et al. How well does the surprise question predict 1-year mortality for patients admitted with COPD? J Gen Intern Med 2021;36(9): 2656–62.

23. Glick J, Gallo MB, Chelluri J, et al. Utility of the "surprise question" in critically ill emergency department patients. Ann Emerg Med 2018;72:S68.

24. Marshall A, Reuter Q, Powell ES, et al. Emergency department-based palliative interventions. Ann Emerg Med 2017;70:S113–4.

25. Richardson A, Medina J, Brown V, et al. Patients' needs assessment in cancer care: a review of assessment tools. Support Care Cancer 2007;15(10):1125–44.

26. Homsi J, Walsh D, Rivera N, et al. Symptom evaluation in palliative medicine: patient report vs systematic assessment. Support Care Cancer 2006;14(5):444–53.
27. National Coalition for Hospice and Palliative Care. Clinical practice guidelines for quality palliative care. 2018. Available at: https://www.nationalcoalitionhpc.org/wp-content/uploads/2018/10/NCHPC-NCPGuidelines_4thED_web_FINAL.pdf. Accessed November 01, 2019.
28. Ma C, Bandukwala S, Burman D, et al. Interconversion of three measures of performance status: an empirical analysis. Eur J Cancer 2010;46(18):3175–83.
29. Yourman LC, Lee SJ, Schonberg MA, Widera EW, Smith AK. Prognostic indices for older adults: a systematic review. JAMA 2012;307(2):182–92.
30. Mirza RD, Ren M, Agarwal A, et al. Assessing patient perspectives on receiving bad news: a survey of 1337 patients with life-changing Diagnoses. AJOB Empir Bioeth 2019;10(1):36–43.
31. Ptacek JT, Eberhardt TL. Breaking bad news. A review of the literature. JAMA 1996;276(6):496–502.
32. Back A, Arnold RM, Tulsky JA. Mastering communication with seriously ill patients : balancing honesty with empathy and hope. Cambridge England New York: Cambridge University Press; 2009.
33. Ouchi K, George N, Schuur JD, et al. Goals-of-Care Conversations for older adults with serious illness in the emergency department: challenges and opportunities. Ann Emerg Med 2019;74(2):276–84.
34. Prachanukool T, Aaronson EL, Lakin JR, et al. Communication training and Code status conversation patterns reported by emergency clinicians. J Pain Symptom Manage 2023;65(1):58–65.
35. Ouchi K, Lawton AJ, Bowman J, et al. Managing Code status Conversations for seriously ill older adults in Respiratory failure. Ann Emerg Med 2020;76(6):751–6.
36. Quill TE, Holloway R. Time-limited trials near the end of life. JAMA 2011;306(13):1483–4.
37. Scherer JS, Holley JL. The role of time-limited trials in Dialysis decision making in critically ill patients. Clin J Am Soc Nephrol 2016;11(2):344–53.
38. Glare P, Miller J, Nikolova T, et al. Treating nausea and vomiting in palliative care: a review. Clin Interv Aging 2011;6:243–59.
39. Kamell A, Marks S, Hallenbeck J. Nausea and Vomiting: Common Etiologies and Management. Fast Facts - Palliative Care Network of Wisconsin. Sept 2021. Accessed Jan 2023.
40. Dzierzanowski T, Larkin P. Proposed criteria for constipation in palliative care patients. A multicenter cohort study. J Clin Med 2020;10(1).
41. Mossman B, Perry LM, Walsh LE, et al. Anxiety, depression, and end-of-life care utilization in adults with metastatic cancer. Psycho Oncol 2021;30(11):1876–83.
42. Watt CL, Momoli F, Ansari MT, et al. The incidence and prevalence of delirium across palliative care settings: a systematic review. Palliat Med 2019;33(8):865–77.
43. Prabhakar A, Smith TJ. Total Pain. Palliative Care Network of Wisconsin. Mar 2021. Available at: https://www.mypcnow.org/fast-fact/total-pain/. Accessed Jan 2023.
44. Friese G. How to use OPQRST as an effective patient assessment tool. EMS1 Online; 2020. Available at: https://www.ems1.com/ems-products/education/articles/how-to-use-opqrst-as-an-effective-patient-assessment-tool-yd2KWgJlBdtd7D5T/. Accessed January 2023.

45. Kematick B, Suliman I, Hood A, et al. The BWH/DFCI pain management tables and guidelines 2020. Available at: https://pinkbook.dfci.org/assets/docs/pinkBook.pdf. Accessed March 2023.

46. Ellison HB, Lau LA, Cook AC, et al. Surgical palliative care: considerations for career development in surgery and hospice and palliative medicine. American College of Surgeons; 2021.

47. Weissman DE. Dyspnea at End-of-Life. Palliative Care Network of Wisconsin. 2015. Available at: www.mypcnow.org/fast-fact/dyspnea-at-end-of-life/. Accessed March 2023.

48. Ahmed A, Graber MA. Approach to the adult with dyspnea in the emergency department. UpToDate 2022. Available at: https://www.uptodate.com/contents/approach-to-the-adult-with-dyspnea-in-the-emergency-department. Accessed March 2023.

49. Hui D, Bohlke K, Bao T, et al. Management of dyspnea in advanced cancer: ASCO guideline. J Clin Oncol 2021;39(12):1389–411. https://doi.org/10.1200/JCO.20.03465.

50. Mularski RA, Reinke LF, Carrieri-Kohlman V, et al. An official American Thoracic Society workshop report: assessment and palliative management of dyspnea crisis. Ann Am Thorac Soc 2013;10(5):S98–106. https://doi.org/10.1513/AnnalsATS.201306-169ST.

51. Quest TE, Lamba S. Palliative for adults in the ED: Concepts, presenting complaints, and symptom management. UpToDate; 2022. Available at: https://www.uptodate.com/contents/palliative-care-for-adults-in-the-ed-concepts-presenting-complaints-and-symptom-management. Accessed March 2023.

52. Prachanukool T, Kanjana K, Lee RS, et al. Acceptability of the palliative dyspnoea protocol by emergency clinicians [published online ahead of print, 2022 Sep 16]. BMJ Support Palliat Care 2022. https://doi.org/10.1136/spcare-2022-003959. spcare-2022-003959.

53. Lamba S, Quest TE. Hospice care and the emergency department: rules, regulations, and referrals. Ann Emerg Med 2011;57(3):282–90.

54. Desandre PL, Quest TE. Management of cancer-related pain. Emerg Med Clin North Am 2009;27(2):179–94.

55. Barbera L, Taylor C, Dudgeon D. Why do patients with cancer visit the emergency department hunear the end of life? CMAJ (Can Med Assoc J) 2010;182(6):563–8.

56. Bailey CJ, Murphy R, Porock D. Dying cases in emergency places: caring for the dying in emergency departments. Soc Sci Med 2011;73(9):1371–7.

57. World Health Organization. Quality health services and palliative care: practical approaches and resources to support policy, strategy and practice. 2021. Available at: https://www.who.int/publications/i/item/9789240035164. Accessed March 2023.

58. Goett R, Isaacs ED, Chan GK, et al. Quality measures for palliative care in the emergency department. Acad Emerg Med 2023;30(1):53–8.

59. De Roo ML, Leemans K, Claessen SJ, et al. Quality indicators for palliative care: update of a systematic review. J Pain Symptom Manage 2013;46(4):556–72.

Optimizing the Care of Persons Living with Dementia in the Emergency Department

Scott M. Dresden, MD, MS

KEYWORDS

- Dementia • Cognitive dysfunction • Emergency medicine
- Mental status and dementia tests • Potentially inappropriate medication list
- Emergency treatment

KEY POINTS

- Persons living with dementia have unique emergency care needs. Standard emergency department (ED) care can be harmful for persons living with dementia (PLWD).
- Identifying patients who may have cognitive impairment or dementia is feasible in the ED using assessments such as the Abbreviated Mental Test-4 or the Ottawa 3DY.
- Behavioral and psychological symptoms of dementia (BPSD) and delirium are important to identify in the ED. The family confusion assessment method (FAM-CAM) can help identify between BPSD and delirium.
- The Assess Diagnose, Evaluate, Prevent, and Treat (ADEPT) framework can help to manage BPSD and delirium in the ED.
- ED processes such as restoring circadian light, limiting, noise, decreasing ED length of stay, improved communication, working with care partners may have, and enhanced care transitions are important for improving outcomes for PLWD in the ED.

INTRODUCTION

In the United States, the number of adults aged 65 and older with Alzheimer's Disease and related dementias is predicted to increase from 4.7 million in 2010 to 13.8 million in 2050.[1] These persons living with dementia (PLWD) have complex medical and social needs with up to 57% of PLWD experiencing at least one emergency department (ED) visit annually,[2] thereby accounting for 20% of all ED visits by individuals 65 and older.[3]

The author has nothing to disclose.
Department of Emergency Medicine, Northwestern University Feinberg School of Medicine, Center for Healthcare Studies and Outcomes Research, 211 East Ontario Street, Suite 200, Chicago, IL 60611, USA
E-mail address: s-dresden@northwestern.edu
Twitter: @SMDresdenMD (S.M.D.)

Clin Geriatr Med 39 (2023) 599–617
https://doi.org/10.1016/j.cger.2023.06.004
0749-0690/23/© 2023 Elsevier Inc. All rights reserved.

geriatric.theclinics.com

ED care focuses on the rapid evaluation and stabilization of acute conditions which typically does not align with the needs of PLWD.[4–6] For example, PLWD are more likely to be given antipsychotics for behavioral and psychological symptoms of dementia (BPSD) in the ED and be hospitalized than older adults without dementia.[7,8] Though often necessary, hospitalization comes with significant risks including delirium, falls, nosocomial infections, functional decline, and higher healthcare costs.[9–14] Therefore, if possible, alternatives to hospitalization should be explored. Conversely, ED discharge is not without risk for PLWD. Discharged PLWD also often suffer high rates of adverse outcomes including repeat ED visits, delirium, falls, increased unsafe behaviors, declines in physical function, and higher mortality compared to older adults without dementia.[2,15,16] These risks reflect the need for effective care coordination and discharge planning.

One example of the mismatch between emergency care and optimal care for PLWD is the evaluation of patients with "altered mental status." Historically, this catchall term for confusion has combined delirium and dementia into one grouping. Though both are important, common ED clinical entities, there is much less published research on ED care for PLWD compared to delirium.[17,18] Additionally, dementia severity is understudied in the ED. Emergency care needs of a patient with mild dementia who has mild but consistent forgetfulness are likely quite different from the needs of a patient with severe dementia who cannot respond to questions or is totally dependent on help for personal care (**Fig. 1**). However, ED studies evaluating care for PLWD have only identified the presence or absence of dementia.

History

In 2013, the Geriatric Emergency Department Guidelines were produced and endorsed by key stakeholder groups to improve the care of older adults in the ED.[19] Recommended care for PLWD included evaluating older adults for cognitive impairment (CI), enhanced care coordination, and limited use of both sedation and physical restraints.[19,20] However, at the time, research surrounding optimal care practices for PLWD in the ED was lacking.

More recently, the United States National Plan to Address Alzheimer's Disease included multiple recommendations which would impact ED care for PLWD.[21] These recommendations include: credentialing the healthcare workforce to deliver dementia-specific care, including the mandatory education of ED clinicians as a condition of federal payment for services, ensuring that PLWD experience safe and effective transitions between care settings and systems, developing and disseminating evidence-based interventions for PLWD and their caregivers. Additionally, the National Plan includes multiple recommendations aimed at decreased ED use for PLWD.

Definitions

Alzheimer's Disease (AD)– a chronic progressive neurodegenerative disorder characterized by 3 primary groups of symptoms, cognitive dysfunction (memory loss, language difficulty, executive dysfunction), psychiatric symptoms and behavioral disturbances (depression, hallucinations, delusions, agitation), difficulties with performing activities of daily living.[22]

Alzheimer's Disease and Related Dementias (ADRD) – the most common causes of dementia including Alzheimer's disease, frontotemporal dementia, Lewy body dementia, vascular contributions to cognitive impairment and dementia, and mixed-etiology dementias.[23]

Behavioral and Psychological Symptoms of Dementia (BPSD)– are a heterogeneous group of non-cognitive symptoms and behaviors occurring in PLWD. BPSD include

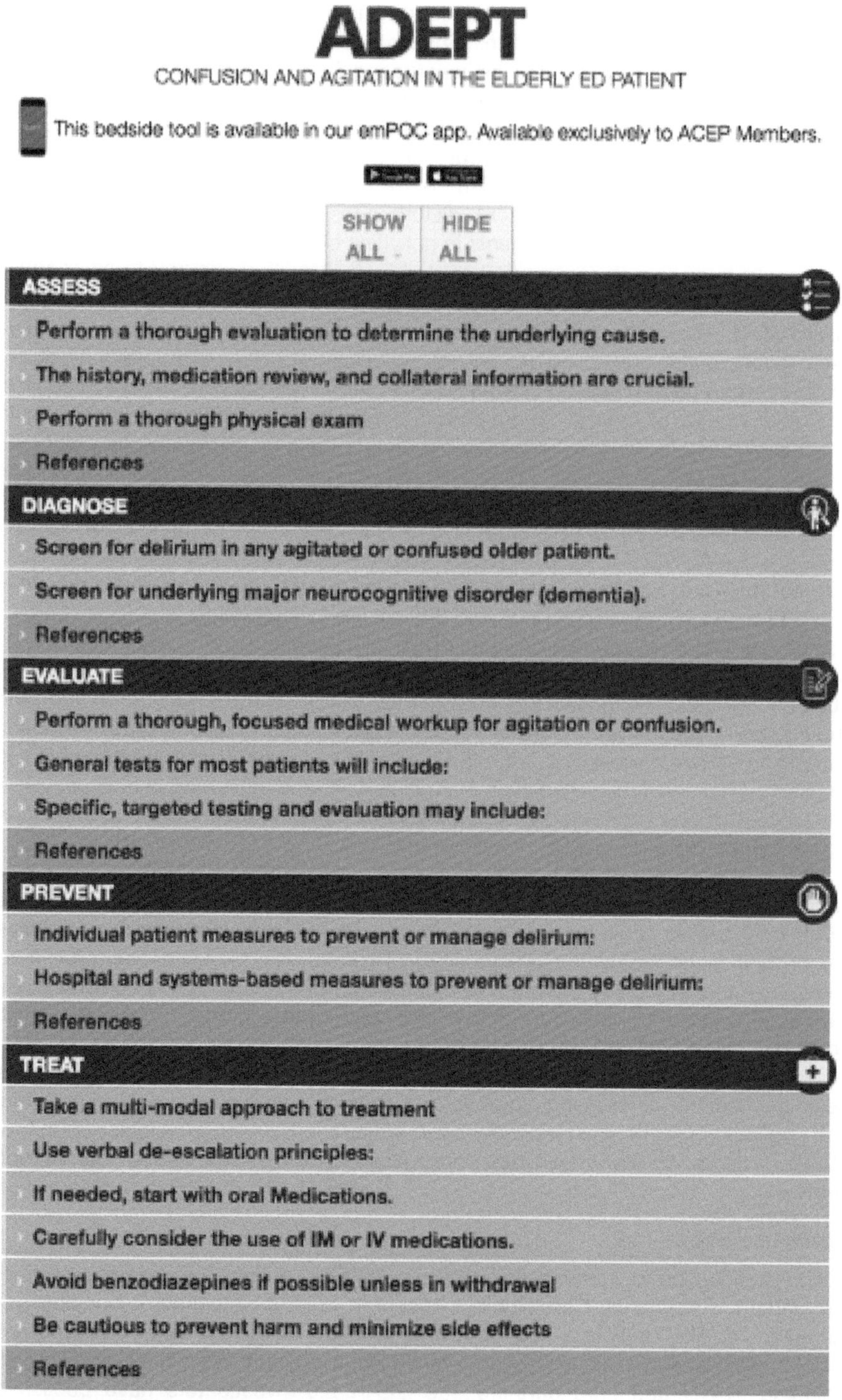

ADEPT

CONFUSION AND AGITATION IN THE ELDERLY ED PATIENT

This bedside tool is available in our emPOC app. Available exclusively to ACEP Members.

| SHOW ALL | HIDE ALL |

ASSESS

Perform a thorough evaluation to determine the underlying cause.

The history, medication review, and collateral information are crucial.

Perform a thorough physical exam

References

DIAGNOSE

Screen for delirium in any agitated or confused older patient.

Screen for underlying major neurocognitive disorder (dementia).

References

EVALUATE

Perform a thorough, focused medical workup for agitation or confusion.

General tests for most patients will include:

Specific, targeted testing and evaluation may include:

References

PREVENT

Individual patient measures to prevent or manage delirium:

Hospital and systems-based measures to prevent or manage delirium:

References

TREAT

Take a multi-modal approach to treatment

Use verbal de-escalation principles:

If needed, start with oral Medications.

Carefully consider the use of IM or IV medications.

Avoid benzodiazepines if possible unless in withdrawal

Be cautious to prevent harm and minimize side effects

References

Fig. 1. The ADEPT tool for managing delirium and agitation.[73] © 2018, American College of Emergency Physicians, Reprinted with Permission.

agitation, aberrant motor behavior, anxiety, elation, irritability, depression, apathy, disinhibition, delusions, hallucinations, and sleep or appetite changes.[24]

Cognitive Impairment (CI) – deficits in neurocognitive domains which can be attributed to either delirium or dementia.[25] Because dementia is not diagnosed during a single encounter, the term cognitive impairment is often used in the ED to refer to global declines in cognition not thought to represent delirium.

Dementia – a clinical syndrome characterized by a cluster of symptoms and signs manifested by difficulties in memory, disturbances in language, psychological and psychiatric changes, and impairments in activities of daily living.[26]

Background

PLWD often initially develop memory impairment, however poor attention, executive dysfunction, behavioral disorders, visual disturbances, sleep disruption, or motor symptoms can be the presenting symptoms. As ADRD progresses, memory declines, and other functions such as language and decision making become more difficult. Eventually, many PLWD are completely reliant on others for assistance with Activities of Daily Living (ADLs) such as eating, dressing, and bathing.[21] PLWD and their care partners endure emotional, physical, and financial stress. Care partners who endure these stressors with PLWD are often unpaid family members or friends who provide most care for PLWD.[27]

In addition to care-giving needs, PLWD often have medical complications which may be related to cognitive impairment, other comorbid conditions such as hypertension or heart disease, or difficulties with ADLs such as dehydration, or aspiration. They are hospitalized more than twice as often as people of the same age who do not have ADRD.[28] However, hospitalization itself comes with significant risks for PLWD, and should be avoided when possible.[9–14] Therefore additional attention to the needs and risks of PLWD is needed in the ED and in the hospital. Common interventions such as dietary restriction, bed alarms, chair alarms, and indwelling urinary catheters are associated with significantly higher rates of delirium and behavioral and psychological symptoms of dementia in the hospital.[29]

Programs such as the Hospital Elder Life Program (HELP) have demonstrated significant improvements in care for elders, including PLWD who are hospitalized.[30] The HELP program involves screening at the time of hospital admission for cognitive impairment, sleep deprivation, immobility, dehydration, and vision or hearing impairment. An interdisciplinary team works closely with primary nurses to address these risk factors with the goal of reducing the incidence of delirium.[31,32] The HELP program has been well studied and has demonstrated reductions in delirium, falls, decline in functional status and decline in cognition.[33] Another similar program has been successful in reducing aggressive behavior, improving cognitive function, and improving functional independence in an inpatient geriatric psychiatric unit for PLWD.[34] However, there have been no published studies of a similar intervention in the ED.

Recommendations

Recommendations for identification and care of PLWD in the ED come primarily from the Geriatric Emergency Care Applied Research (GEAR) Network's Advancing Dementia Care (ADC) initiative, also known as GEAR 2.0 – ADC.[35] After conducting 4 scoping reviews and a consensus conference including multidisciplinary stakeholders including PLWD and care partners, the GEAR 2.0 investigators have published research priorities on detection, communication, ED care practices, and care transitions for PLWD in the ED.[18,36–39]

Identification of patients with cognitive impairment in the emergency department
To better care for PLWD in the ED, first these patients need to be identified. Often, dementia goes unrecognized in the ED which can lead to diagnostic inaccuracy.[40] Additionally, failure to identify and address the complexity of caring for PLWD in the ED may lead to prolonged ED length of stay, increased hospitalization rates, subsequent ED returns, hospital readmissions, and higher mortality.[8,15,41]

Though quick and accurate screens for dementia such as the Abbreviated Mental Test-4 (AMT-4) and Ottawa 3DY (O3DY) have been described for ED use, these screens are not frequently implemented in ED care.[42–46] Of five instruments studied in a systematic review and meta-analysis by Carpenter and colleagues, (AMT-4, caregiver Alzheimer's Disease-8, O3DY, Short Blessed Test, and Six Item Screener), the AMT-4 was best at identifying increased likelihood of dementia with a pooled LR+ of 7.69 (95% CI 3.47–17.10), while the O3DY was best at ruling out dementia with a pooled LR- (0.17[95% CI: 0.009–0.39]).[46] Both are feasible to implement, consisting of 4 simple questions. The AMT-4 takes under 5 minutes to complete.

Ottawa 3DY
What is the *D*ay?
What is the *D*ate?
Spell WORL*D* backwards
What is the *Y*ear?
Any incorrect answer indicates cognitive impairment
Abbreviated Mental Test-4
Age
Date of birth
Place
Year
Any incorrect answer indicates abnormal cognition

Routine screening for dementia among patients with ED aged 65 and older is recommended under the parameters set by Carpenter and colleagues They recommend screening using the O3DY or the AMT-4 in the ED when the pre-test probability of dementia is between 15% and 40%. ED-based observational studies using validated cognitive screening instruments suggest a dementia prevalence ranging from 12% to 43% with a weighted mean prevalence of 31%. With this pre-test probability, the potential benefits of screening are likely to outweigh the risks of potential "misdiagnosis" of dementia or potential delay to definitive emergency care. However, it is important to note that no screening test in the ED can definitively diagnose someone with dementia. Rather, when concern for cognitive impairment is identified, patients should either undergo comprehensive geriatric assessment (CGA) in the ED, be referred for outpatient evaluation for possible cognitive impairment, or both.[39] Therefore, even a false positive is not a "misdiagnosis." Rather a positive screen indicates a potentially life-altering diagnosis which needs to be further evaluated.

For patients who screen positive, it is important to ascertain whether the abnormal cognition truly represents a change in mental status. Performing validated screening tests for delirium with a screen such as the brief Confusion Assessment Method (bCAM), or FAMily Confusion Assessment Method (FAM-CAM).[47,48] If there is a concern for delirium, it is important to evaluate for causes of delirium as described later in this article. However, not all patients with impaired cognition require admission for "altered mental status." Patients who are at their baseline, with no evidence of delirium, with appropriate home support and connection to outpatient care may be safely discharged home as hospitalization is unlikely to benefit them, and in fact may induce delirium, deconditioning, or other hazards.

Acute care needs for persons living with dementia in the emergency department

PLWD may have different emergency care needs from of other elders in the ED. Common reasons for ED visits by PLWD include pain, falls or injury, "altered mental status," fluid or electrolyte imbalance, infection, immobility, medication side effects, respiratory, digestive, or cardiovascular issues, stroke, worsening dementia severity, and non-specific symptoms.[49–55] Urinary tract infections (UTIs) are commonly identified in an estimated 33% of all ED encounters for PLWD, compared to 13.4% in older adults without dementia.[54] However, PLWD who were diagnosed with UTI had a higher prevalence of non-specific signs of UTI and lower prevalence of urinary specific signs and symptoms than older adults without dementia. Given the frequency non-specific signs of UTI and the frequency of asymptomatic bacteriuria in older adults, it is difficult to determine how many of these diagnosed UTIs are true infections and how many represent bacterial colonization of the lower urinary tract.

Pain is a common and undertreated problem for PLWD in the ED.[56–59] Pain is a contributing factor for an estimated 45% of PLWD who visit the ED.[58] However, it is often difficult to identify and treat pain for PLWD because of communication difficulties regarding pain and pain relief.[56] PLWD are less likely to be assessed using a standardized pain assessment tool, have longer delay to first pain assessment, and have longer time between pain assessments than other patients in the ED.[60] They are less likely to receive parenteral analgesia and receive lower doses of analgesia than persons without ADRD.[61] To address these disparities in analgesia, the Pain Assessment IN Advanced Dementia (PAINAD) scale was developed.[62–64] The PAINAD scale evaluates breathing, vocalizations, facial expression, body language, and consolability. It is well accepted by ED RNs, the results in earlier and more complete assessments of pain, but did not impact time to analgesia for PLWD. Because pain is so common among PLWD in the ED, it is important to evaluate patients' pain frequently and systematically, particularly if they develop agitation or other Behavioral and Psychological Symptoms of Dementia (BPSD).

When treating pain acetaminophen should be considered first line except in patients who have contraindications, because many other analgesics are potentially inappropriate for older adults.[65] Local analgesia such as lidocaine patches, or diclofenac gel may be considered in pain which is localizable. Systemic non-steroidal anti-inflammatory drugs (NSAIDs) should be used with caution particularly in patients with impaired creatinine clearance, history of gastric ulcers, or gastritis. Muscle relaxants (including benzodiazepines) should be avoided because of risk of sedation and delirium. Weak opioids such as tramadol or codeine are not effective and carry significant adverse reactions. Oftentimes low dose opioids are necessary, such as 2.5mg oxycodone PO, 0.2mg IV hydromorphone or 2mg of morphine. Hydromorphone may be preferred over morphine because morphine's metabolites are renally cleared and may contribute to delirium.[66]

Difficulties with Activities of Daily Living (ADLs) and Instrumental Activities of Daily Living (IADLs) may also contribute to ED visits. PLWD's are often dependent on assistance to complete their ADLs and IADLs.[57,67–69] Commonly, patients with ED with moderate dementia require assistance with dressing and taking their own medications.[67] For PLWD who used the ED in the last month of life, 70% had more than three ADL impairments.[57] Unfortunately, PLWD often experience a worsening of functional status after an ED visit.[68] It is important to assess patients' abilities to complete ADLs and IADLs, as well as their support systems for helping them if they have difficulties with ADLs and IADLs. Interdisciplinary consultations from social work, occupational therapy, or physical therapy may help to evaluate patients' abilities to conduct ADLs and IADLs safely and effectively or to help provide support when needed.

Behavioral and psychological symptoms of dementia (BPSD) are a significant problem for PLWD in the ED with a range in prevalence from 3% to 39%.[55,58,70,71] PLWD may have BPSD at home or in a skilled nursing facility which leads to their ED visit. Symptoms such as wandering, physical aggression, sleep disturbance, verbal aggression, and suspicious/paranoid thoughts may present themselves during a crisis.[55] Additionally, PLWD may have BPSD while in the ED. Many factors including pain can precipitate or exacerbate BPSD. An estimated 36% of patients with ED with CI and pain in the ED experienced BPSD.[70]

In addition to BPSD, PLWD are at increased risk of developing delirium. Oftentimes it is difficult to can be difficult to decipher the difference between BPSD and delirium for PLWD in the ED, however the ADEPT tool by Shenvi and colleagues provides a systematic way to *A*ssess, *D*iagnose, *E*valuate, *P*revent, and *T*reat delirium and BPSD (**Fig. 2**).[72,73] To assess, emergency clinicians should begin by evaluating for immediate treatable causes such as hypoglycemia or ST-elevation MI, and ensure patient and staff safety. Next, determining the patient's baseline cognitive and functional status is key to identify any changes from baseline. If the symptoms represent an acute change, evaluating for causes of delirium such as infection, electrolyte alteration, or adverse medication effect. To assess for the presence of delirium, the brief Confusion Assessment Method is a feasible, sensitive, and specific test for delirium. It takes approximately 1 minute to administer, is 78% to 84% sensitive, and 96% to 97% specific.[47] In PLWD, the Family Confusion Assessment Method (FAM-CAM) and the Richmond Agitation and Sedation Scale also have demonstrated utility in identifying delirium.[48,74] The FAM-CAM demonstrated a sensitivity of 61%, specificity of 74% and positive likelihood ratio (LR+) of 2.2 for PLWD in the ED and was with increased hospitalization, ED visit, and mortality. The Richmond Agitation and Sedation Scale demonstrated a 92.5% sensitivity, 83.0% specificity, LR+ of 5.44, and negative likelihood ratio of 0.09.[75] Regardless of the strategy chosen, a systematic way to identify delirium in PLWD is of upmost importance for ED care.

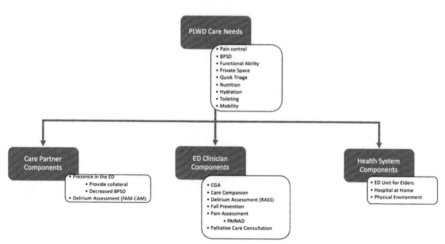

Fig. 2. Emergency Care needs and Components of Emergency Care for Persons Living with Dementia.[18]

When delirium is diagnosed, an evaluation to identify the cause might include core (rectal) temperature, blood glucose, complete cell count, basic metabolic panel, urinalysis and culture, and electrocardiogram. Additional testing might include X rays, blood cultures, CT of the brain, or abdomen, drug levels, blood gas, cardiac markers, thyroid stimulating hormone.

For both delirium and BPSD, it is important to prevent or manage additional behavioral and psychological symptoms. Clinicians should treat symptoms such as pain, nausea, and constipation. Home medications should be continued (or restarted if missed) in the ED. Potentially inappropriate medications such as antihistamines, other anticholinergics, and benzodiazepines should be avoided. Daily function should be normalized. Patients should have food, water, access to toileting, mobility, visual, and hearing assists. Mobility such as guided ambulation around the ED can often be effective in managing restlessness. Sitting in a recliner chair instead of a gurney may be more comfortable for many patients. Pillows and warm blankets may be helpful for patient comfort. Activities such as newspapers or magazines, word puzzles, fidgets, dolls, or playing cards may be helpful.[76,77] Unless medically indicated, tethers including blood pressure cuffs, telemetry monitoring, and pulse oximeters should be removed. Foley catheters should be avoided. Continuous IV infusions should be limited and disconnected when not in use. Day/night signals should be normalized with outside lighting if possible, or artificial diurnal lighting. At the very least, the lights should be turned off in the patient's room at night. PLWD who are being hospitalized should be prioritized for inpatient beds. Despite many improvements, the ED environment continues to present difficulties for PLWD and length of stay should be minimized. PLWD should not board in hallway spaces.[78]

When treating delirium or BPSD in the ED it is important to first try the non-pharmacological treatments suggested above. Additionally, if the patient becomes agitated verbal de-escalation, distraction, and reassurance from family or staff can prevent dangerous situations and can minimize the need for pharmacologic therapy.[79] If pharmacologic therapy is necessary, as mentioned previously, it is important to note that benzodiazepines should generally be avoided because they may worsen delirium.[80] Antipsychotics should be used with caution as they are known to cause increased mortality in PLWD. However, many patients PLWD are prescribed antipsychotics as an outpatient. If they will take their home oral medication, that would be a good first pharmacologic step. Other oral options include risperidone 1mg or less. Olanzapine 2.5 to 5 mg, quetiapine 25 to 50mg. If patients require IM or IV mediations ziprasidone 10 to 20mg IM, olanzapine 2.5-5mg IM, or haloperidol 1mg-2.5mg IM may be considered. IV haloperidol should be used with caution at low doses (0.25-1mg) because of potential adverse events. Additionally, antipsychotics particularly haloperidol should be avoided in patients with Parkinson's disease or Lewy Body dementia.

Process improvements for persons living with dementia

PLWD are particularly vulnerable to delirium and BPSD while in the unfamiliar, crowded, noisy ED, with no circadian cues.[81–85] This may be even worse in the waiting room. Often, patients are told they cannot eat or drink until they see a doctor, and even then, the NPO status is not immediately revoked. PLWD can be "under triaged" due to their inability to effectively communicate.[86] To address this communication issue and to prevent BPSD and delirium, PLWD should be triaged quickly, and their dementia should be considered in the triage process with the goal of minimizing time in the waiting room. Though, there are no studies demonstrating the effectiveness in prioritizing PLWD in the triage process, understanding of the effects of unfamiliar environments, increased stimulation, dehydration, and malnourishment justify allowing PLWD to "skip the line" rather than languishing in the waiting room.

The busy, noisy, crowded environment of the ED can result in sensory overload and BPSD.[87] Because of the difficulties in the ED environment, care partners sometimes feel the need to "keep vigil" and act as an advocate to ensure needs including basic human needs such as nutrition, hydration, toileting, and mobility are appropriately met.[85] Unfortunately ED clinicians have pressure from conflicting priorities and acknowledge they often cannot provide optimal care for PLWD in the ED. This mismatch in needs of PLWD and ED clinician priority was exacerbated by the COVID-19 pandemic. During this time many ED's restricted "visitors" access to the emergency department. This is particularly detrimental for PLWD, as their care partners are not just visiting, but are a very important part of the patient's healthcare team.[88] In times of restricted access to the ED such as safety concerns from violence, or infectious disease, care partners should be recognized as distinct from visitors and should have additional access to being with PLWD. Additionally, clinicians should value care partners as a valuable information source who can help clinicians better understand their patients. Care partners can provide valuable information on changes from baseline, successful techniques to address BPSD, they may also help reduce confusion and agitation and modify agitated behavior.[89,90] When care partners are unavailable to be with PLWD in the ED, care companions, hospital staff members serving as a companion for PLWD, should be used. Care companions are different from a "sitter," they engage the patient in activities, advocate and help with feeding and hydration, help with guided mobility, and can address BPSD and delirium early with non-pharmacologic methods. The use of care companions in the ED has been associated with a reduction in falls and BPSD.[91]

Many changes to ED physical environment have been described in the geriatric ED guidelines and are advocated for by the Geriatric Emergency Department Accreditation program through the American College of Emergency Physicians and are described in Donald L. Melady and John G. Schumacher's article, "Developing a Geriatric Emergency Department: People, Processes, and Place," in this issue. Many of those modifications are likely to be beneficial to PLWD in the ED. Specific changes to the ED environment which have demonstrated improved care for PLWD include creating dedicated treatment space for PLWD closer to nursing staff with soothing colors and adjustable lighting.[92] Noise-dampening doors or curtains can help decrease stimulation. Additional space and chairs can make the space more comfortable for care partners to stay with patients. Another way to decrease stimulation is the use of non-contact monitoring systems. One study of a non-contact monitoring system and tent-like "Charite Dome" designed to decrease stimulation demonstrated that 53% of PLWD experienced decreased agitation or improved overall wellbeing in a geriatric-gerontopsychiatric ward.[93] Similar interventions might be helpful for PLWD in the ED.

Of the many different models of GED care, a French study lends support to the Geriatric ED Unit Model.[94,95] Bosetti and colleagues demonstrated a reduction in 30-day admissions for PLWD after the index ED visit. Their program used a dedicated GED space and a comprehensive geriatric assessment and a multidisciplinary team in the ED including geriatricians, nurses trained in gerontology, and social workers specializing in the care of elderly patients. This program involved a medical assessment by a geriatrician, a social assessment, the development of individual healthcare plans, and guidance in choosing appropriate care facilities or home care services.[95] Though 30-day readmissions decreased, this intervention led to an increase in hospitalizations during the index ED visit. Though many GEDs use different techniques to provide care to elders, many rely on nurses or emergency physicians to identify those at higher risk for poor outcomes. The Bosetti study suggests that PLWD should be an important population to receive specialized GED care in whatever model is implemented.

Because of the risks of hospitalization discussed above, caring for patients in a familiar space is generally preferred for PLWD when feasible. As an extension of high-quality ED care for PLWD, a hospital at home program can be used to provide inpatient level care in a more familiar environment. Hospital at home has been shown to reduce sleeping disorders, agitation and aggressiveness, feeding disorders, and the use of antipsychotic medications for PLWD.[96]

Communication

Communication with PLWD and their care partners is critical in the ED; however, it often takes more time and requires additional considerations when caring for PLWD than other patients because of impairment in memory, comprehension, and communication. Oftentimes, emergency clinicians have insufficient communication with PLWD and their care partners because of competing priorities or lack of understanding of necessary communication techniques. ED communication with PLWD and care partners can be more difficult than other settings because of unfamiliar clinicians and unfamiliar setting. In ED studies, PLWD and care partners have described multiple communication problems in the ED. They noted feeling that communication is lacking and rushed and that messaging between physicians in the ED, hospital, and outpatient settings are discordant and confusing.[97,98] PLWD are more likely to misunderstand ED diagnoses, return precautions, and follow-up instructions.[40] Poor communication is also associated with a decreased willingness to return to the ED for future care.[99] **Fig. 3** describes the complex interplay of factors related to the patient, care partner, ED medical team, and health care system which impact communication in the ED. Unfortunately, there is little evidence to guide communication with PLWD in the ED.[37,100]

Studies on communication with PLWD are limited to specific scenarios of advanced care planning discussions. The We DECide training for PLWD living in dementia care

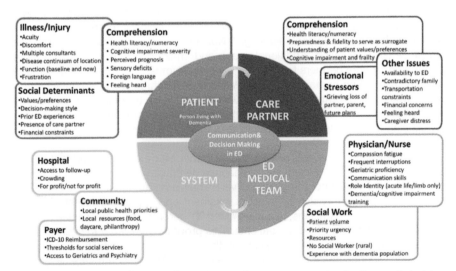

Fig. 3. Multi-level complexities of emergency department communication and decision-making with persons living with dementia.[37]

units.[37] This model applies the Elwyn Three-Step Model for Shared Decision Making: the "Choice talk" (acknowledging that choices exist), the "Option talk" (discussing different options), and the "Decision talk" (making a decision).[101] The Goals of Care Intervention consists of an 18-min video decision aid for care partners, and a structured discussion with nursing home staff.[102] Both the We DECide training and the Goals of Care Intervention both show improved goals of care discussions with PLWD and care partners in nursing homes. However, neither has been studied in the ED.

In lieu of specific studies on ED communication with PLWD, the guidelines by Limpahan and colleagues provide structure to communication with PLWD and care partners.[103] This discussion should involve both the patient and designated care partner. Additionally, written instructions can be particularly helpful for patients who have impaired memory. The discussion should address:

1. Diagnosis
2. Condition-specific red flags to inform the patient when and from whom to seek medical treatment
3. When and who to contact for follow-up appointments
4. Medication changes and the reasons for the change
5. Assessment of patient (and care-partner) understanding, incorporating concepts of health literacy and cultural competency
6. Name of ED clinician and telephone number (and name if known) to call for questions
7. Written discharge instructions reviewing these topics given to the patient or care partner.

Transitions of Care

The ED-to community care transition, where a patient is transferred from the ED to a personal residence, independent, or congregate living setting, is a particularly important aspect of care for PLWD in the ED with little medical oversite and high patient vulnerability.[38] PLWD and care partners frequently cite concerns regarding transitions of care (TOC) such as: difficulty with medication management, self-care, difficulty with outpatient follow up, loss of independence, home safety, costs-of long term care, and falls.[98,104] These difficulties may contribute to the high rates of ED revisits and rehospitalizations for PLWD. As described above, Bosetti and colleagues demonstrated improvements in TOC for PLWD by using a multidisciplinary team in the ED including geriatricians, nurses trained in gerontology, and social workers specializing in the care of elderly patients. This program involved a medical assessment by a geriatrician, a social assessment, development of individual healthcare plans, and guidance in choosing appropriate care facilities or home care services.[95]

In two US EDs, a paramedic-delivered ED-to-home Care Transitions Intervention (CTI) **(Fig. 4)** delivered by paramedics showed a significant reduction in repeat ED visits within 30 days.[105–107] This intervention involved a home visit 24 to 48 hours after discharge from the ED, and three follow up calls after the home visit by paramedics who underwent CTI coach training. PLWD who received the CTI had an odds ratio of 0.25 (95% CI: 0.07–0.90) for return to the ED within 30 days. The CTI works by developing self-management behaviors for PLWD and their care partners. This intervention improved outpatient follow-up, medication self-management, and knowledge of red flags.

Other interventions including comprehensive geriatric assessment (GCA),[108] GCA and a homecare visit,[109] focused geriatrics assessment and geriatrics followup,[110] and outpatient rehabilitation services and case management all showed improvement in transitions of care for older adults including PLWD, but the effects on PLWD were not specifically measured.[111]

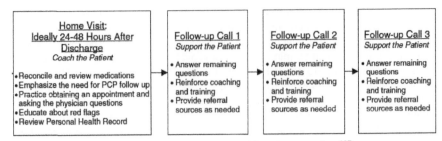

Fig. 4. Emergency department-to-home care transitions intervention.[107]

DISCUSSION
Future Directions

In 2022, the Geriatric Emergency Department Applied Research Network 2.0 Advancing Dementia Care (GEAR 2.0-ADC) recommendations for future research were published based on 4 scoping reviews and a consensus conference. These recommendations were created by a diverse group of stakeholders including PLWD, their care partners, researchers, emergency physicians, geriatricians, neuropsychologists, pharmacists, nurses, and social workers. In addition to the interventions described above, research priorities for each domain were developed.

Members of the consensus conference felt it important to address ED care for PLWD by changing the paradigm of emergency care for PLWD at the system and policy level, rather than relying on improving individual clinician performance. This includes the development and use of new technologies, financial incentives for improved ED care, and other implementation science techniques to ensure that changes are durable. It is critical to include the voices and perspectives of PLWD and care partners. Currently, they feel that they do not have a voice in emergency care.[81–85] This breeds a lack of trust with clinicians, researchers, administrators, and policymakers involved in ED care.

SUMMARY

ED care for PLWD involves the identification of dementia or cognitive impairment, in ED medical care which is sensitive to the specific needs of PLWD, effective communication with PLWD, their care partners, and outpatient clinicians who the patient and care-partner know and trust, and care-transitions from the ED to other health care settings. The recommendations above are made based on wide-ranging heterogeneous studies of various interventions which have been studied primarily in single-site studies. Future research should work to incorporate promising findings from interventions such as hospital at home, or ED to home Care Transitions Intervention.

CLINICS CARE POINTS

- *Identification* – Validated screening instruments should be used to identify patients in the ED with diagnosed and undiagnosed dementia who may benefit from referral to geriatrics, psychiatry, or neurology for formal evaluation and management.

- *Behavioral and Psychological Symptoms of Dementia (BPSD)* can be identified and systematically managed using resources such as the ADEPT tool.

- *Delirium* can be identified in PLWD using the brief Confusion Assessment Method (bCAM) or FAMily Confusion Assessment Method (FAM-CAM) and should be systematically managed using resources such as the ADEPT tool.
- *Pain* should be evaluated systematically for considered in patients with BPSD or delirium, evaluated systematically, and treated with acetaminophen as first line.
- *Activities of Daily Living (ADLs) and Instrumental Activities of Daily Living (IADLs)* should be assessed in the ED and appropriate referrals should be made.
- *Nutrition and hydration* should be promoted in the ED by the elimination of nil per os (NPO) status as default for patients with ED.
- *Toileting* should be addressed understanding the patient's baseline toileting routine and any limitations presented by the acute illness or injury.
- *Mobility* should be encouraged in the ED with guidance for safety.
- *Care partners* are key members of the care team and should be allowed and encouraged to stay with the patient, provide context for the clinical history, and help identify and manage BPSD and delirium.
- *Communication and decision* making are complex and should involve both patients and care partners as appropriate.
- *Care transitions* can be improved using interventions such as hospital at home and the ED-to-home Care Transitions Intervention.

FUNDING

Much of the work published in this article was supported by the National Institute on Aging of the National Institutes of Health under Award Number R21/R33AG058926.

REFERENCES

1. Hebert LE, Weuve J, Scherr PA, et al. Alzheimer disease in the United States (2010-2050) estimated using the 2010 census. Neurology 2013;80(19):1778–83.
2. Hunt LJ, Coombs LA, Stephens CE. Emergency department use by community-dwelling individuals with dementia in the United States: an integrative review. J Gerontol Nurs 2018;44(3):23–30.
3. Kent T, Lesser A, Israni J, et al. 30-Day emergency department revisit rates among older adults with documented dementia. J Am Geriatr Soc 2019; 67(11):2254–9.
4. Hwang U, Morrison RS. The geriatric emergency department. J Am Geriatr Soc 2007;55(11):1873–6.
5. Ostir GV, Schenkel SM, Berges IM, et al. Cognitive health and risk of ED revisit in underserved older adults. Am J Emerg Med 2016;34(10):1973–6.
6. Kales HC, Gitlin LN, Lyketsos CG. Assessment and management of behavioral and psychological symptoms of dementia. Bmj 2015;350:h369.
7. Kennedy M, Ciampa K, Koehl J, et al. 95 Use of antipsychotic and sedative medications in older patients in the emergency department. Ann Emerg Med 2020;76(4):S37–8.
8. LaMantia MA, Stump TE, Messina FC, et al. Emergency department use among older adults with dementia. Alzheimer Dis Assoc Disord 2016;30(1):35.
9. Covinsky KE, Palmer RM, Fortinsky RH, et al. Loss of independence in activities of daily living in older adults hospitalized with medical illnesses: increased vulnerability with age. J Am Geriatr Soc 2003;51(4):451–8.

10. Hibbard JH, Greene J, Sacks RM, et al. Improving population health management strategies: identifying patients who are more likely to be users of avoidable costly care and those more likely to develop a new chronic disease. Health Serv Res 2017;52(4):1297–309.

11. Morrison J, Palumbo MV, Rambur B. Reducing preventable hospitalizations with two models of transitional care. J Nurs Scholarsh 2016;48(3):322–9.

12. Galarraga JE, Pines JM. Costs of ED episodes of care in the United States. Am J Emerg Med 2016;34(3):357–65.

13. Basu S, Jack HE, Arabadjis SD, et al. Benchmarks for reducing emergency department visits and hospitalizations through community health workers integrated into primary care: a cost-benefit analysis. Medical care 2017;55(2):140–7.

14. Aminzadeh F, Dalziel WB. Older adults in the emergency department: a systematic review of patterns of use, adverse outcomes, and effectiveness of interventions. Ann Emerg Med 2002;39(3):238–47.

15. de Gelder J, Lucke JA, de Groot B, et al. Predictors and outcomes of revisits in older adults discharged from the emergency department. J Am Geriatr Soc 2018;66(4):735–41.

16. Gagnon-Roy M, Hami B, Généreux M, et al. Preventing emergency department (ED) visits and hospitalisations of older adults with cognitive impairment compared with the general senior population: what do we know about avoidable incidents? Results from a scoping review. BMJ Open 2018;8(4):e019908.

17. Carpenter CR, Hammouda N, Linton EA, et al. Delirium prevention, detection, and treatment in emergency medicine settings: a geriatric emergency care applied research (GEAR) network scoping review and consensus statement. Acad Emerg Med 2021;28(1):19–35.

18. Dresden SM, Taylor Z, Serina P, et al. Optimal emergency department care practices for persons living with dementia: a scoping review. J Am Med Dir Assoc 2022;23(8). 1314.e1311-29.

19. Carpenter CR, Bromley M, Caterino JM, et al. Optimal older adult emergency care: introducing multidisciplinary geriatric emergency department guidelines from the American College of emergency physicians, American geriatrics society, emergency nurses association, and society for Academic emergency medicine. J Am Geriatr Soc 2014;62(7):1360–3.

20. Han JH, Wilber ST. Altered mental status in older patients in the emergency department. Clin Geriatr Med 2013;29(1):101–36.

21. Health Udo, Services H. National plan to address Alzheimer's disease: 2021 Update. 2022. https://aspe.hhs.gov/reports/national-plan-2021-update.

22. Burns A, Iliffe S. Alzheimer's disease. BMJ Br Med J (Clin Res Ed) 2009;338(7692):467–71.

23. Jain S, Rosenbaum PR, Reiter JG, et al. Using Medicare claims in identifying Alzheimer's disease and related dementias. Alzheimer's Dementia 2021;17(3):515–24.

24. Cerejeira J, Lagarto L, Mukaetova-Ladinska EB. Behavioral and psychological symptoms of dementia. Front Neurol 2012;3:73.

25. Richey L, Peters MMD. Cognitive Impairment 2022;. https://www.hopkinsguides.com/hopkins/view/Johns_Hopkins_Psychiatry_Guide/787027/all/Cognitive_Impairment.

26. Burns A, Iliffe S. Dementia. BMJ 2009;338(7691):405–9.

27. Mahoney R, Regan C, Katona C, et al. Anxiety and depression in family care-givers of people with Alzheimer disease: the LASER-AD study. Am J Geriatr Psychiatry 2005;13(9):795–801.
28. Phelan EA, Borson S, Grothaus L, et al. Association of incident dementia with hospitalizations. JAMA 2012;307(2):165–72.
29. Tannenbaum R, Boltz M, Ilyas A, et al. Hospital practices and clinical outcomes associated with behavioral symptoms in persons with dementia. J Hosp Med 2022;17(9):702–9.
30. Inouye SK, Bogardus ST Jr, Baker DI, et al. The Hospital Elder Life Program: a model of care to prevent cognitive and functional decline in older hospitalized patients. Hospital Elder Life Program. J Am Geriatr Soc 2000;48(12):1697–706.
31. Reuben DB, Inouye SK, Bogardus ST Jr, et al. MODELS of geriatrics practice; the hospital elder life program: a model of care to prevent cognitive and functional decline in older hospitalized patients. J Am Geriatr Soc 2000;48(12):1697–706.
32. Inouye SK, Bogardus ST Jr, Charpentier PA, et al. A multicomponent intervention to prevent delirium in hospitalized older patients. N Engl J Med 1999;340(9):669–76.
33. Hshieh TT, Yang T, Gartaganis SL, et al. Hospital elder life program: systematic review and meta-analysis of effectiveness. Am J Geriatr Psychiatr 2018;26(10):1015–33.
34. Holm A, Michel M, Stern GA, et al. The outcomes of an inpatient treatment program for geriatric patients with dementia and dysfunctional behaviors. Gerontol 1999;39(6):668–76.
35. Research Priorities GEAR 2.0 - GEAR Network. GEAR Network. Available at: https://gearnetwork.org/about-gear-2/research-priorities-gear2/. Accessed April 13, 2023, 2023.
36. Hwang U, Carpenter C, Dresden S, et al. The Geriatric Emergency Care Applied Research (GEAR) network approach: a protocol to advance stakeholder consensus and research priorities in geriatrics and dementia care in the emergency department. BMJ Open 2022;12(4):e060974.
37. Carpenter CR, Leggett J, Bellolio F, et al. Emergency department communication in persons living with dementia and care partners: a scoping review. J Am Med Dir Assoc 2022;23(8). 1313.e1315-46.
38. Gettel CJ, Falvey JR, Gifford A, et al. Emergency department care transitions for patients with cognitive impairment: a scoping review. J Am Med Dir Assoc 2022;23(8):1313.e1–13.
39. Nowroozpoor A, Dussetschleger J, Perry W, et al. Detecting cognitive impairment and dementia in the emergency department: a scoping review. J Am Med Dir Assoc 2022;23(8). 1314.e1331-88.
40. Han JH, Bryce SN, Ely EW, et al. The effect of cognitive impairment on the accuracy of the presenting complaint and discharge instruction comprehension in older emergency department patients. Ann Emerg Med 2011;57(6):662–71, e662.
41. Sax DR, Mark DG, Hsia RY, et al. Short-term outcomes and factors associated with adverse events among adults discharged from the emergency department after treatment for acute heart failure. Circ Heart Fail 2017;10(12):e004144.
42. Dyer AH, Nabeel S, Briggs R, et al. Cognitive assessment of older adults at the acute care interface: the informant history. Postgrad Med 2016;92(1087):255–9.

43. Barbic D, Kim B, Salehmohamed Q, et al. Diagnostic accuracy of the Ottawa 3DY and Short Blessed Test to detect cognitive dysfunction in geriatric patients presenting to the emergency department. BMJ Open 2018;8(3):e019652.

44. Carpenter CR, DesPain B, Keeling TN, et al. The Six-Item Screener and AD8 for the detection of cognitive impairment in geriatric emergency department patients. Ann Emerg Med 2011;57(6):653–61.

45. Wilding L, Eagles D, Molnar F, et al. Prospective validation of the Ottawa 3DY scale by geriatric emergency management nurses to identify impaired cognition in older emergency department patients. Ann Emerg Med 2016;67(2):157–63.

46. Carpenter CR, Banerjee J, Keyes D, et al. Accuracy of dementia screening instruments in emergency medicine: a diagnostic meta-analysis. Acad Emerg Med 2019;26(2):226–45.

47. Han JH, Wilson A, Vasilevskis EE, et al. Diagnosing delirium in older emergency department patients: validity and reliability of the delirium triage screen and the brief confusion assessment method. Ann Emerg Med 2013;62(5):457–65.

48. Mailhot T, Darling C, Ela J, et al. Family identification of delirium in the emergency department in patients with and without dementia: validity of the family confusion assessment method (FAM-CAM). J Am Geriatr Soc 2020;68(5):983–90.

49. Benner M, Steiner V, Pierce LL. Family caregivers' reports of hospitalizations and emergency department visits in community-dwelling individuals with dementia. Dementia 2018;17(5):585–95.

50. Björck M, Wijk H. Is hospitalisation necessary? A survey of frail older persons with cognitive impairment transferred from nursing homes to the emergency department. Scand J Caring Sci 2018;32(3):1138–47.

51. Holden TR, Shah MN, Gibson TA, et al. Outcomes of patients with syncope and suspected dementia. Acad Emerg Med 2018;25(8):880–90.

52. Lin P-C, Lin L-C, Hsieh H-F, et al. Primary diagnoses and outcomes of emergency department visits in older people with dementia: a hospital-based retrospective study in Taiwan. Int Psychogeriatr 2020;32(1):97–104.

53. Tadokoro K, Sasaki R, Wakutani Y, et al. Clinical characteristics of patients with dementia in a local emergency clinic in Japan. Geriatr Gerontol Int 2018;18(9):1383–7.

54. Yourman LC, Kent TJ, Israni JS, et al. Association of dementia diagnosis with urinary tract infection in the emergency department. J Am Coll Emerg Phys Open 2020;1(6):1291–6.

55. Ledgerd R, Hoe J, Hoare Z, et al. Identifying the causes, prevention and management of crises in dementia. An online survey of stakeholders. Int J Geriatr Psychiatr 2016;31(6):638–47.

56. Fry M, Chenoweth L, Arendts G. Assessment and management of acute pain in the older person with cognitive impairment: a qualitative study. Int Emerg Nurs 2016;24:54–60.

57. Hunt LJ, Ritchie CS, Cataldo JK, et al. Pain and emergency department use in the last month of life among older adults with dementia. J Pain Symptom Manag 2018;56(6):871–7, e877.

58. Schnitker LM, Beattie ER, Martin-Khan M, et al. Characteristics of older people with cognitive impairment attending emergency departments: a descriptive study. Australas Emerg Nurs J 2016;19(2):118–26.

59. Seffo N, Senorski EH, Westin O, et al. Communication and assessment of pain in hip fracture patients with dementia-experiences of healthcare professionals at

an accident and emergency department in Sweden. Med Glas 2020;17(1): e019908.

60. Jones J, Sim TF, Parsons R, et al. Influence of cognitive impairment on pain assessment and management in the emergency department: a retrospective cross-sectional study. Emerg Med Australasia (EMA) 2019;31(6):989–96.

61. Chang AK, Edwards RR, Morrison RS, et al. Disparities in acute pain treatment by cognitive status in older adults with hip fracture. J Gerontol: Series A 2020; 75(10):2003–7.

62. Fry M, Arendts G, Chenoweth L. Emergency nurses' evaluation of observational pain assessment tools for older people with cognitive impairment. J Clin Nurs 2017;26(9–10):1281–90.

63. Fry M, Chenoweth L, Arendts G. Can an observational pain assessment tool improve time to analgesia for cognitively impaired older persons? A cluster randomised controlled trial. Emerg Med J 2018;35(1):33–8.

64. Fry M, Elliott R. Pragmatic evaluation of an observational pain assessment scale in the emergency department: the Pain Assessment in Advanced Dementia (PAINAD) scale. Australas Emerg Care 2018;21(4):131–6.

65. Panel BtAGSBCUE. American Geriatrics Society 2023 updated AGS Beers Criteria® for potentially inappropriate medication use in older adults. J Am Geriatr Soc 2023. https://doi.org/10.1111/jgs.18372.

66. Smith M. Neuroexcitatory effects of morphine and hydromorphone: evidence implicating the 3-glucuronide metabolites. Clin Exp Pharmacol Physiol 2000; 27(7):524–8.

67. Chiovenda P, Vincentelli GM, Alegiani F. Cognitive impairment in elderly ED patients: need for multidimensional assessment for better management after discharge. Am J Emerg Med 2002;20(4):332–5.

68. Provencher V, Sirois MJ, Ouellet MC, et al. Decline in activities of daily living after a visit to a Canadian emergency department for minor injuries in independent older adults: are frail older adults with cognitive impairment at greater risk? J Am Geriatr Soc 2015;63(5):860–8.

69. Kelly S, Rivera-Reyes L, Levy S, et al. The association between cognitive function and functional status in older adults in the emergency department setting: 503. Acad Emerg Med 2016;23.

70. Erel M, Shapira Z, Volicer L. Behavioral problems of seniors in an emergency department. J Emerg Med 2013;45(1):13–8.

71. Tropea J, LoGiudice D, Kelly L. People with dementia in the emergency department: behavioural symptoms and use of restraint. Emerg Med Australas 2017; 29(5):605–6.

72. Kennedy M, Koehl J, Shenvi CL, et al. The agitated older adult in the emergency department: a narrative review of common causes and management strategies. J Am Coll Emerg Phys Open 2020;1(5):812–23.

73. Shenvi C, Kennedy M, Austin CA, et al. Managing delirium and agitation in the older emergency department patient: the ADEPT tool. Ann Emerg Med 2020; 75(2):136–45.

74. Yeon H, Saczynski J. Comparison of delirium detection rates in dementia vs. non-dementia elderly population using FAM-CAM in the emergency department. Paper presented at: PHARMACOTHERAPY2017.

75. Morandi A, Han JH, Meagher D, et al. Detecting delirium superimposed on dementia: evaluation of the diagnostic performance of the Richmond Agitation and Sedation Scale. J Am Med Dir Assoc 2016;17(9):828–33.

76. Lichen IM, Berning MJ, Bower SM, et al. Non-pharmacologic interventions improve comfort and experience among older adults in the Emergency Department. Am J Emerg Med 2021;39:15–20.

77. Sanon M, Baumlin KM, Kaplan SS, et al. Care and respect for elders in emergencies program: a preliminary report of a volunteer approach to enhance care in the emergency department. J Am Geriatr Soc 2014;62(2):365–70.

78. Casey CP, Lindroth H, Mohanty R, et al. Postoperative delirium is associated with increased plasma neurofilament light. Brain 2020;143(1):47–54.

79. Cohen-Mansfield J, Werner P. Management of verbally disruptive behaviors in nursing home residents. J Gerontol A Biol Sci Med Sci 1997;52(6):M369–77.

80. Zaal IJ, Devlin JW, Hazelbag M, et al. Benzodiazepine-associated delirium in critically ill adults. Intensive Care Med 2015;41:2130–7.

81. Watkins S, Murphy F, Kennedy C, et al. Caring for older people with dementia in the emergency department. Br J Nurs 2020;29(12):692–9.

82. Parke B, Hunter KF, Strain LA, et al. Facilitators and barriers to safe emergency department transitions for community dwelling older people with dementia and their caregivers: a social ecological study. Int J Nurs Stud 2013;50(9):1206–18.

83. Parke B, Hunter KF, Schulz ME, et al. Know me–A new person-centered approach for dementia-friendly emergency department care. Dementia 2019; 18(2):432–47.

84. Jacobsohn GC, Hollander M, Beck AP, et al. Factors influencing emergency care by persons with dementia: stakeholder perceptions and unmet needs. J Am Geriatr Soc 2019;67(4):711–8.

85. Hunter K, Parke B, Babb M, et al. Balancing safety and harm for older adults with dementia in rural emergency departments: healthcare professionals' perspectives. Rural Rem Health 2017;17(1):4055.

86. Platts-Mills TF, Travers D, Biese K, et al. Accuracy of the Emergency Severity Index triage instrument for identifying elder emergency department patients receiving an immediate life-saving intervention. Acad Emerg Med 2010;17(3): 238–43.

87. Manning SN. Managing behaviour that challenges in people with dementia in the emergency department. Emerg Nurse 2021;29(3).

88. Lo AX, Wedel LK, Liu SW, et al. COVID-19 hospital and emergency department visitor policies in the United States: impact on persons with cognitive or physical impairment or receiving end-of-life care. J Am Coll Emerg Phys Open 2022;3(1): e12622.

89. Fry M, Chenoweth L, MacGregor C, et al. Emergency nurses perceptions of the role of family/carers in caring for cognitively impaired older persons in pain: a descriptive qualitative study. Int J Nurs Stud 2015;52(8):1323–31.

90. Chary AN, Castilla-Ojo N, Joshi C, et al. Evaluating older adults with cognitive dysfunction: a qualitative study with emergency clinicians. J Am Geriatr Soc 2022;70(2):341–51.

91. Graham E, Loughran M, Monaghan M. 071An innovation to delivering person-centred dementia care in the acute hospital setting: dementia companion role. Age Ageing 2017;46(Suppl_3).

92. Bracken-Scally M, Keogh B, Daly L, et al. Assessing the impact of dementia inclusive environmental adjustment in the emergency department. Dementia 2021;20(1):28–46.

93. Kroll L, Böhning N, Müßigbrodt H, et al. Non-contact monitoring of agitation and use of a sheltering device in patients with dementia in emergency departments: a feasibility study. BMC Psychiatr 2020;20(1):1–8.

94. Southerland LT, Lo AX, Biese K, et al. Concepts in practice: geriatric emergency departments. Ann Emerg Med 2020;75(2):162–70.
95. Bosetti A, Gayot C, Preux P-M, et al. Effectiveness of a geriatric emergency medicine unit for the management of neurocognitive disorders in older patients: results of the MUPACog study. Dement Geriatr Cognit Disord 2020;49(4):394–400.
96. Tibaldi V, Aimonino N, Ponzetto M, et al. A randomized controlled trial of a home hospital intervention for frail elderly demented patients: behavioral disturbances and caregiver's stress. Arch Gerontol Geriatr Suppl 2004;(9):431–6.
97. Baraff LJ, Bernstein E, Bradley K, et al. Perceptions of emergency care by the elderly: results of multicenter focus group interviews. Ann Emerg Med 1992; 21(7):814–8.
98. Gettel CJ, Hayes K, Shield RR, et al. Care transition decisions after a fall-related emergency department visit: a qualitative study of patients' and caregivers' experiences. Acad Emerg Med 2020;27(9):876–86.
99. McCusker J, Cetin-Sahin D, Cossette S, et al. How older adults experience an emergency department visit: development and validation of measures. Ann Emerg Med 2018;71(6):755–66.e754.
100. Clevenger CK, Chu TA, Yang Z, et al. Clinical care of persons with dementia in the emergency department: a review of the literature and agenda for research. J Am Geriatr Soc 2012;60(9):1742–8.
101. Elwyn G, Frosch D, Thomson R, et al. Shared decision making: a model for clinical practice. J Gen Intern Med 2012;27:1361–7.
102. Hanson LC, Zimmerman S, Song M-K, et al. Effect of the goals of care intervention for advanced dementia: a randomized clinical trial. JAMA Intern Med 2017; 177(1):24–31.
103. Limpahan LP, Baier RR, Gravenstein S, et al. Closing the loop: best practices for cross-setting communication at ED discharge. Am J Emerg Med 2013;31(9): 1297–301.
104. Foulon V, Wuyts J, Desplenter F, et al. Problems in continuity of medication management upon transition between primary and secondary care: patients' and professionals' experiences. Acta Clin Belg 2019;74(4):263–71.
105. Shah MN, Jacobsohn GC, Jones CM, et al. Care transitions intervention reduces ED revisits in cognitively impaired patients. Alzheimers Dement (N Y) 2022;8(1): e12261.
106. Coleman EA, Smith JD, Frank JC, et al. Preparing patients and caregivers to participate in care delivered across settings: the Care Transitions Intervention. J Am Geriatr Soc 2004;52(11):1817–25.
107. Mi R, Hollander MM, Jones CMC, et al. A randomized controlled trial testing the effectiveness of a paramedic-delivered care transitions intervention to reduce emergency department revisits. BMC Geriatr 2018;18(1):104.
108. Ballabio C, Bergamaschini L, Mauri S, et al. A comprehensive evaluation of elderly people discharged from an Emergency Department. Int Emerg Med 2008;3(3):245–9.
109. Pedersen LH, Gregersen M, Barat I, et al. Early geriatric follow-up after discharge reduces mortality among patients living in their own home. A randomised controlled trial. European Geriatric Medicine 2017;8(4):330–6.
110. MacDonald Z, Stiell IG, Genovezos I, et al. Adherence of older emergency department patients to community-based specialized geriatric services. Cjem 2019;21(5):659–66.
111. O'Riordan Y, Bernard P, Maloney P, et al. Safer transitions: optimising care and function from hospital to home. Int J Integrated Care 2017;17(5):1–8.

Emergency Department Pain Management in the Older Adult

Natalie M. Elder, MD, PharmD[a], Sean F. Heavey, MD[b],
Katren R. Tyler, MD[b],*

KEYWORDS

- Pain • Pharmacology • Older adults • Older patients

KEY POINTS

- Adequate pain control in older adults is more complicated to achieve than in younger adults.
- Drug–drug and drug–disease interactions are particularly important in older adults.
- Fragility fractures, especially hip fractures, should have established pathways of care within emergency departments to help prevent complications such as delirium.

INTRODUCTION

Acute pain is a common reason for seeking emergency care.[1] The prevalence of both acute and chronic pain in older adults seeking care in the emergency department (ED) is likely higher, with 40% of adults aged older than 75 years reporting daily pain.[2] Older adults are less likely to receive pain medication than younger patients in the ED.[3,4]

Given many older adults have complex living arrangement and multiple comorbidities, using a biopsychosocial model may be helpful in managing pain in this vulnerable population. Older adults in residential care facilities depend on others for medication administration. Untreated or undertreated pain is a risk factor for many adverse events, including increased anxiety and depression, sleep disturbance, and development of delirium.[5] This can be especially problematic in older adults already prone to delirium due to age-related neurocognitive changes or dementia. Pain can reduce mobility, further increasing the risk of deconditioning and falls.[5]

The complex issues managing older adults with pain have been addressed by multiple professional societies.[6–8] The American Geriatrics Society published and updated

[a] University of Vermont, 111 Colchester Avenue, Burlington, VT 05401, USA; [b] University of California Davis, 4150 V Street, Sacramento, CA 95817, USA
* Corresponding author.
E-mail address: krtyler@ucdavis.edu

Clin Geriatr Med 39 (2023) 619–634
https://doi.org/10.1016/j.cger.2023.05.012
0749-0690/23/© 2023 Elsevier Inc. All rights reserved.

the Beers' Criteria for Potentially Inappropriate Medications.[9,10] Many older patients already have substantial medication burdens.[11] The risks of undertreating pain must be balanced with the potential side effects of medication administration. Many analgesic medications increase the risk of delirium in older adults.[10] Opioid analgesics, neuropathic medications and other sedative agents increase the risk of falls.[12–14]

This article summarizes key principles of acute pharmacologic pain management in older adults, including a review of pathological processes, pharmacologic and non-pharmacologic strategies, and adjunctive or alternative therapies.[15]

GENERAL APPROACH TO PAIN IN OLDER ADULTS
Assessment of Pain

Acute pain management in older adults necessitates emergency providers perform a thorough pain assessment and frequently reassess patients for their response to treatment. There are currently no clinically useful biomarkers for assessing the presence or degree of pain.[16] The most reliable assessment of pain involves patient self-reporting of pain, which can be facilitated with validated screening tools.[17,18]

However, communication barriers and cognitive changes may prevent self-reported pain assessment in older adults. Communication barriers include older patients' reluctance to disclose pain, neurologic disorders such as dysphasia or aphasia, and changes in motor ability and sensory perception.[18] Patients with significant cognitive impairment require physiological and behavioral evaluations of pain such as the Pain in Advanced Dementia score.[7,19,20]

Pharmacologic and Physiological Changes in Older Adults

Pharmacokinetics and pharmacodynamics are affected in older adults. Physiologic changes associated with aging include decreased muscle mass and total body water and an increase in body fat. This can increase the distribution of lipophilic drugs, resulting in prolonged effects.[21] Additionally, changes in hepatic metabolism and renal function can increase drug and active metabolite concentrations.[21,22] Polypharmacy is also common in older adults, with higher incidence of comorbid disease compared with younger patients. Prescribers must be cautious of potential drug–drug interactions or drug-related renal injury that may alter a patient's response to pain medication.[23]

Medication Strategies

When considering pain management strategies for older adults in the ED, the benefit of treatment must be balanced with the risk of adverse effects. It is worth discussing these risks with patients and their families and establishing expectations that resolution of pain may not be feasible. Geriatric prescribing principles recommend starting with the lowest effective dose for the shortest duration of time to control pain episodes. Typically, longer acting medications should be avoided for the management of acute pain episodes to avoid combined effects of multiple administrations or medications. Additionally, when using multiple medications, careful consideration should be given to the synergistic or complementary effects of certain medications.[24]

Types of Pain

Pain is a complex phenomenon, with physical, emotional, and psychosocial components. Patients' responses to pain or painful stimuli are variable.[25] When discussing pain management, it is useful to classify pain based on physiologic mechanisms—receptor pain (nociceptive pain) or nonreceptor (neuropathic) pain.

Nociceptive pain is mediated by specialized nerve endings that transmit information about chemical, thermal, or mechanical tissue damage or potential tissue damage, which is interpreted as pain.[25] This can be either somatic or visceral in nature. This pain is usually improved with both opioid and nonopioid pain medications and treatment of inciting cause/injury.

Neuropathic pain is pain due to injury or disease to peripheral nerves, spinal cord, or brain stem involved in the somatosensory pathway.[26] Clinically, neuropathic pain is harder to describe or quantify and may present as burning, tingling, allodynia, or temperature sensitivity. There are many conditions that can cause neuropathic pain including postherpetic neuralgia, diabetes mellitus, arthritis, cancer, and cancer treatments.[26] Additionally, there is a high degree of comorbid psychiatric disease such as depression or mood disorder, associated with neuropathic pain that may increase chronicity or intensity of this pain. Management of neuropathic pain is challenging and frequently requires the use of nonopioid adjuvant medications. Even with treatment, up to 50% of patients with neuropathic pain will have no clinically meaningful improvement. In those patients that do see improvement in pain, they commonly report only partial relief of symptoms.[26] Additionally, there are significant adverse effects of many neuropathic pain agents, limiting patients' ability to tolerate treatment.

PHARMACOLOGIC TREATMENTS
Acetaminophen (Paracetamol)

Acetaminophen is effective for treating symptoms associated with musculoskeletal pain, headaches, and osteoarthritis but less effective for inflammatory pain because it lacks anti-inflammatory qualities.[8,25,27] Acetaminophen, when taken at the recommended dose, is the first-line agent for the treatment of mild-to-moderate pain in older adults owing to its safety profile when compared with other analgesics.

The maximum daily dose is 4 g. In patients with hepatic dysfunction or those who consume more than 3 alcoholic beverages daily, doses should be reduced by 50% to 70%. Dose reduction should be considered in those taking medications primarily metabolized in the liver such as warfarin and anticonvulsants, those with heavy alcohol use, and for people weighing less than 50 kg.[28] It is crucial clinicians educate patients about acetaminophen-containing products because there are hundreds of these available over-the-counter (such as cold and flu medications) as well as prescription medications (such as opioid combination products with oxycodone, hydrocodone).

Nonsteroidal Anti-inflammatory Drugs

Oral nonsteroidal anti-inflammatory drugs (NSAIDs) are mostly used for localized pain, such as headache, gout, or renal and biliary colic. They can be administered in addition to acetaminophen or if acetaminophen fails to control the patient's pain. Owing to their anti-inflammatory properties, NSAIDs are particularly useful in the treatment of inflammatory type of pain. However, NSAIDs should be given at low doses for short periods of time and with extreme caution to geriatric patients due to their side effects and drug–drug interactions.[29,30] NSAIDs are included in the Beers criteria for potentially inappropriate medication (PIM) in older adults and the American Geriatric Society generally recommend against their use in older adults.[10] NSAIDs are often not recommended for analgesia in acute fractures because of concerns regarding fracture healing. In older adults with osteoporosis, this may be of more concern.[31] NSAIDs may be more effective for spine-related pain than acetaminophen.[30]

The association between oral NSAID use and gastrointestinal complications in the older adult is well known. The risk increases with age, dose and duration, and concomitant use of corticosteroids, or anticoagulants/antiplatelet agents.[32] There is strong evidence that prophylaxis with a proton pump inhibitor may decrease bleeding risk; however, this medication class is also associated with adverse events and drug–drug interactions.[33] Electrolyte imbalances and acute or chronic renal failure can also occur with oral NSAID use. Cardiovascular adverse events include fluid retention, hypertension, myocardial infarction, and cerebral vascular accidents.[34]

Factors that should be considered when deciding to prescribe oral NSAIDs to older adults include comorbidities, concomitant medications, and duration of NSAID use. Because this population is at higher risk of complications, shared decision-making should be used to minimize potential risks and maximize outcomes. Assuming no existing renal impairment, active heart failure exacerbation or gastrointestinal distress, a trial of a low dose of NSAIDs for 5 to 7 days is reasonable especially if acetaminophen has been already tried.[30] Stress ulcer prophylaxis with a proton pump inhibitor should be standard.

Topical Nonsteroidal Anti-inflammatory Drugs

Topical NSAIDs are used for acute musculoskeletal pain and osteoarthritis-related joint pain. Topical NSAIDs are unlikely to provide pain relief for fractures. Preparations include gel, patch, and liquid. In the United States, diclofenac gel is available over the counter and as a prescription. Compounding pharmacies can compound topical solutions of ibuprofen, ketoprofen, indomethacin, and piroxicam.

Compared with oral NSAIDs, topical NSAIDs provide equivalent pain relief with decreased systemic side effects but there is increased skin irritation at the site of application.[35–37] There are limited data to support its use in older adults with renal impairment or those at an increased risk of drug–drug interactions mentioned above. In addition, caution should be taken for individuals with joint pain at multiple sites to not exceed the maximum recommended dose. For patients who cannot or will not take oral NSAIDs, topical NSAIDs can be considered first-line.

OPIOIDS

In older adults, opioids are used to manage acute moderate-to-severe pain or pain that other treatment modalities failed to manage.[6] Dosing should be individualized considering changes in pharmacodynamics, comorbidities, and polypharmacy. For opiate-naïve older patients starting with 25% to 50%, usual adult dosages are recommended.[6,38] For older patients with a long-term use of opioids or other central nervous system (CNS) depressants (alcohol, benzodiazepines, barbiturates), there is a risk of augmented medication effects. Common adverse effects of opioids in the geriatric population include respiratory depression, constipation, nausea, vomiting, sedation, and confusion.[39] Pain can also contribute to the development of delirium.[40]

In the ED, oral, subcutaneous, intranasal, and intravenous formulations of short-acting or intermediate-acting opioids are preferred. Intramuscular administration should be avoided because decreased muscle mass will prolong drug absorption and delay pain relief.[6] Pain should be reassessed when effects are expected to take place, approximately 15 to 30 minutes after intravenous and 30 to 60 minutes after oral opioids are given. If needed, the dose may be titrated in balance with limiting side effects.

If the patient is taking opiates around the clock, it is recommended to determine the daily dosage of the opioid by converting to oral morphine milligram equivalents using the equianalgesic dose conversion listed in **Table 1**.

OPIOID USE DISORDER

The prevalence of opioid use disorder in older adults tripled from 2013 and 2018 and continues to increase.[41] Older adults have higher rates of death following opioid

Table 1
Opiates agents available for treatment of moderate-to-severe pain

Medication	Recommended Starting Dosage	Approximate Equianalgesic Dose		Side Effects/Monitoring	Special Considerations
		Oral	Parenteral		
Morphine	2.5–5 mg PO Q4H 2–4 mg IV Q1–2H	15 mg	5 mg	Constipation, nausea, headache, drowsiness, dizziness Transient pruritus and hives	• Metabolites may accumulate in patients with renal impairment leading to an increased risk of adverse events
Hydromorphone	1–2 mg PO Q4H 0.2–0.4 mg IV Q1–2H	3 mg	1 mg	Constipation, nausea, headache, drowsiness, dizziness	• Metabolites may accumulate in patients with renal impairment leading to an increased risk of adverse events • Considered safer than morphine in renal insufficiency • Less gastrointestinal side effects than other opioids
Oxycodone	2.5–5 mg PO Q4–6H	10 mg	N/A	Constipation, nausea, headache, drowsiness, dizziness	• Long-acting product (oxycontin) should not be used for the treatment of acute pain • Contraindicated in patients on dialysis
Fentanyl	12.5–25mcg IV Q1–2H	N/A	50 mcg	Constipation, nausea, headache, drowsiness, dizziness	• May be used in renal impairment • Faster onset than most opiates • Can be used safely in patients with morphine allergy
Hydrocodone	2.5–5 mg PO Q4–6H	15 mg	N/A	Constipation, nausea, headache, drowsiness, dizziness	• Only available in combination with acetaminophen
Tramadol	25 mg Q4–6H	150 mg	N/A	Constipation, nausea, headache, drowsiness, dizziness	• Weak inhibitor of serotonin and norepinephrine reuptake, avoid in patients are serotonergic medications • Lowers seizure threshold, avoid in patients with history of seizures • May increase suicide risk, avoid in patients with history of suicidal ideation or suicidal attempt • Generally, not recommended for older adults

(continued on next page)

Table 1
(continued)

Medication	Recommended Starting Dosage	Approximate Equianalgesic Dose		Side Effects/Monitoring	Special Considerations
		Oral	Parenteral		
Methadone	Consult with pharmacist or pain specialist			Constipation, nausea, headache, drowsiness, dizziness	• Multiple potential drug–drug interactions • May be used in renal impairment • Prolongs QT interval • Not recommended for opioid-naïve patients
Buprenorphine	Consult with pharmacist or pain specialist			Constipation, nausea, headache, drowsiness, dizziness	• May be used in renal impairment • As of 2023, X-waiver is no longer a requirement to prescribe in the United States

Approximate equianalgesic dose should be used for patients with long-term opiate use.

overdose compared with younger adults.[42] Medication for opiate use disorder is effective in preventing overdose deaths and involves maintenance therapy with either methadone, buprenorphine, or naltrexone.[43] There are no clinical trials evaluating effectiveness in patients aged older than 65 years.[44]

For opioid withdrawal and subsequent maintenance treatment, either methadone or buprenorphine are recommended as first-line treatment because they have both been shown to be equally effective and superior to nonopioid medication treatment.[45] Both can reduce withdrawal symptoms, opioid cravings, and risk of relapse and overdose.[45] Buprenorphine is preferred to methadone because it is less likely to cause withdrawal symptoms and prolonged QT interval; buprenorphine is safer in overdose and less likely than methadone to cause respiratory depression or respiratory arrest.[43]

Initiation of treatment is patient-specific and depends on other substance use, medications, and comorbidities. Involvement of a clinical pharmacist, substance use disorder specialist, pain management specialist, and/or a geriatric psychiatrist is recommended to ensure proper starting doses and close follow-up.

NEUROPATHIC AGENTS

In the ED setting, there is a paucity of data on the use of neuropathic agents for the management of acute pain complaints. With an increasing number of older adults with chronic pain seeking ED care and both local and national attention to opioid prescribing patterns, many older adults may present while taking neuropathic medications. **Table 2** summarizes commonly used neuropathic agents.

The most widely used neuropathic pain agent is gabapentin.[46,47] Pregabalin is a gabapentin prodrug and often used as an alternative to gabapentin if there is insufficient response or significant side effects.[46] Both agents can cause lethargy, vertigo, visual disturbances, and respiratory depression.[48] They may interact synergistically with opioid medications, decreasing overall opioid consumption; however, this potential benefit must be balanced against increased side effects with combined use, most notably respiratory depression.[49]

Several classes of antidepressant medications have been used for the management of neuropathic pain. Both tricyclic antidepressants (TCAs) and serotonin-norepinephrine reuptake inhibitors (SNRIs) have been shown to provide pain relief separate from their antidepressant effects and in patients without depressive symptoms.[50] Both TCAs and SNRIs can cause anticholinergic side effects and adverse cardiac events.[50] The use of these antidepressant medications for acute pain is limited as analgesic effects may take 2 to 4 weeks. However, older patients may be taking these medications at home complicating prescribing decisions in the ED.

SKELETAL MUSCLE RELAXANTS

Skeletal muscle relaxants are a heterogenous group of medications that fall into 2 broad categories: antispasmodics and antispasticity (or spasmolytics). Antispasmodics are used for the treatment of acute muscle spasm, whereas antispasticity agents are used for conditions where there is increased muscle spasticity or clonus.[51] Both classes of agents are used as adjuncts for the management of acute musculoskeletal pain.

Skeletal muscle relaxants can cause CNS depression and are considered a PIM.[10,24] Despite this, some studies suggest that up to 15% of prescriptions for skeletal muscle relaxers are given to patients aged older than 65 years.[52]

Although routine use of skeletal muscle relaxers is not recommended in older adults, emergency providers should still be familiar with these agents because they are likely

Table 2
Agents for neuropathic pain

Category	Starting Dose	Target Dose	Special Considerations
Gabapentinoids			
Gabapentin Pregabalin	100–300 mg 1–3 time daily 50–150 mg/d in 2–3 divided doses • Increase by 25–150 mg/d weekly	300 mg to 1200 mg 3 times daily 300–600 mg/d in 2–3 divided doses	Dose dependent CNS depression, somnolence, and dizziness may occur Increased risk of respiratory depression when combined with other CNS depressants Dose adjustment recommended for patients with renal impairment
TCAs			
Amitriptyline	10–25 mg daily at bedtime • Increase by 10–25 mg weekly	150 mg/d at bedtime	Anticholinergic effects such as constipation, blurry vision, urinary retention Cardiac conduction abnormalities (sinus tachycardia, heart block, ventricular arrhythmias)
SNRIs			
Venlafaxine	37.5 or 75 mg once daily. • Increase by 75mg weekly	225 mg once daily	May cause or worsen hypertension Limited data suggest associated with an increased risk of fragility fractures Dose adjustment may be required for renal impairment

Table 3
Skeletal muscle relaxants

Category	Starting Dose	Target Dose	Special Considerations
Antispasticity			
Baclofen	5-10 mg 3 times daily as needed		May cause significant CNS depression Dose adjustment recommended for impaired renal function. Use of medication not recommended for severe renal impairment
Antispasmodics			
Cyclobenzaprine	Immediate release: 5–10 mg three times daily. Extended release: 15–30mg daily		Anticholinergic effects Limit duration of use to <3 wk
methocarbamol	500mg or 750mg qhs 1500–2000 mg 4 times daily for 2–3 d	Maintenance dosing 750–1000 mg 3 times daily	May cause sedation, vertigo, insomnia Increased risk of respiratory depression when used in combination with benzodiazepines or opioids

to encounter older adults who are taking these medications. Common skeletal muscle relaxants, dosing, and side effects are listed in **Table 3**.

Regional Anesthesia

Regional anesthesia is an important component of acute pain management of older patients and should be offered routinely to patients with hip fractures. Patients with hip fractures are at high risk of delirium, and long hospital stays. The benefits of regional anesthesia of the femoral nerve in the management of hip fractures include improved pain management, reduced opiate use, decreased delirium, and decreased in-patient length of stay; preoperative regional anesthesia is strongly recommended by orthopedic professional societies.[53–56] In general, complications of regional anesthesia can be broadly grouped as block failure requiring alternative analgesia (or anesthesia in the operating room environment), bleeding/hematomas, neurologic injury, and local anesthetic systemic toxicity (LAST).[57]

Regional anesthesia of the femoral nerve can be accomplished by multiple techniques. The Fascia Iliaca Compartment Block (FICB) is favored for multiple reasons.[58] It is straightforward to teach and learn and can be performed under ultrasound guidance, using a landmark approach, or using a hybrid-landmark approach.[54,59] As a compartment block, the injection site is remote from the vascular bundle with a corresponding lower risk of bleeding, hematomas, and LAST. Ropivacaine, an isomer of bupivacaine, is preferred to minimize the risk of cardiovascular collapse in the unlikely event of systemic toxicity. Intralipid should always be available if large volume regional anesthesia is being performed. Many older patients are medically anticoagulated or on antiplatelet agents; proximal regional anesthesia should be avoided in these patients in the ED.[60] Similar other compartment blocks, directly targeting the nerve itself is avoided, minimizing direct injury to nerves.

Special Considerations in Older Adult Pain Management

Fragility fractures

Fractures that occur in patients with osteoporosis following minor or minimal trauma are referred to as fragility fractures. Osteoporosis is most often seen in older patients, particularly women. Fragility fractures are diagnostic for osteoporosis and often occur in older women. Generally, fragility fractures occur after ground level falls but they can also be seen with other minor traumatic events. Fragility fractures include rib, hip, pubic rami, and vertebral compression fractures (VCFs) and distal radius fractures.[61] Proximal and midshaft humerus fractures may be fragility fractures given an appropriate mechanism such as a ground level fall. VCFs can be seen without any inciting trauma. All these fractures may be seen following high-velocity traumas but the management, comorbidities, and prognoses are different for fragility fractures. This section focuses on the pain management of fragility fractures in older adults.

Hip fractures

Hip fractures are a common injury in older patients and are associated with a high 30-day and 12-month mortality.[62] Women account for about 75% of hip fractures in the United States and other high-income countries. Men who break their hips following a ground level fall usually have significant underlying comorbidities, and the 12-month mortality for a hip fracture in older men approaches 45%.[62] For many older adults, a hip fracture is a turning point in their independence, with only about 50% able to return to their prefracture mobility and 10% to 20% requiring long-term residential care.[63]

In the ED, our role is to identify the fracture, provide multimodal analgesia, and expedite surgical management.[64] Even for patients with limited mobility at baseline, operative fixation provides the best analgesia and should be offered to most patients.

Pain in the fractured hip ranges from minimal to severe and occasionally patients have been weight-bearing on a hip fracture for some time. Many patients with hip fractures are relatively pain-free at rest, experiencing pain only with movement. For this reason, it is essential to gently move the suspected leg as part of the physical examination, ideally with a rotational component. Most hip fractures are identified on plain films of the hip and pelvis. If the plain films are negative or nondiagnostic and the patient still experiences pain with weight-bearing, advanced imaging is recommended. Selective MRI after CT scan is a possible solution for identifying occult hip fractures if the initial plain films and CT scan are negative.[65]

Preoperative regional anesthesia of the femoral nerve has been recommended by the professional orthopedic societies as integral to care of patients with hip fractures.[56] Preoperative regional anesthesia may reduce the risk of delirium in hip fracture patients; this effect is tempered in patients with baseline cognitive impairment.[66,67] As mentioned above, of the multiple approaches to regional anesthesia of the femoral nerve the FICB is one of the simplest and safest methods.[54,68,69]

Multimodal analgesia is a method of improving pain control while reducing adverse drug reactions. Many health systems and EDs have care coordination pathways for hip fractures.[56] Hip fracture pathways include multimodal analgesia with acetaminophen (including intravenous administration), opioid analgesics, and regional anesthesia of the femoral nerve.

Vertebral compression fractures

VCFs can be spontaneous, progressive, or occur following a low-velocity trauma such as a fall. In general, if VCFs are subacute and not directly associated with trauma, they may be relatively painless. If traumatic, VCFs may be significantly painful. Management is determined by the degree of compression, pain, and general mobility of the patient. Spinal cord compression or other neurological impairment is uncommon with vertebral compression fractures. Acute fractures associated with greater than 50% loss of vertebral height are operatively managed with kyphoplasty or vertebroplasty.[70] Subacute fractures with less than 50% loss of vertebral height are usually managed nonoperatively. Pain control includes acetaminophen, topical lidocaine, judicious use of opioids, and intranasal calcitonin. Intranasal calcitonin is underutilized despite high efficacy and minimal side effects with one systematic review reporting a number needed to treat of 2.[71] Thoracolumbar bracing may help with pain but should not be used long term because of atrophy of core musculature and older patients may have difficulty tolerating thoracolumbar bracing.

Rib fractures

The location of ribs makes them vulnerable to fractures following a ground level fall. As pneumonia is the most common complication of rib fractures after low velocity injuries, management should include analgesia sufficient to allow respiration and mobility. Pain limiting overall mobility and specifically deep inspiration, increases the risk of atelectasis and subsequent pneumonia. Analgesic requirements may range from acetaminophen to regional anesthesia including serratus anterior blocks.

Pelvic fragility fractures

The pelvis is another location vulnerable to osteoporosis and fractures. Nondisplaced acetabular and pubic rami fractures are commonly seen in older patients following a ground level fall. Pubic rami fractures are often identified when a patient is being evaluated for hip or groin pain following a fall. Management is usually nonoperative.

SUMMARY

Pain assessment and management in older adults is complex and requires evaluation and consideration of the type of pain, the acuity of the condition, comorbidities, and medications. Many older adults do not receive appropriate therapy for painful conditions, including fractures. This review is focused on pharmacologic agents, drug–drug interactions, drug–disease interactions, and approaches in the management of painful conditions seen in older adults in the emergency department.

CLINICS CARE POINTS

- Acute pain is undertreated in older adults.
- Assess for pain and response to interventions frequently in the emergency department.
- A step-wise approach to pain medications is best, starting with oral acetaminophen and escalating as needed.
- Use the lowest effective dose for the shortest amount of time.
- Special consideration is required for polypharmacy, medication interactions, and opiate use disorder.

DISCLOSURE

No authors have any commercial or financial conflicts of interest.

FUNDING

There is no funding source for these authors.

REFERENCES

1. Chang HY, Daubresse M, Kruszewski SP, et al. Prevalence and treatment of pain in EDs in the United States, 2000 to 2010. Am J Emerg Med 2014;32(5): 421–31.
2. Gray LC, Peel NM, Costa AP, et al. Profiles of older patients in the emergency department: findings from the interRAI Multinational Emergency Department Study. Ann Emerg Med 2013;62(5):467–74.
3. Hwang U, Richardson LD, Harris B, et al. The quality of emergency department pain care for older adult patients. J Am Geriatr Soc 2010;58(11):2122–8.
4. Platts-Mills TF, Esserman DA, Brown DL, et al. Older US emergency department patients are less likely to receive pain medication than younger patients: results from a national survey. Research Support, N.I.H., Extramural. Ann Emerg Med 2012;60(2):199–206.
5. Patel KV, Guralnik JM, Dansie EJ, et al. Prevalence and impact of pain among older adults in the United States: findings from the 2011 National Health and Aging Trends Study. Pain 2013;154(12):2649–57.
6. Abdulla A, Adams N, Bone M, et al. Guidance on the management of pain in older people. Age Ageing 2013;42(Suppl 1):i1–57.

7. Schofield P. The assessment of pain in older people: UK national guidelines. Age Ageing 2018;47(suppl_1):i1–22.

8. American geriatrics society Panel on pharmacological management of persistent pain in older persons. J Am Geriatr Soc 2009;57(8):1331–46.

9. American Geriatrics Society updated Beers Criteria for potentially inappropriate medication use in older adults. Review. J Am Geriatr Soc 2012;60(4):616–31.

10. American geriatrics society 2019 updated AGS Beers Criteria® for potentially inappropriate medication Use in older adults. J Am Geriatr Soc 2019;67(4): 674–94.

11. Mangin D, Bahat G, Golomb BA, et al. International group for reducing inappropriate medication Use & Polypharmacy (IGRIMUP): Position statement and 10 Recommendations for action. Drugs Aging 2018;35(7):575–87.

12. Schmader KE, Baron R, Haanpää ML, et al. Treatment considerations for elderly and frail patients with neuropathic pain. Mayo Clin Proc 2010;85(3 Suppl):S26–32.

13. Virnes RE, Tiihonen M, Karttunen N, et al. Opioids and falls risk in older adults: a narrative review. Drugs Aging 2022;39(3):199–207.

14. Bloomer A, Wally M, Bailey G, et al. Balancing safety, Comfort, and fall risk: an Intervention to Limit opioid and benzodiazepine prescriptions for geriatric patients. Geriatr Orthop Surg Rehabil 2022;13. 21514593221125616.

15. Makris UE, Abrams RC, Gurland B, et al. Management of persistent pain in the older patient: a clinical review. JAMA 2014;312(8):825–36.

16. Tracey I, Woolf CJ, Andrews NA. Composite pain biomarker Signatures for Objective assessment and effective treatment. Neuron 2019;101(5):783–800.

17. Karcioglu O, Topacoglu H, Dikme O, et al. A systematic review of the pain scales in adults: which to use? Am J Emerg Med 2018;36(4):707–14.

18. Hadjistavropoulos T, Herr K, Turk DC, et al. An interdisciplinary expert consensus statement on assessment of pain in older persons. Clin J Pain 2007;23(1 Suppl): S1–43.

19. Malara A, De Biase GA, Bettarini F, et al. Pain assessment in elderly with behavioral and Psychological symptoms of Dementia. J Alzheimers Dis 2016;50(4): 1217–25.

20. Warden V, Hurley AC, Volicer L. Development and psychometric evaluation of the pain assessment in advanced Dementia (PAINAD) scale. J Am Med Dir Assoc 2003;4(1):9–15.

21. Bowie MW, Slattum PW. Pharmacodynamics in older adults: a review. Am J Geriatr Pharmacother 2007;5(3):263–303.

22. Hanlon JT, Aspinall SL, Semla TP, et al. Consensus guidelines for oral dosing of primarily renally cleared medications in older adults. J Am Geriatr Soc 2009; 57(2):335–40.

23. Dresden SM, Allen K, Lyden AE. Common medication management approaches for older adults in the emergency department. Clin Geriatr Med 2018;34(3): 415–33.

24. Khan NF, Bykov K, Barnett ML, et al. Comparative risk of opioid overdose with concomitant Use of prescription opioids and skeletal muscle relaxants. Neurology 2022;99(13):e1432–42.

25. Chan HKI, Chan CPI. Managing chronic pain in older people. Clin Med 2022; 22(4):292–4.

26. Pickering G, Marcoux M, Chapiro S, et al. An Algorithm for neuropathic pain management in older people. Drugs Aging 2016;33(8):575–83.

27. Graham GG, Davies MJ, Day RO, et al. The modern pharmacology of paracetamol: therapeutic actions, mechanism of action, metabolism, toxicity and recent pharmacological findings. Inflammopharmacology 2013;21(3):201–32.
28. What dose of paracetamol for older people? Drug Ther Bull 2018;56(6):69–72.
29. Pharmacological management of persistent pain in older persons. Pain Med 2009;10(6):1062–83.
30. Fu JL, Perloff MD. Pharmacotherapy for spine-related pain in older adults. Drugs Aging 2022;39(7):523–50.
31. Al Farii H, Farahdel L, Frazer A, et al. The effect of NSAIDs on postfracture bone healing: a meta-analysis of randomized controlled trials. OTA Int 2021;4(2):e092.
32. Vascular and upper gastrointestinal effects of non-steroidal anti-inflammatory drugs: meta-analyses of individual participant data from randomised trials. Lancet 2013;382(9894):769–79.
33. Savarino V, Marabotto E, Zentilin P, et al. Proton pump inhibitors: use and misuse in the clinical setting. Expert Rev Clin Pharmacol 2018;11(11):1123–34.
34. Wang K, Li X. Comparison of cardiorenal safety of nonsteroidal anti-inflammatory drugs in the treatment of arthritis: a network meta-analysis. Ann Transl Med 2022; 10(24):1388.
35. Derry S, Conaghan P, Da Silva JAP, et al. Topical NSAIDs for chronic musculoskeletal pain in adults. Cochrane Database Syst Rev 2016;4. https://doi.org/10. 1002/14651858.CD007400.pub3.
36. Derry S, Moore RA, Gaskell H, et al. Topical NSAIDs for acute musculoskeletal pain in adults. Cochrane Database Syst Rev 2015;6. https://doi.org/10.1002/ 14651858.CD007402.pub3.
37. Derry S, Wiffen PJ, Kalso EA, et al. Topical analgesics for acute and chronic pain in adults - an overview of Cochrane Reviews. Cochrane Database Syst Rev 2017; 5(5):CD008609.
38. Tracy B, Sean Morrison R. Pain management in older adults. Clin Therapeut 2013; 35(11):1659–68.
39. McLachlan AJ, Bath S, Naganathan V, et al. Clinical pharmacology of analgesic medicines in older people: impact of frailty and cognitive impairment. Br J Clin Pharmacol 2011;71(3):351–64.
40. Daoust R, Paquet J, Boucher V, et al. Relationship between pain, opioid treatment, and delirium in older emergency department patients. Acad Emerg Med 2020;27(8):708–16.
41. Shoff C, Yang TC, Shaw BA. Trends in opioid use disorder among older adults: analyzing medicare data, 2013-2018. Am J Prev Med 2021;60(6):850–5.
42. Mason M, Soliman R, Kim HS, et al. Disparities by Sex and Race and Ethnicity in death rates due to opioid overdose among adults 55 Years or older, 1999 to 2019. JAMA Netw Open 2022;5(1). e2142982.
43. Wakeman SE, Larochelle MR, Ameli O, et al. Comparative effectiveness of different treatment pathways for opioid Use disorder. JAMA Netw Open 2020; 3(2). e1920622.
44. Carew AM, Comiskey C. Treatment for opioid use and outcomes in older adults: a systematic literature review. Drug Alcohol Depend 2018;182:48–57.
45. Rieb LM, Samaan Z, Furlan AD, et al. Canadian guidelines on opioid Use disorder among older adults. Can Geriatr J 2020;23(1):123–34.
46. Dworkin RH, O'Connor AB, Audette J, et al. Recommendations for the pharmacological management of neuropathic pain: an overview and literature update. Mayo Clin Proc 2010;85(3 Suppl):S3–14.

47. Moore A, Derry S, Wiffen P. Gabapentin for chronic neuropathic pain. JAMA 2018; 319(8):818–9.
48. Cavalli E, Mammana S, Nicoletti F, et al. The neuropathic pain: an overview of the current treatment and future therapeutic approaches. Int J Immunopathol Pharmacol 2019;33. 2058738419838383.
49. Goodman CW, Brett AS. A clinical overview of Off-label Use of gabapentinoid drugs. JAMA Intern Med 2019;179(5):695–701.
50. Urits I, Peck J, Orhurhu MS, et al. Off-label antidepressant Use for treatment and management of chronic pain: Evolving Understanding and Comprehensive review. Curr Pain Headache Rep 2019;23(9):66.
51. See S, Ginzburg R. Skeletal muscle relaxants. Pharmacotherapy 2008;28(2):207–13.
52. Witenko C, Moorman-Li R, Motycka C, et al. Considerations for the appropriate use of skeletal muscle relaxants for the management of acute low back pain. P t 2014;39(6):427–35.
53. Ritcey B, Pageau P, Woo MY, et al. Regional nerve blocks for hip and femoral Neck fractures in the emergency department: a systematic review. Cjem 2016; 18(1):37–47.
54. Kolodychuk N, Krebs JC, Stenberg R, et al. Fascia iliaca blocks performed in the emergency department decrease opioid consumption and length of stay in patients with hip fracture. J Orthop Trauma 2022;36(3):142–6.
55. Wennberg P, Norlin R, Herlitz J, et al. Pre-operative pain management with nerve block in patients with hip fractures: a randomized, controlled trial. Int J Orthop Trauma Nurs 2019;33:35–43.
56. Switzer JA, O'Connor MI. AAOS management of hip fractures in older adults evidence-based clinical Practice Guideline. J Am Acad Orthop Surg 2022; 30(20):e1297–301.
57. Shams D, Sachse K, Statzer N, et al. Regional anesthesia complications and Contraindications. Clin Sports Med 2022;41(2):329–43.
58. O'Reilly N, Desmet M, Kearns R. Fascia iliaca compartment block. BJA Educ 2019;19(6):191–7.
59. Steenberg J, Møller AM. Systematic review of the effects of fascia iliaca compartment block on hip fracture patients before operation. Br J Anaesth 2018;120(6): 1368–80.
60. Kietaibl S, Ferrandis R, Godier A, et al. Regional anaesthesia in patients on antithrombotic drugs: joint ESAIC/ESRA guidelines. Eur J Anaesthesiol 2022;39(2): 100–32.
61. Sahota O, van Berkel D, Ong T, et al. Pelvic fragility fractures-the forgotten osteoporotic fracture. Osteoporosis international 2021;32(4):785–6.
62. Guzon-Illescas O, Perez Fernandez E, Crespí Villarias N, et al. Mortality after osteoporotic hip fracture: incidence, trends, and associated factors. J Orthop Surg Res 2019;14(1):203.
63. Dyer SM, Crotty M, Fairhall N, et al. A critical review of the long-term disability outcomes following hip fracture. BMC Geriatr 2016;16(1):158.
64. Accelerated surgery versus standard care in hip fracture (HIP ATTACK): an international, randomised, controlled trial. Lancet 2020;395(10225):698–708.
65. Davidson A, Silver N, Cohen D, et al. Justifying CT prior to MRI in cases of suspected occult hip fracture. A proposed diagnostic protocol. Injury 2021;52(6): 1429–33.

66. Casey SD, Stevenson DE, Mumma BE, et al. Emergency department pain management following Implementation of a geriatric hip fracture Program. West J Emerg Med 2017;0(0).

67. Kim CH, Yang JY, Min CH, et al. The effect of regional nerve block on perioperative delirium in hip fracture surgery for the elderly: a systematic review and meta-analysis of randomized controlled trials. Orthop Traumatol Surg Res 2022;108(1):103151.

68. Schulte SS, Fernandez I, Van Tienderen R, et al. Impact of the fascia iliaca block on pain, opioid consumption, and Ambulation for patients with hip fractures: a Prospective, randomized Study. J Orthop Trauma 2020;34(10):533–8.

69. Garlich JM, Pujari A, Moak Z, et al. Pain management with Early regional anesthesia in geriatric hip fracture patients. J Am Geriatr Soc 2020;68(9):2043–50.

70. Patel D, Liu J, Ebraheim NA. Managements of osteoporotic vertebral compression fractures: a narrative review. World J Orthop 2022;13(6):564–73.

71. Boucher E, Rosgen B, Lang E. Efficacy of calcitonin for treating acute pain associated with osteoporotic vertebral compression fracture: an updated systematic review. Cjem 2020;22(3):359–67.

Adverse Drug Event Prevention and Detection in Older Emergency Department Patients

Jennifer L. Koehl, PharmD, BCPS

KEYWORDS

- Polypharmacy • Prescribing cascade • Adverse drug event • Medication review
- Deprescribe • Potentially inappropriate medication

KEY POINTS

- Multimorbidity, changes in physiologic function, and polypharmacy make older adults seven times more likely to have an adverse drug event requiring hospitalization.
- About 45% of older patients are discharged from the emergency department (ED) with at least one new prescription medication with 11.6% being potentially inappropriate.
- Existing prescribing references can be classified as explicit (criterion-based) or implicit (judgment based), however, they are not comprehensive nor ED-specific, and must be put in context of the individual patient.
- Medication review, reconciliation, and deprescribing are important components of geriatric assessments in the ED.
- Adverse drug events that are misinterpreted as a sign or symptom of a new disorder results in prescribing cascades.

INTRODUCTION

Across the globe, people are living longer and the medical field continues to develop and prescribe therapies to enhance the quality and longevity of life in our growing geriatric population. With the benefits of medication therapy also comes the potential for adverse drug events (ADEs). There are five categories of ADEs: adverse medication reactions, medication errors, therapeutic failures, adverse medication withdrawal events, and overdoses.[1] Adverse medication reactions are the most common, accounting for three-fourths of hospitalizations from ADEs, with the remainder caused by nonadherence, omission, or cessation of treatment.[2] This article will refer to

Department of Pharmacy, Emergency Medicine, Massachusetts General Hospital, 55 Fruit Street, Boston, MA 02114, USA
E-mail address: jkoehl@mgh.harvard.edu

Clin Geriatr Med 39 (2023) 635–645
https://doi.org/10.1016/j.cger.2023.04.008
0749-0690/23/© 2023 Elsevier Inc. All rights reserved.

ADEs as any unintended or undesired effect of a medication due to multimorbidity, polypharmacy, or modified physiologic function.

Older adults are nearly seven times more likely to have an ADE requiring hospitalization that commonly results from polypharmacy, as 39% of adults aged 65 or older take more than five medications.[3–5] Antiplatelets, diuretics, nonsteroidal anti-inflammatory medications (NSAIDs), and anticoagulants account for > 50% of preventable medication-related hospital admissions. The most common consequences of ADEs include falls, orthostatic hypotension, heart and/or renal failure, gastrointestinal and internal bleeding, and delirium.[6]

Studies have shown that more than one-half of the ADEs in the outpatient setting are potentially preventable and inevitably increase health care costs to both the patient and the health care system.[7] As a result, improving prescribing of medications from the emergency department (ED) is paramount as nearly 45% of older patients are discharged from the ED with at least one new prescription medication,[8] and of these, 11.6% are medications recommended to avoid in older adults.[9,10]

DISCUSSION
Adverse Drug Events as a Geriatric Syndrome

A broad approach is needed to address ADEs in older adults and medication-related harm should be treated as a geriatric syndrome. ED clinicians must have a high index of suspicion for medication-related ADEs as they are often difficult to recognize due to nonspecific presenting clinical symptoms. Clinical suspicion should be heightened if a patient has a change in activities of daily living due to cognitive or functional decline, has new symptoms after starting a medication or dose titration, or changes in physiologic function that could alter pharmacokinetics and pharmacodynamics of the medication. Lack of identifying medication-related ADEs increases the risk of propagating prescribing cascades. A prescribing cascade occurs when the ADE is misinterpreted as a sign or symptom of a new disorder and then a new medication is prescribed to treat it. This is problematic as several ADEs resemble symptoms of disorders common in older adults or changes due to aging. For example, cholinesterase inhibitors (donepezil, rivastigmine) may cause urinary frequency or urge incontinence which if thought to be a new condition may then be treated with anticholinergic medications or antibiotics rather than deprescribing the offending agent. Another common example is dihydropyridine calcium channel blockers (eg, nifedipine, felodipine, and amlodipine) causing peripheral edema that is confused for volume overload leading to addition of unnecessary diuretic therapy. Prescribing cascades have become more common, especially in settings such as the ED where the treating team often knows the least about the patient's medical and prescriptive history.

Aging Effects on Pharmacokinetics

With biological aging, we experience a decline in organ and body functions that alter the pharmacokinetics (PK) and pharmacodynamics (PD) of many medications (Table 1). PK refers to the movement of the medication into, around, and out of the body including its absorption, distribution, metabolism, and excretion, whereas PD refers to the physiologic effects that the medication has on our body.[11] In short, PK are what the body does to the drug and PD are what the drug does to the body. Older adults tend to have smaller body compositions, less water, and larger proportions of fat. This impacts many medications differently depending on their hydrophilic or lipophilic properties resulting in either enhanced or diminished medication exposure and distribution throughout the body. Systemic circulation and blood flow throughout

Table 1
Physiologic changes in geriatric patients

PK Process	Physiologic Change	Impact on Drug Exposure
Absorption	↓ GI motility ↓ Splanchnic blood flow ↓ Mucosal surface area ↓ Perfusion to cutaneous tissue	↑ GI absorption time: ↑ time to therapeutic effect and ↑ serum drug concentrations ↓ Passive diffusion in GI tract: ↓ serum drug concentrations ↓ GI metabolism: ↑ serum drug concentrations ↑ Erratic intramuscular, subcutaneous, and transdermal absorption
Distribution	↑ Total body fat ↓ Lean body mass ↓ Total body water ↓ Serum proteins	↑ Distribution of fat-soluble drugs: ↓ serum concentration of lipophilic drugs and ↑ total body accumulation with repeat dosing–> ↑ duration of therapeutic effect ↓ Distribution of water-soluble drug: ↑ serum concentrations of hydrophilic drugs and risk of toxicity ↓ Binding of acidic drugs to albumin: ↑ concentrations of free drug and risk of toxicity
Metabolism	↓ Liver mass ↓ Hepatic blood flow	↓ Hepatic metabolism: ↑ serum drug concentrations and risk of toxicity ↓ Conversion of pro-drug to active drug: ↓ pharmacologic effect
Elimination	↓ Nephron size ↓ Renal blood flow	↓ Glomerular filtration of medications: ↓ elimination of drug from the body and ↑ risk of accumulation

the body decreases with age including blood flow to the gastrointestinal tract, liver, and kidneys that impact medication absorption, metabolism, and excretion.[12] The volume of the liver and kidney also change with reduced nephrons and hepatocytes resulting in impaired organ function and ability to process and excrete medications. Many medications have a high first-pass metabolism through the liver where a portion of the medication is metabolized before reaching systemic circulation, and without this, there can be significant increases in medication bioavailability and risk of toxicity. Additionally, some medications are pro-drugs and require first-pass metabolism for activation resulting in lower concentrations of active drug in the setting of liver dysfunction. Decreased blood flow to the kidneys and impaired kidney function lead to reduced elimination of drug from the body and risk of accumulation. These physiologic changes in body size and altered body composition (more fat, less water), along with decreased gastrointestinal, liver, and kidney function cause many medications to accumulate in older people's bodies at higher levels and for longer durations resulting in drug-related ADEs. This is compounded by older adults being more frail and vulnerable to ADEs with reduced ability to maintain their blood pressure and temperature, having more diseases that affect response to medications, and increased sensitivity to the therapeutic effects of certain medications including those that work on the central nervous system due to increased permeability of the blood–brain barrier.[13]

As a result, physiologic changes are patient- and medication-specific and may result in increased or decreased medication exposure, duration of pharmacologic effect, and toxicity. For this reason, it is best to select a medication with a large therapeutic index so that there is a wider range between therapeutic and toxic doses.[11] The mantra of "start low and go slow" is an important principal for dose selection and titration, however, ADEs can occur at any dosage and effective dosages of medications must be prescribed to prevent medication failure.

Implicit and Explicit Prescribing and Deprescribing Tools

Several prescribing/deprescribing references have been created to improve our prescribing practices in older adults. Prescribing/deprescribing tools are classified as explicit (criterion-based) or implicit (judgment-based). Explicit tools such as the Beers Criteria, Screening Tool of Older Persons' potentially inappropriate Prescriptions (STOPP)/Screening Tool to Alert to Right Treatment (START) criteria, and European Union (EU) (7) criteria contain lists of medications or medication classes that are felt to expose older adults to potential harms.[14–16] The most historic and widely used reference assigning medications as potentially harmful is the Beers Criteria. The Beers Criteria were developed with the purpose of identifying medications for which potential harm outweighed the expected benefit and that should be avoided in nursing home residents. In addition to highlighting risk of medications as monotherapy, the Beers Criteria more recent updates also recognize the risks associated with concurrent use of medications with similar side effect profiles such as additive anticholinergic burden. This concept of cumulative side effect burden is complex but mirrors real-world practice.

The STOPP criteria were developed due to several criticisms surrounding realistic use of the Beers Criteria and the fact that several large studies have not found an association between prescribing of medications on the Beers Criteria and the occurrence of ADEs.[17] Unlike the Beers Criteria, the STOPP criteria are organized by physiologic system, contain only medications that are in widespread use, identify potentially inappropriate drug–drug interactions, and discuss the risk of duplicate medication class prescribing. STOPP criteria are designed to be used in conjunction with the START criteria which describe inappropriate omission of potentially beneficial medications that likely should be prescribed but are not for various reasons, including perceived high-level frailty.[14]

The risk of employing explicit tools such as the Beers Criteria and STOPP/START criteria is that the recommendations can be applied with little clinical judgment, do not address individual differences between patients, and generally do not take into account comorbidities. Explicit tools also do not incorporate patient preferences or previous treatment successes or failures. Although important references for prescribing, more research is needed to know whether routine application of the Beers Criteria and STOPP/START criteria leads to meaningful clinical benefits and significant reductions in health care costs. Moreover, as these tools were not developed for use in the ED specifically, research is needed to look at their utility in the ED setting. One study reported that among 400 older adults discharged from their ED, 304 patients (76%) received a medication deemed potentially inappropriate by the Beers Criteria, however, none of these patients returned within 7 days with an identified medication-related adverse event.[15]

Conversely, implicit prescribing assessment tools such as the Medication Appropriateness Index (MAI) require knowledge of individual treatment goals and comorbidities in the context of each prescribed medication by incorporating clinical information from the individual patient assessment.[16] MAI assesses 10 elements of prescribing: indication, effectiveness, dose, correct directions, practical directions, drug–drug and drug–disease interactions, dual therapy, duration of therapy, and cost. Assessing these elements results in a weighted score that serves as a guide to determine if the medication is appropriate for the individual patient.[16] Although the MAI is patient-centered, it is more time-consuming and highly user-dependent.

Patient- and Medication-Specific Considerations

Although these prescribing tools are helpful in reducing ADEs in older adults, they are not comprehensive, and adults are frequently admitted to hospitals with ADEs from medications not listed in any of these prescribing references. Additionally, these references miss several important patient-level considerations nuanced to the geriatric population. For example, older adults have the likelihood of being prescribed the same medication multiple times throughout their lifespan which for some medications increases the risk of medication-related harm. An example of this is the commonly prescribed antibiotic nitrofurantoin (Macrobid) used to treat urinary tract infections. With repeat exposures to nitrofurantoin, there is an increased risk of pulmonary toxicity in the form of diffuse interstitial pneumonitis and bronchiolitis, thought to reflect an allergic or toxic response.[18,19] In addition to multiple exposures to medications, duration of exposure is also important. For example, first- and second-generation antipsychotics carry black box warnings that their use in elderly patients with dementia-related psychosis results in an increased risk of death based on several epidemiological studies in the outpatient- or long-term care setting.[20,21] This association was further explored in the inpatient setting where it was found that typical and atypical antipsychotics were associated with increased risk of mortality or cardiopulmonary arrest, however, the chronicity of exposure was not detailed.[22] One-time administration of these medications to manage severe agitation in the ED setting may not carry the same risks. What is more important in this scenario are patient-specific characteristics such as the presence of Parkinson's disease or Lewy body dementia which should steer us away from first-generation antipsychotic use due to their high degree of dopamine receptor blockade, which may worsen movement disorders in these patients.[23] These examples highlight the fact that it is impossible to create a comprehensive list of medications that should not be prescribed to older adults, and decisions should be made based on the patient and clinical scenario with continuous review of the medication list for optimization and deprescribing opportunities.

When we review prescribing/deprescribing references, a major focus is on reducing the use of medications that have central-nervous-system-related effects including over-sedation, confusion, delirium, and hallucinations. Delirium, or acute confusional states, affects up to 7 million (30–40%) hospitalized older adults annually,[24] and is associated with increased risk of mortality, institutionalization, and cognitive and functional impairment.[25] Medications have been cited as one of the most common causes of delirium and potentially one of the most preventable and treatable. In fact, medications are the sole precipitant for delirium in up to 39% of cases.[26] Despite this, few studies have investigated this topic and so the role of many medications in the development of delirium remains unclear. A recent systematic review found only 14 studies examining the association between medications and delirium, with half examining only a single medication class, and all being low to moderate quality.[27] Increased risk was found for opioids, benzodiazepines, and dihydropyridine calcium channel blockers, but not with several other medications widely thought to be delirogenic in the Beers Criteria and STOPP criteria.

In addition to physiologic changes, older adults have complex living situations that must be considered. When prescribing medications, it is important to discuss who will be administering the medications, how many times a day the individual is able to take medications, and how they are taking their medications. More in-depth consideration must be made when considering the dangers of a mistaken overdose, missed dose, and incorrect method of administration that may change the PK and PD of the drug.

PRESCRIBING AND DEPRESCRIBING ELECTRONIC TOOLS

To enhance the safety of prescribing new medications, computerized clinical decision support systems that utilize ADE predictor variables have been created to help identify patients who may be at increased risk. To date, three validated predictive tools have been created, but none have been found to have sufficient predictive value.[28] A large number of variables contribute to ADE occurrence in older patients, thus rendering it difficult to develop a robust ADE prediction tool that is applicable to a heterogeneous population.[29]

There has also been a dedicated effort to design and implement electronic prescribing support systems with improved sensitivity to detect inappropriate prescribing of medications with greater specificity to reduce prescriber alert fatigue. Although many electronic health record software companies have released platforms that alert providers if available patient data do not align with the safe use of certain medications, there are several deficiencies in these systems. First, chronic medications may be missing from the patient's electronic medical record resulting in a missed alert. Second, many of these detection systems are exclusive to inpatient prescribing and do not assess medication prescribing at the time of inpatient or ED discharge. Third, these detection systems are not complex enough to identify meaningful drug–disease interactions that may result from multi-organ involvement. Fourth, alert fatigue remains a problem with a high percentage of alerts bypassed with little review.

The Veterans Health Administration (VA) has developed programs to enhance the quality of prescribing and deprescribing practices that have been successfully implemented in academic health systems. The Enhancing the Quality of Prescribing Practices for Older Adults Discharged from the Emergency Department (EQUIPPED) medication safety program aims at reducing provider prescribing of potentially inappropriate medications (PIM) for older adults at the time of ED discharge. EQUIPPED involves three core components including provider education, clinical decision support in the form of discharge medication order sets, and provider audit and feedback using the American Geriatrics Society Beers Criteria to determine.[9] VA-based EQUIPPED programs have shown a significant reduction in PIM prescribing at the time of ED discharge and although exporting this program to non-VA academic medical centers did not show similar impact consistently, the core components of provider education and implementation of geriatric-friendly order sets universally improves prescribing practices.[30]

The VA also has created an electronic deprescribing medication management tool called VIONE that places medications into categories of necessity including Vital (V), Important (I), Optional (O), and Not indicated (N). When reviewing each medication on the home medication list, the provider or pharmacist places each medication into the appropriate VIONE category electronically with subsequent deprescribing if appropriate. Upon medication discontinuation, a dropdown menu delineates reasons for discontinuation: dose decrease, no diagnosis, not indicated/treatment complete, discontinue alternate medication prescribed, and patient reported no longer taking that improves information sharing across transitions of care.[31]

INTEGRATING INTO EMERGENCY DEPARTMENT WORKFLOW

Optimal geriatric care in the ED requires a multispecialty, multidisciplinary approach rooted in comprehensive patient assessments, effective team communication, shared goals of care, and leveraging informatics when applicable.[32]

The American College of Emergency Physicians launched a Geriatric ED Accreditation (GEDA) program consisting of accreditation levels based on adherence to policies and protocols that improve emergency care of older ED patients. Specific to pharmacotherapy, the GEDA program recommends establishing a pharmacist-led medication reconciliation process and designing a program to minimize the use of PIMs with the incorporation of geriatric-specific order sets.[33]

As recommended by GEDA, a structured, comprehensive geriatric assessment that includes medication review and reconciliation is vital to assess medication-related ADEs as the presenting diagnoses and has shown to reduce length of stay and in-hospital mortality.[34] Furthermore, medication lists should not be propagated from prior encounters, and an accurate medication list should be obtained at every ED visit as it has been found that up to 94% of geriatric patients have a medication discrepancy following review.[35]

Many organizations take a multidisciplinary approach to complete medication history taking and subsequent reconciliation, utilizing pharmacists, physicians, and nurses, based on resource allocation. Pharmacists are an incredible resource within the medical team able to obtain accurate medication histories, update home medication lists, and review prescriber orders before administration. The presence of a pharmacist on the care team has shown to increase the quality of patient care while positively affecting the workload of the interprofessional team.[36] However, as clinical pharmacy services continue to expand in the ED, it is not always feasible for the pharmacist to perform the medication history. As a result, utilizing pharmacy extenders (pharmacy technicians, pharmacy students, etc.) to perform the medication histories has resulted in improved allocation of resources and retained accuracy of medication review.[37] In addition to medication history taking, extending the pharmacists' role to include ordering home medications for hospital administration has been shown to increase prescribing accuracy and efficiency.[38]

Although reviewing the home medication list, the medical team should actively evaluate the appropriateness of each medication. Particular attention should be given when assessing high-risk medications present on the medication list (**Box 1**). There are many guidelines and recommendations that identify different medications and medication classes as potentially inappropriate depending on the patient population, with no widely used or streamlined approach to review or deprescribe those medications in the ED. The most straightforward recommendation is that the medication list should serve as the problem list and if there is a medication that does not treat a

---

Box 1
High-risk medications

- Anticoagulants and anti-platelet medications
- Anti-hyperglycemics
- Cardiac medications including digoxin, amiodarone, B-blockers, Ca channel blockers
- Diuretics
- Narcotics
- Antipsychotics and other psychiatric medications
- Immunosuppressant medications, including chemotherapy agents
- Anticholinergic agents
- Sedatives and sedative-hypnotics

Table 2	
Mnemonics for safe and appropriate medication prescribing	
DRUGS	*D: Discuss goals of care with the patient keeping in mind* that quality-of-life most valued by the patient should take precedence over the routine implementation of practice guidelines *R:* Review all medications *U:* Use available reference tools to help guide prescribing decisions *G:* Geriatric appropriate to dosage and titrations *S:* Stop the medication when appropriate
ARMOR	*A:* Assess (medications) *R:* Review (interactions: drug–drug, drug–disease, ADR) *M:* Minimize (number of drugs and functional status) *O:* Optimize (for renal/hepatic clearance) *R:* Re-assess (functional/cognitive/clinical status; compliance) to improve functional status

current problem or does not align with the patient's adherence, compliance, or preference it should be deprescribed.

When a new medication is prescribed in the ED or at the time of discharge, electronic order sets and clinical decision support can help guide prescribing. However, implementing evidence-based medication safety programs across institutions is challenging due to clinical and environmental differences and prioritization of electronic health record (EHR) advancement. Without integrated EHR upgrades, ED pharmacists can facilitate widespread teaching of geriatric psychopharmacology and guideline recommendations, and dissemination order sets outside of the EHR.[39] One study found that when pharmacists were part of the geriatric assessment team, there was a 16% reduction in all visits to the hospital, a 47% reduction in visits to the ED, and an 80% reduction in medication-related readmissions. These improvements led to a lower total cost per patient of $230 compared to the care team without pharmacist involvement.[40]

New medications should be prescribed cautiously with clear therapeutic goals and recognition of the impact a medication can have on multiple organ systems. There are several mnemonics aimed at improving *prescribing of new medications to older adults* **(Table 2)**. Furthermore, empiric medication trials should include a target date when effectiveness and potential ADEs are reviewed *along with direct communication to outpatient providers and the ambulatory care team that outlines medication changes and reassessment plans whereby improving safe medication use across the care continuum.*

SUMMARY

Avoiding ADEs has become a national health priority identified as having a substantial impact on health outcomes and health care costs, and the presence of multimorbidity, changes in physiologic function, and polypharmacy make older adults more vulnerable to medication-related ADEs. Criteria used to identify PIM are not meant to replace clinical judgment; rather, they are designed to create educational guidelines. The decision to prescribe any medication, the choice of medication, and the way it is prescribed are all factors that are under the control of the provider as not all PIM can or should be avoided. Therefore, prescribing decisions must be individualized based on medical, functional, and social conditions; quality-o- life; and prognosis, and should involve shared decision-making.

CLINICS CARE POINT

- An individualized, multidisciplinary, and multifaceted approach should be taken when assessing the appropriateness of pharmacotherapy and risk of ADEs with continued emphasis on medication review and deprescribing

- Obtaining an accurate medication list is of upmost importance and should be a primary step in the comprehensive geriatric assessment

- The medication list should serve as the problem list and if there is a medication that does not treat a current problem or does not align with the patient's adherence, compliance, or preference, it should be deprescribed

- When prescribing a new medication, only one new medication should be added at a time with clear concise information given to the patient and their caregivers describing the purpose of the medication, dose titrations, monitoring requirements, and potential ADEs

- Interactive support tools in the form of geriatric-friendly medication order sets and multidisciplinary geriatric consultations with subsequent provider education lead to the greatest sustainable improvement in prescribing medications to older adults

DISCLOSURE

This author has no relationships to disclose.

REFERENCES

1. Nebeker JR, Barach P, Samore MH. Clarifying adverse drug events: a clinician's guide to terminology, documentation, and reporting. Ann Intern Med 2004; 140(10):795–801.
2. Chan M, Nicklason F, Vial JH. Adverse drug events as a cause of hospital admission in the elderly. Intern Med J 2001;31(4):199–205.
3. Budnitz DS, Pollock DA, Weidenbach KN, et al. National surveillance of emergency department visits for outpatient adverse drug events. JAMA 2006; 296(15):1858–66.
4. Khezrian M, McNeil CJ, Murray AD, et al. An overview of prevalence, determinants and health outcomes of polypharmacy. Ther Adv Drug Saf 2020;11. https://doi.org/10.1177/2042098620933741. 2042098620933741.
5. Kantor ED, Rehm CD, Haas JS, et al. Trends in prescription drug use among adults in the United States from 1999-2012. JAMA 2015;314(17):1818–31.
6. Lavan AH, Gallagher P. Predicting risk of adverse drug reactions in older adults. Ther Adv Drug Saf 2016;7(1):11–22.
7. Pretorius RW, Gataric G, Swedlund SK, et al. Reducing the risk of adverse drug events in older adults. Am Fam Physician 2013;87(5):331–6.
8. Shehab N, Lovegrove MC, Geller AI, et al. US emergency department visits for outpatient adverse drug events, 2013-2014. JAMA 2016;316(20):2115–25.
9. Stevens M, Hastings SN, Markland AD, et al. Enhancing quality of provider practices for older adults in the emergency department (EQUiPPED). J Am Geriatr Soc 2017;65(7):1609–14.
10. Hastings SN, Schmader KE, Sloane RJ, et al. Quality of pharmacotherapy and outcomes for older veterans discharged from the emergency department. J Am Geriatr Soc 2008;56(5):875–80.
11. Drenth-van Maanen AC, Wilting I, Jansen PAF. Prescribing medicines to older people-How to consider the impact of ageing on human organ and body functions. Br J Clin Pharmacol 2020;86(10):1921–30.

12. Kirkwood TB. A systematic look at an old problem. Nature 2008;451(7179):644–7.

13. Reeve E, Wiese MD, Mangoni AA. Alterations in drug disposition in older adults. Expert Opin Drug Metab Toxicol 2015;11(4):491–508.

14. Barry PJ, Gallagher P, Ryan C, et al. START (screening tool to alert doctors to the right treatment)–an evidence-based screening tool to detect prescribing omissions in elderly patients. Age Ageing 2007;36(6):632–8.

15. Harrison L, O'Connor E, Jie C, et al. Potentially inappropriate medication prescribing in the elderly: is the beers criteria relevant in the emergency department today? Am J Emerg Med 2019;37(9):1734–7.

16. Hanlon JT, Schmader KE. The medication appropriateness index at 20: where it started, where it has been, and where it may be going. Drugs Aging 2013;30(11): 893–900.

17. Hamilton H, Gallagher P, Ryan C, et al. Potentially inappropriate medications defined by STOPP criteria and the risk of adverse drug events in older hospitalized patients. Arch Intern Med 2011;171(11):1013–9.

18. Cameron RJ, Kolbe J, Wilsher ML, et al. Bronchiolitis obliterans organising pneumonia associated with the use of nitrofurantoin. Thorax 2000;55(3):249–51.

19. Weir M, Daly GJ. Lung toxicity and Nitrofurantoin: the tip of the iceberg? QJM 2013;106(3):271–2.

20. Schneider LS, Dagerman KS, Insel P. Risk of death with atypical antipsychotic drug treatment for dementia: meta-analysis of randomized placebo-controlled trials. JAMA 2005;294(15):1934–43.

21. Schneider LS, Dagerman K, Insel PS. Efficacy and adverse effects of atypical antipsychotics for dementia: meta-analysis of randomized, placebo-controlled trials. Am J Geriatr Psychiatry 2006;14(3):191–210.

22. Basciotta M, Zhou W, Ngo L, et al. Antipsychotics and the risk of mortality or cardiopulmonary arrest in hospitalized adults. J Am Geriatr Soc 2020;68(3):544–50.

23. Meltzer HY. Clinical studies on the mechanism of action of clozapine: the dopamine-serotonin hypothesis of schizophrenia. Psychopharmacology (Berl) 1989;99(Suppl):S18–27.

24. Fong TG, Tulebaev SR, Inouye SK. Delirium in elderly adults: diagnosis, prevention and treatment. Nat Rev Neurol 2009;5(4):210–20.

25. Maldonado JR. Acute brain failure: pathophysiology, diagnosis, management, and sequelae of delirium. Crit Care Clin 2017;33(3):461–519.

26. Alagiakrishnan K, Wiens CA. An approach to drug induced delirium in the elderly. Postgrad Med J 2004;80(945):388–93.

27. Clegg A, Young JB. Which medications to avoid in people at risk of delirium: a systematic review. Age Ageing 2011;40(1):23–9.

28. Onder G, Petrovic M, Tangiisuran B, et al. Development and validation of a score to assess risk of adverse drug reactions among in-hospital patients 65 years or older: the GerontoNet ADR risk score. Arch Intern Med 2010;170(13):1142–8.

29. Tangiisuran B, Wright J, Van der Cammen T, et al. Adverse drug reactions in elderly: challenges in identification and improving preventative strategies. Age Ageing 2009;38(4):358–9.

30. Vaughan CP, Hwang U, Vandenberg AE, et al. Early prescribing outcomes after exporting the EQUIPPED medication safety improvement programme. BMJ Open Qual 2021;10(4).

31. Battar S, Watson Dickerson KR, Sedgwick C, et al. Understanding principles of high reliability organizations through the eyes of VIONE: a clinical program to improve patient safety by deprescribing potentially inappropriate medications and reducing polypharmacy. Fed Pract 2019;36(12):564–8.

32. Carpenter CR, Bromley M, Caterino JM, et al. Optimal older adult emergency care: introducing multidisciplinary geriatric emergency department guidelines from the American College of emergency physicians, American geriatrics society, emergency nurses association, and society for academic emergency medicine. J Am Geriatr Soc 2014;62(7):1360–3.
33. Kennedy M, Lesser A, Israni J, et al. Reach and adoption of a geriatric emergency department accreditation program in the United States. Ann Emerg Med 2022;79(4):367–73.
34. Marshall J, Hayes BD, Koehl J, et al. Effects of a pharmacy-driven medication history program on patient outcomes. Am J Health Syst Pharm 2022;79(19):1652–62.
35. Rose O, Jaehde U, Köberlein-Neu J. Discrepancies between home medication and patient documentation in primary care. Res Social Adm Pharm 2018;14(4):340–6.
36. Balsom C, Pittman N, King R, et al. Impact of a pharmacist-administered deprescribing intervention on nursing home residents: a randomized controlled trial. Int J Clin Pharmacol 2020;42(4):1153–67.
37. Arrison W, Merritt E, Powell A. Comparing medication histories obtained by pharmacy technicians and nursing staff in the emergency department. Res Social Adm Pharm 2020;16(10):1398–400.
38. Koehl J, Steffenhagen A, Halfpap J. Implementation and impact of pharmacist-initiated home medication ordering in an emergency department observation unit. J Pharm Pract 2021;34(3):459–64.
39. Ali S, Salahudeen MS, Bereznicki LRE, et al. Pharmacist-led interventions to reduce adverse drug events in older people living in residential aged care facilities: a systematic review. Br J Clin Pharmacol 2021;87(10):3672–89.
40. Gillespie U, Alassaad A, Henrohn D, et al. A comprehensive pharmacist intervention to reduce morbidity in patients 80 years or older: a randomized controlled trial. Arch Intern Med 2009;169(9):894–900.

Developing a Geriatric Emergency Department
People, Processes, and Place

Don Melady, MD, MSc(Ed)[a,b,*], John G. Schumacher, MA, PhD[c,d]

KEYWORDS

- Geriatric emergency department • Processes • Structures • Interdisciplinary team
- Physical environment

KEY POINTS

- Creating a Geriatric Emergency Department (GED) involves changes in the people, processes, and physical place of a general ED.
- A GED can produce improvements in clinical outcomes, patient and carer experience, financial status of the ED, and staff morale and retention.
- People are at the core of a GED: doctors and nurses with enhanced education and practice; geriatric nurse care coordinator; access to physical and occupational therapy, social workers, and pharmacists. Any one of these interdisciplinary collaborators enhances care.
- GED processes include changing general approaches to care; screening for high-risk conditions; enhanced assessment; workflow alterations; and transitions of care.
- In the GED place, minimal low-cost additions and changes in the physical space (eg, extra chairs, a clock, walkers) can make a large improvement.

INTRODUCTION

Consider the last year in any emergency department (ED) in the world—urban or rural, large or small. More older people were seen there that year than in any previous year due to sustained global population aging. If concrete proof is need, send a simple data request for the number of patients with ED age 65 and older for the past 5 years. If you

[a] Department of Family and Community Medicine, Faculty of Medicine, University of Toronto, 500 University Avenue, Toronto, Ontario M5G 1V7, Canada; [b] Schwartz-Reisman Emergency Medicine Institute, Mount Sinai Hospital, 600 University Avenue, Toronto, Ontario, M5G 1X5, Canada; [c] Department of Sociology, Anthropology, and Public Health, University of Maryland, Baltimore County (UMBC), 104 Fairfield Drive, Baltimore, MD 21228, USA; [d] Department of Epidemiology and Public Health, School of Medicine, University of Maryland, Baltimore (UMB), Baltimore, MD, USA
* Corresponding author. Department of Family and Community Medicine, Faculty of Medicine, University of Toronto, 500 University Avenue, Toronto, Ontario M5G 1V7, Canada
E-mail address: don.melady@utoronto.ca

Clin Geriatr Med 39 (2023) 647–658
https://doi.org/10.1016/j.cger.2023.05.008
geriatric.theclinics.com

are like most EDs you will learn you are seeing increasing numbers of older people each year. In fact, the most recent national ED data in the US shows a 30% increase in the number of age 65+ patients with ED between 2015 and 2019.[1,2] Older people now make nearly 28 million ED visits annually representing an all-time high of 18.4% of all U.S. ED visits.[1] Your staff can also report their experience of treating older people: listen for challenges they face. With your information in mind, ask yourself: How is your ED responding to these changes in the number and complexity of older patients with ED? Continuing with business as usual is probably not an option for you or your organization.

This article provides a brief overview of key concepts in the current literature that describes models for geriatric care in the ED. The umbrella term "Geriatric Emergency Department (GED)" is used in this article to refer to the emerging models and individual practices implemented in EDs that are consistent with and informed by principles of geriatric medicine. Our use of the term GED refers to any general ED that "has made the decision to intentionally implement changes in its people, processes, and place in order to improve the quality of care it provides to older people–regardless of physical space or resources."[3]

This article highlights key points from the co-authors' recent book "Creating A Geriatric Emergency Department: A Practical Guide" published by Cambridge University Press.[3] For a more in-depth treatment of the GED concepts briefly introduced in this article, we refer you to this highly accessible and readable book.

Brief History of Geriatric Emergency Medicine

Surprising to many, there is a more than a 30-year history of research on geriatric emergency medicine and models of care.[3–7] The first reported dedicated geriatric emergency departments were opened at Holy Cross Hospital in Maryland (2008)[3] and St. Joseph's Medical Center in New Jersey (2009).[3] Internationally, early geriatric emergency medicine efforts developed simultaneously in Canada, Australia, and the United Kingdom.[8–10]

Key milestones in GEDs' development included Sanders' (1996) book *Elder Care in the Emergency Department*, Hwang and Morrison's[11] description of the geriatric emergency department and Hogan's[12] articulation of geriatric emergency medicine competencies for emergency medicine residents. On these foundations were built the 2013 Geriatric Emergency Department (GED) Guidelines[13] endorsed by four major professional associations: the American Geriatrics Society, American College of Emergency Physicians, Society for Academic Emergency Medicine, and the Emergency Nurses Association. Building on the GED guidelines, the Geriatric Emergency Department Accreditation program was launched by the American College of Emergency Physicians in 2018.[14]

Approaches to Implementing a Geriatric Emergency Department

The general concept of a GED goes by numerous names: Geriatric Emergency Department, Senior Emergency Center, Geriatric Observation Unit, Frailty Unit, Age-Friendly Emergency Department among others. Common to this concept and its implementation is the decision regarding the physical space of the GED. An early decision regarding creating a GED is whether your ED takes (1) an integrated space approach; or (2) a separate space approach.[3] The more common GED approach is the integrated space approach where geriatric services are available wherever the older person is in the general ED–triage, acute, trauma bay, boarding. In contrast, the separate space GED approach creates a dedicated, purpose-built physical space where older ED people are treated apart from the general ED population which could include a hospital's observation unit.[15]

Essential Elements of a Geriatric Emergency Department: the 3 Ps

While GEDs vary widely, most are characterized by three core elements which we identify as the "3 Ps": People, Processes, and Place.[3] The People of the GED include the champions, physicians, nurses, advance practice nurses, social workers, pharmacists, physical and occupational therapists, clinical assistants, and administrators. The Processes of the GED include processes tailored to the care of older people including intake, assessment, screenings, delirium assessment, prevention, and treatment, falls assessment and prevention, medications, nutrition, disposition planning and follow-up. Finally, the Place of the GED includes the ED's physical space, wayfinding, access to hard material such as walkers and canes, lighting, sound, bedding, and room features. The 3Ps represent a holistic approach to developing a GED. Each will be described in detail in the sections later in discussion.

Geriatric Emergency Department: People

The first P–People–focuses on identifying the needed changes in human resources. These people include: (1) GED Champions; and (2) GED Clinicians. Organizationally, the GED Champions are the influential people who will advocate for the creation and maintenance of your GED and usually include a triad of an emergency physician champion, an emergency nurse champion, and a hospital executive champion. Together these champions advance the GED project and build the organizational momentum to implementation and continuation.

Complementing the triad of GED champions, the People also refers to the clinical staff who will be the workforce providing the GED care. These core roles include: (1) GED medical director, (2) GED nurse care coordinator, (3) GED physical and/or occupational therapist, (4) GED social worker, and (5) GED pharmacist. These roles may vary in terms of full-time/part-time; background and experience; and educational qualifications/certifications. Typically, the GED medical director and GED nurse care coordinator collaborate to design and implement the mission of the GED. The GED nurse care coordinator is a linchpin role that is divided between providing frontline clinical care/consultation and GED capacity development. These coordinators ensure the delivery of specialized GED nursing services, care coordination, as well as building capacity through staff education and advocacy within the larger hospital. Beyond the GED medical director, the composition of the GED workforce is heterogeneous depending on the ED goals, culture, existing staff, and resources. For example, while many organizations commonly have a GED nurse care coordinator, some organizations may designate a GED social worker in a leadership GED coordinator role serving to bring together the clinical and social services that make up a GED.

Geriatric Emergency Department Staff Education and Training

Developing and implementing a sustainable GED education and training program for the unit's ongoing workforce is a critical planning consideration. Successful education programs build on and extend the existing skills, knowledge, and attitudes staff possess. Integrating geriatric content into existing in-service and self-study is a proven strategy. Educational resources for GEDs are rapidly expanding and include articles, textbooks, websites, webinars, online education programs, dedicated in-service programming, and bootcamp style training. **Box 1** provides a summary of key resources.

Box 1
Key Geriatric Emergency Department educational resources

Hogan, T. et. al. Competences Development of Geriatric Competencies for Emergency Medicine Residents Using an Expert Consensus Process. Academic Emergency Medicine. 2010; 17:316 to 32

https://onlinelibrary.wiley.com/doi/10.1111/j.1553-2712.2010.00684.x[12]

Carpenter C. et al. Optimal older adult emergency care: introducing multidisciplinary geriatric emergency department guidelines from the American College of Emergency Physicians, American Geriatrics Society, Emergency Nurses Association, and Society for Academic Emergency Medicine. Acad Emerg Med. 2014 Jul;21(7):806 to 9. doi: 10.1111/acem.12415. Epub 2014 Aug 12. PMID: 2,117,158.[13]

Geriatric Emergency Department Collaborative.https://gedcollaborative.com/[16]

Emergency Nurses Association. Geriatric Emergency Department Readiness Toolkit.

https://www.ena.org/shop/catalog/education/toolkits/geriatric-emergency-department-readiness-toolkit/c-23/c-94/p-361

Geriatric Emergency Department Intervention Tool Kit. https://clinicalexcellence.qld.gov.au/resources/gedi-toolkit

A Practical Guide to Implementing a Geriatric Emergency Department by West Health and UC San Diego Health. https://www.westhealth.org/resource/ged-implementation-guide/

Geriatric Emergency Medicine Textbooks and Volumes

Conroy, S. et al. (2021). The Silver Book II: Quality care for older people with urgent and emergency care needs. British Geriatrics Society.

Chapter 6 https://www.bgs.org.uk/resources/silver-book-ii-training-and-development

Malone, M. and Biese, K. (2018). Care for the Older Adult in the Emergency Department. Clinics in Geriatric Medicine. Elsevier, Philadelphia, PA.[17]

Mattu, A., Grossman, S. and Rosen, P. (2016). Geriatric Emergencies. A Discussion-Based Review. Wiley-Blackwell. West Sussex, UK.[18]

Kahn, J. et al. (2016). Current Trends in Geriatric Emergency Medicine. Emergency Medicine Clinics, Volume 34.[19]

Meldon, S., Ma, O., Woolard, R. (2004). Geriatric Emergency Medicine. American College of Emergency Physicians. McGraw-Hill.[5]

Sanders, A. (1996). Emergency Care of the Elder Person. Beverely-Cracom Publications. St. Louis, MO.[4]

On-Line Geriatric Emergency Medicine Education Resources

The Geriatric Emergency Department Collaborative (GEDC) hosts a growing set of online education module and resources. It is an open-access non-fee-paying site with interactive modules, which are accredited for both nursing and medical continuing education credits. The topics include: cognitive Impairment; atypical presentations; medication management; frailty; falls assessment and management; major trauma resuscitation; functional assessment and discharge planning; elder mistreatment; and end of life issues and symptom management. https://gedcollaborative.com/online-learning/

GEMCast is a geriatric emergency medicine podcast on clinical topics. Each episode includes references, show notes, and downloadable resources. https://gedcollaborative.com/resources/gemcast/

The Emergency Nurses Association (ENA) created the Geriatric Emergency Nursing Education program delivered as an online program https://www.ena.org/shop/catalog/

education/online-learning/the-geriatric-emergency-nursing-education-(gene)/c-23/c-100/p-200. It focuses on recognizing the presentation of illness and effective nursing intervention and care strategies. Completion of this fee-paying program provides Continuing Nursing Education (CNE) credit and a certificate.

Geriatric Emergency Department: Processes

The GED's second "P" is for processes. The care processes represent all the activities and actions which happen within the structure of an ED and carried out by its staff. Collectively the care processes represent an important area for change or addition that moves a general ED toward being a GED. In this section, we present 25 different care processes that could be implemented in a general ED. Any one of them will improve care. Implementing all of them would transform a general ED into a world-class GED.

We segment these care processes into five thematic groupings outlined in **Box 2** They are consistent with the 2013 GED Guidelines and the 2018 GED Accreditation criteria: (1) General approaches to care; (2) Screening for high-risk conditions; (3) Enhanced assessment; (4) Workflow alterations; and (5) Transitions of care.

We have placed general approaches to care in the first position with the belief that these components, which could reasonably be thought of as fundamental to

---

Box 2
Geriatric Emergency Department Processes

1. General approaches to care
   Access to food and drink
   Pain management
   Mobility promotion
   Physical restraints
   Volunteer engagement

2. Screening for high-risk conditions
   Cognitive impairment/Delirium
   Cognitive impairment/Dementia
   Polypharmacy
   Fall risk
   Frailty and functional decline
   Elder abuse
   Unmet palliative care needs

3. Enhanced assessments
   Delirium assessment
   Fall assessment
   Standardized assessment of common geriatric presentations

4. Workflow alterations
   Assessment by geriatric nurse care coordinator
   Assessment by physical and occupational therapist
   Assessment by pharmacist
   Assessment by specialist consultants: Geriatric Psychiatry; Palliative Medicine; Wound Care

5. Managing transitions of care
   Protocol for discharge instructions
   Protocol for transfers from residential care facilities
   Direct access to palliative care and acute rehabilitation beds
   Patient transportation
   Access to telehealth interventions and/or hospital-at-home
   Links to community paramedicine

providing good care and therefore "routine," are sometimes overlooked despite their impact on the quality of care provided to and experienced by older people. To become a GED, every ED should have easy access to food and drink for all patients but definitely for those who are most at risk for hunger and thirst during the often-prolonged stays while undergoing multiple tests, investigations, and assessments; or while waiting for a disposition plan or bed. Every ED should have processes that ensure early, proactive, and effective management of pain that may include strategies for assessing pain in people with cognitive impairment[20]; or innovations that prioritize older patient issues such as nerve blocks for hips fractures. Since mobility is such an important component of well-being for older people—and essential for preventing delirium and slowing functional decline–every ED should have processes that permit, promote, and enhance mobility. They can include simple interventions such as: having ready access to gait aids such as walkers and canes; minimizing the use of unnecessary continuous monitoring, avoiding urinary catheters and other tethering devices; engaging volunteers or family members to actively mobilize patients; and even having a chair in the room where she can be "up for meals" or while waiting for investigations. These changes have an impact during short ED stays (eg, having a walker to assess safe ambulation for discharge) and long ones produced by ED boarding where physical de-conditioning is a real risk. A final example of enhancements to routine care would be the addition of a volunteer program.[21] A cohort of specially trained non-clinical supporters can provide additional care–providing warm blankets, setting up for eating, distractions, mobility–that enhance care, avoid bad outcomes, and unload duties from the RN and MD staff.

Older people in an ED often have serious conditions that are not easily detected unless routine screening for high-risk conditions is implemented. These would include screening for.

- Cognitive impairment (both dementia and delirium);
- Frailty and functional decline;
- Polypharmacy;
- Increased risk of falls;
- Elder abuse; and
- Unmet palliative care needs.

For each of these conditions, there are ample tools, validated for ED use highlighted here.

Older people have a high incidence of *dementia* with roughly a quarter of all the population over 80 having some cognitive impairment. Chronic brain failure is often not identified or diagnosed before the ED visit which offers an opportunity for screening for a condition that has an impact on all other ED processes (such as informed consent, communication, participation in care, and disposition planning.) Dementia screening tools used in the ED can include the Mini Cog and the AMT-4.[22,23]

All older people, particularly frail or polymorbid ones, have an increased risk of acute brain failure or *delirium*–an important and consequential syndrome that is a serious medical condition. However, since its components can be subtle (eg, a bit drowsier) or difficult for a clinician to identify (eg, more confused than usual in a person with dementia at baseline), a process of standardized screening for all the at-risk population (which means basically everyone over 65 in an emergency department) will help to identify people with delirium.[24]

There is an increasing body of evidence that identifying functional status or *level of frailty* can lead to multiple other helpful ED interventions–enhanced assessments, linking with community services, establishing prognosis, and durable disposition planning.[25–27] The GED should have some screening process to establish baseline function or frailty level and changes. Multiple tools to do so–the Clinical Frailty Score,[28] the Identifying Seniors at Risk[29] tool, among others–are available.

Older people often take many different *medications* to manage their multiple chronic conditions–with an impact on presenting symptoms, adverse interactions, withdrawal, or toxicity. A GED should have a well-established process for gathering accurate information about a patient's medication use and for ensuring that information informs assessments and planning. Ideally there would be a process to involve a pharmacist to assist in screening the medication list of each older person or of those with pre-established cut-offs (age, or number or medications, or presence of falls, or re-visits.) Tools used in the ED include STOPP and START[30] as well as the EQUiPPed program.[31]

Some older people are in the ED as a result of a fall. Others are there for non-fall related problems but are still at high risk of falls. Both groups can benefit from screening for their *risk of recurrent falls*, among the most consequential of the geriatric syndromes.[32] Such a process may include in-ED assessment of mobility, strength, and gait. It may involve the possibility of an assessment by a physical therapist. It should permit a referral for post-ED, community-based strategies for fall risk mitigation (home assessment, fall clinic, exercise program.) Anything less would be analogous to identifying someone as high-risk for severe coronary artery disease. . . and then doing nothing to modify that risk!

Unseen *elder abuse and neglect* is a reality for many older people visiting EDs. There are no ED-specific tools for identifying those at risk for or experiencing the various kinds of abuse or neglect. However, one tool, the EASI, developed for primary care may help inform ED care.[33] A GED will have some strategies (standardized screening for all patients, targeted questions by social work colleagues, heightened awareness by staff through education) to help see the problem and strategies for follow up and support.

EDs see older people at many points along the trajectory of serious illness, chronic organ failure, and frailty. All those people likely have *unmet palliative care* needs–symptom management, improving function, establishing goals of care.[34] The GED should have a process for identifying those people and facilitating access to palliative care expertise.

If there are processes in place for screening, then there needs to be processes in place for extended or enhanced assessment and management of the outcomes of that screening.[35] The GED will have strategies in place (eg, an order set, a best practice guide) for standardized investigation of the cause of delirium once it has been identified as well as strategies for reducing the severity of the symptoms of delirium. Similarly, there should be a process for assessment in the ED by appropriate members of an interdisciplinary team (see next section "People") who can target some or all of the conditions that are going to impact the quality of care and promote a durable discharge plan. This recognizes the reality that older people are rarely in the ED with a single isolated problem: their complex web of interconnected medical, psychological, social, and functional conditions is usually too much for a single practitioner to fully assess. To this end, a GED may choose to establish locally appropriate standardized approaches to the investigation and management of common presentations in the form of order sets, or best practice guides, or pick menus–that encourage good practices and avoid common pitfalls. Examples would include the management of geriatric sepsis, hip fracture, or the imminently dying patient.

Adding or changing some of these approaches leads inevitably to workflow alterations which will need to be clarified in the GED.[36] It will be valuable to implement some protocols that clarify the role of the various professionals involved. For example, if a geriatric nurse care coordinator is added to the team, it will be essential to establish how this clinician is involved in the ED workflow: At what point do they see the patient? Which patients? Using what criteria? What is their scope of practice? To whom do they report? How is that information communicated? A similar approach will be required for all the interdisciplinary team–physical therapist, occupational therapist, pharmacist, and any specialized consultants such as geriatrician, geriatric psychiatrist, palliative care team, or wound care practitioner.

Because older people are so complex and typically have multiple care providers and sites of care involved, one of the core competencies of Geriatric Emergency Medicine is the management of transitions of care.[37] And yet, it is remarkable that many patients, including high-functioning cognitively intact patients, leave an ED and report little understanding of what has happened, what is going to happen next, what they are expected to do. The GED will have clear policies about this most important point of care transition. Many departments have pre-established texts to explain and provide advice about common ED presentations–lacerations, fractures, head injuries, viral illnesses. It will probably be necessary to go much further to ensure that a frail older person understands the complexities of post-ED care. Discharge instructions should certainly involve printed-in-large-font, clear-language explanation–which are placed directly into the hands of the patient. Caregivers should be involved in this exchange of information so that all the people who need to know about next steps are aware. This will include primary care providers, community-based services that the patient may access, specialist consultants, and specialized geriatric referrals. Other transitions that are fraught with complexity are those to and from residential long-term-care homes, palliative care hospices, or in-patient rehabilitation facilities. A carefully considered protocol should exist for all of them, including a strategy for transportation.

Geriatric Emergency Department: Place

The GED's third "P" is for Place. This is the physical space where the GED services are delivered. This could use, as noted above, an integrated space approach where services are provided through the general ED; or a separate space approach, where a separate, dedicated, purpose-built GED space is created. Regardless of the space decision, the concept of the GED Place focuses on the design features of the ED

Box 3
Equipment and supplies

Equipment	Furniture	Safety Enhancements	Visual Orientation	Acoustic Enhancements
Hearing amplifiers	Beds at safe transfer level	Doors with levers	Soft lighting	Noise reducing drapes
Walkers, canes, nonslip socks	Chairs with arms	Enhanced signage	Matte colors	Music availability
Commode	Reclining exam chairs		Minimize patterns	Reducing alarm volume
Nonslip fall mats	Pressure reducing mattresses		Clocks	
Blanket Warmers			Communication boards	

room and ED unit that are "age-friendly." A good starting question is: "What is your desired ED patient experience like?"[38] or more specifically "How do you want to make your patients with GED feel?" Briefly answering these questions for a specific ED setting and culture will provide guidance on specific design decisions regarding Place in a GED.

The GED Place involves the specific items in the GED that relate to an older ED person's sensory experience, mobility, and overall comfort. Two resources that inform decisions regarding GED Place include the: (1) GED Guidelines[13]; and (2) Geriatric Emergency Department Accreditation Standards.[14] Specific equipment and supplies are listed in **Box 3**.

Geriatric Focused Observation Unit

ED Observation Units with 23-h monitoring are emerging in some hospitals that are consistent with Medicare billing guidelines before triggering an inpatient billing code.[15] The design of these observation units can incorporate elements of GED Place to provide a flexible and supportive space for older people who need enhanced assessment while the appropriate disposition plan is established.

SUMMARY

The decision to create a GED model of care is a significant one that requires a clear and convincing answer to the question: Why do it? There are at least two themes to our response: it is good for older patients and it's good for health care systems.

People around the world, especially in wealthy nations, are living longer with complications of chronic diseases, and with a concomitant increase in rates of dementia and often-fraying social support networks. Just about everywhere in the world, growing numbers of older people are visiting EDs with ever-increasing frequency. Once they are at an ED, they use more resources per visit, are more likely to get expensive tests with advanced imaging, are more likely to be admitted, and are more likely to suffer healthcare-related harms.[39] Adopting and accelerating[40] a new approach to their care–using this People, Processes, and Place model[3] or another one–can have a big impact in terms of improved outcomes for patients while saving money.[41] As the demographic Silver Boom continues over the next two decades, the changes presented in this article are essential both on moral and clinical grounds and to achieve financial sustainability and ongoing quality of care in your ED.

By enhancing the structures and processes of your ED to better assess and manage older patients, there is ever more emphasis on providing increased value. A team approach and standardized protocols give the patient what she needs. She gets not just a splint for a broken wrist and a pat on the back as she leaves. She also gets an assessment of her fall that considers her medication list; that provides PT assessment for strength conditioning to prevent the next fall; and coordinated links to necessary social services. By providing alternatives to hospital admission through enhanced assessments and improved transitions of care, a GED may also contribute to decrease the boarding of medical patients in EDs, a population which is disproportionately older. The hospital thus avoids an unnecessary admission of this frail older person who might otherwise be admitted "for further assessment" just because she is not "safe for discharge" and the emergency doctor has no alternatives available. This approach ensures both that she does well at home and that the hospital is not financially penalized for an avoidable ED re-visit. Fortunately, based on a recent large study, there is strong evidence that creating a GED is associated with cost savings to the health system of up to US$3000 per patient.[42]

This article provides options for making changes in an ED's people, processes, and place that can lead to enhancements in the ED experience of older people and the quality of their outcomes. Our recent book[3] expands on these 3 Ps and gives ample guidance to their implementation–including making the financial case and overcoming resistance to change. Whatever your ED chooses to do, these will provide starting points to preparing for improved care of the most rapidly expanding demographic in our society and our EDs.

DISCLOSURE

D.L. Melady receives an annual stipend from the Geriatric ED Collaborative. One of his job requirements in that role is to promote the dissemination and implementation of Geriatric ED models of care. He also sits, on a voluntary basis, on the Board of Governors of the Geriatric ED Accreditation Program which is not-for-profit offering of the American College of Emergency Physicians. J.G. Schumacher has no disclosures.

REFERENCES

1. Cairns C, Kang K. National hospital ambulatory medical care survey: 2019 emergency department summary tables. U.S: National Center for Health Statistics; 2022. https://doi.org/10.15620/cdc:115748.
2. Rui P, Kang K. National hospital ambulatory medical care survey: 2015 emergency department summary tables. Centers for Disease Control National Center for Health Statistics 2016;. http://www.cdc.gov/nchs/data/ahcd/nhamcs_emergency/2015_ed_web_tables.pdf.
3. Schumacher JG, Melady D. Creating a geriatric emergency department a practical guide. Cambridge, UK: Cambridge University Press; 2022.
4. Sanders AB. Emergency care of the elder person. Beverly Cracom Publications 1996.
5. Meldon S, Ma OJ, Woolard R. Geriatric Emergency Medicine. (Meldon S, ed.). McGraw-Hill, Medical Pub Division; 2004. http://survey.hshsl.umaryland.edu/?url=http://search.ebscohost.com/login.aspx?direct=true&db=cat01362a&AN=hshs.003076762&site=eds-live.
6. Bosker G, Michael S. Geriatric emergency medicine. St. Louis, MO, USA: Mosby; 1990.
7. Mooijaart SP, Carpenter CR, Conroy SP. Geriatric emergency medicine—a model for frailty friendly healthcare. Age Ageing 2022;51(3):afab280.
8. Conroy SP, Banerjee J, Carpenter CR. Silver Book II: Quality Urgent Care For Older People.; 2021. https://www.bgs.org.uk/resources/resource-series/silver-book-ii.
9. Australian College of Emergency Physicians. Care of older persons in the emergency department. Published April 2020. https://acem.org.au/getmedia/bfd84f83-fcb2-492a-9e66-47b7896e5c70/P51_Care_Elderly_Patients_in_ED_Sep-15.aspx. Accessed January 31, 2023.
10. Melady D. Geriatric emergency medicine: research priorities to respond to "The Silver Boom.". CJEM 2018;20(3):327–8.
11. Hwang U, Morrison S. The geriatric emergency department. J Am Geriatr Soc 2007;55(11):1873–6.
12. Hogan TM, Losman ED, Carpenter CR, et al. Development of geriatric competencies for emergency medicine residents using an expert consensus process. Acad Emerg Med 2010;17(3):316–24.
13. Carpenter CR, Bromley M, Caterino J, et al. Optimal older adult emergency care: introducing multidisciplinary geriatric emergency department guidelines from the

American college of emergency physicians, American geriatrics society, emergency nurses association, and society for academic emergency medicine. Ann Emerg Med 2014;63(5):1–3.

14. Geriatric Emergency Department Accreditation (GEDA). Accessed January 30, 2023. https://www.acep.org/geda.
15. Southerland LT, Vargas AJ, Nagaraj L, et al. An emergency department observation unit is a feasible setting for multidisciplinary geriatric assessments in compliance with the geriatric emergency department guidelines. Acad Emerg Med 2018;25(1):76–82.
16. Home - GEDC. Published November 3, 2022 https://gedcollaborative.com/, https://gedcollaborative.com/. Accessed January 28, 2023.
17. Malone ML, Beise K. Care for the older adult in the emergency department, vol. 34. Amsterdam, The Netherlands: Elsevier; 2018.
18. Mattu A, Grossman S, Rosen P. Geriatric Emergencies: A Discussion-Based Review. Hoboken, NJ, USA: John Wiley & Sons; 2016.
19. Kahn JH, Magauran BG, Olshaker JS. Geriatric emergency medicine: principles and practice. Cambridge, UK: Cambridge University Press; 2014.
20. Warden V, Hurley AC, Volicer L. Development and psychometric evaluation of the pain assessment in advanced dementia (PAINAD) scale. J Am Med Dir Assoc 2003;4(1):9–15.
21. Ellis B, Melady D, Foster N, et al. Using volunteers to improve the experience of older patients in the emergency department. CJEM 2020;22(4):514–8.
22. Mini-Cog© – Quick Screening for Early Dementia Detection. Accessed January 28, 2023. https://mini-cog.com/.
23. Dyer AH, Briggs R, Nabeel S, et al. The Abbreviated Mental Test 4 for cognitive screening of older adults presenting to the emergency department. Eur J Emerg Med 2017;24(6):417–22.
24. Han JH, Suyama J. Delirium and dementia. Clin Geriatr Med 2018;34(3):327–54.
25. Mowbray F, Brousseau AA, Mercier E, et al. Examining the relationship between triage acuity and frailty to inform the care of older emergency department patients: findings from a large Canadian multisite cohort study. CJEM 2020;22(1): 74–81.
26. Rueegg M, Nissen SK, Brabrand M, et al. The clinical frailty scale predicts 1-year mortality in emergency department patients aged 65 years and older. Acad Emerg Med 2022;29(5):572–80.
27. Ng CJ, Chien LT, Huang CH, et al. Integrating the clinical frailty scale with emergency department triage systems for elder patients: a prospective study. Am J Emerg Med 2023;66:16–21.
28. Rockwood K, Song X, MacKnight C, et al. A global clinical measure of fitness and frailty in elderly people. CMAJ (Can Med Assoc J) 2005;173(5):489.
29. Asomaning N, Loftus C. Identification of Seniors at risk (ISAR) screening tool in the emergency department: implementation using the plan-do-study-act model and validation results. J Emerg Nurs 2014;40(4):357–64.
30. Hill-Taylor B, Walsh KA, Stewart S, et al. Effectiveness of the STOPP/START (Screening Tool of Older Persons' potentially inappropriate Prescriptions/ Screening Tool to Alert doctors to the Right Treatment) criteria: systematic review and meta-analysis of randomized controlled studies. J Clin Pharm Therapeut 2016;41(2):158–69.
31. Vandenberg AE, Stevens M, Echt KV, et al. Implementing the EQUiPPED medication management program at 5 VA emergency departments. Fed Pract 2016; 33(4):29–33.

32. Carpenter CR, Cameron A, Ganz DA, et al. Older adult falls in emergency medicine. Clin Geriatr Med 2019;35(2):205–19.

33. Rosen T, Platts-Mills TF, Fulmer T. Screening for elder mistreatment in emergency departments: current progress and recommendations for next steps. J Elder Abuse Negl 2020;32(3):295–315.

34. Aaronson EL, Petrillo L, Stoltenberg M, et al. The experience of emergency department providers with embedded palliative care during COVID. J Pain Symptom Manage 2020;60(5):35–43.

35. Dresden S, Courtney DM, Lindquist L. Geriatric emergency department assessments and association with hospitalization. J Am Geriatr Soc 2018;66:248–9.

36. Stern M, Mulcare M. The geriatric ED and clinical protocols for the emergency care of older adults. Emerg Med 2014;46(6):263–74.

37. Bambach K, Southerland LT. Applying geriatric principles to transitions of care in the emergency department. Emerg Med Clin 2021. https://doi.org/10.1016/j.emc.2021.01.006.

38. Huddy J, Sanson T. Emergency Department Design : A Practical Guide to Planning for the Future. 2nd edition American College of Emergency Physicians; 2016.

39. Grief CL. Patterns of ED use and perceptions of the elderly regarding their emergency care: a synthesis of recent research. J Emerg Nurs 2003;29(2):122–6.

40. Hastings, Nicole. Research to accelerate practice change in geriatric emergency medicine. 2022;3(3):1–3.

41. Marsden E, Craswell A, Taylor A, et al. Translation of the geriatric emergency department intervention into other emergency departments: a post implementation evaluation of outcomes for older adults. BMC Geriatr 2022;22(1):290.

42. Hwang U, Dresden SM, Vargas-Torres C, et al. Association of a geriatric emergency department innovation program with cost outcomes among Medicare beneficiaries. JAMA Netw Open 2021;4(3):e2037334.

Emergency Department-to-Community Transitions of Care

Best Practices for the Older Adult Population

Cameron J. Gettel, MD, MHS[a,b,]*,
Susan N. Hastings, MD, MHS[c,d,e,f,g], Kevin J. Biese, MD[h,i],
Elizabeth M. Goldberg, MD, ScM[j]

KEYWORDS

- Emergency department • Transitions of care • Older adult

KEY POINTS

- Opportunities for improved communication with older adults and their care partners during ED-to-community care transitions may help overcome common adverse events after ED discharge.
- Older adults experiencing social isolation and those with impaired mobility or cognition represent unique populations that are particularly at risk during ED-to-community transitions of care.
- Care transition interventions to date have had variable efficacy and effectiveness in reducing ED revisit rates, yet promising solutions that target at-risk populations exist.
- Investment in transitional care management services in EDs could position ED clinicians, patients, and their care partners to reduce adverse events during this care transition.

[a] Department of Emergency Medicine, Yale School of Medicine, 464 Congress Avenue, Suite 260, New Haven, CT 06519, USA; [b] Center for Outcomes Research and Evaluation, Yale School of Medicine, New Haven, CT 06519, USA; [c] Center of Innovation to Accelerate Discovery and Practice Transformation (ADAPT), Durham VA Health Care System, Durham, NC, USA; [d] Department of Medicine, Duke University School of Medicine, Box 3003, Durham, NC 27710, USA; [e] Geriatric Research, Education, Clinical Center, Durham VA Health Care System, Durham, NC, USA; [f] Center for the Study of Human Aging and Development, Duke University School of Medicine, Durham, NC, USA; [g] Department of Population Health Sciences, Duke University School of Medicine, Durham, NC, USA; [h] Department of Emergency Medicine, University of North Carolina, 170 Manning Drive, CB #7594, Chapel Hill, NC 27599, USA; [i] Department of Medicine, Center for Aging and Health, University of North Carolina at Chapel Hill, Chapel Hill, NC, USA; [j] Department of Emergency Medicine, School of Medicine, University of Colorado, Anschutz Medical Campus, 13001 East 17th Place, CB #C290, Aurora, CO 80045, USA
* Corresponding author. 464 Congress Avenue, Suite 260, New Haven, CT 06519.
E-mail address: cameron.gettel@yale.edu

Clin Geriatr Med 39 (2023) 659–672
https://doi.org/10.1016/j.cger.2023.05.009
0749-0690/23/© 2023 Elsevier Inc. All rights reserved.
geriatric.theclinics.com

INTRODUCTION

Older adults, defined as those aged 65 years or older, are an increasing population in emergency departments (EDs) worldwide, with visit volumes increasing at a rate beyond that expected from demographic change alone.[1] Within the United States, older adults account for over 27 million ED visits annually, representing over 18% of all ED visits.[2] ED care-seeking among older adults has increased because of the aging population, an increased prevalence of loneliness and lack of social support, changes in the organization of primary care, and expectations for convenient medical care by emergency medicine "availablists" within a 24-hour one-stop shop environment.[3,4]

Older adults requiring ED care are more likely to suffer from chronic illnesses, multiple chronic conditions, and cognitive and functional impairments potentially limiting their ability to communicate symptoms and preexisting social problems.[5,6]

ED visits often reflect a critical inflection point in older person's health trajectory, with many factors contributing to care-seeking and several outcomes commonly deemed important to older adults (**Fig. 1**).[7] Approximately 65% of older adult ED patients are discharged home,[8] and prior studies show the ED-to-community care transition is fraught with inadequate communication and poor patient comprehension of their medical condition.[9,10] Consequences include a higher likelihood of adverse health outcomes such as decline in mobility and function, ED revisits, hospital admission, and mortality.[11–13] Highlighting the importance of the problem, repeat ED visit rates for older adults after ED discharge are 7.8% at 3 days,[14] 10%–16% at 1 month, 24% at 3 months, and up to 44% at 6 months.[15] The 2014 consensus geriatric ED guidelines and the 2018 launch of the geriatric ED accreditation process have attempted to improve these outcomes in older adults by prioritizing high-quality ED-to-community care transitions.[16–18] This article describes ED-to-community care transitions for older adults and associated challenges, measurement, efficacious and effective interventions, and policy considerations.

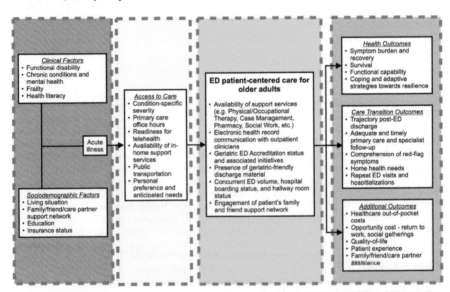

Fig. 1. Conceptual model and framework for ED-to-community care transitions among older adults (*From* Gettel CJ, Serina PT, Uzamere I, et al. Emergency department-to-community care transition barriers: A qualitative study of older adults. *J Am Geriatr Soc.* Published online July 2, 2022. https://onlinelibrary.wiley.com/doi/10.1111/jgs.17950. *With permission.*)

What Do the Guidelines Say?

Published in 2014, the geriatric ED guidelines provide a standardized set of best practices aimed at improving the care of the geriatric population within the ED.[18] Pertaining to care transitions, the published guidelines recommend ensuring adequate communication of clinically relevant information (eg, working discharge diagnosis, new prescription, physician note, follow-up plan) to the patient/family and outpatient care providers, including nursing homes. They also suggest large-font discharge instructions, ensuring a process in place to obtain follow-up clinical evaluation (with consideration for telemedicine), and maintaining relationships with community organizations to facilitate necessary future care.

How to Identify Who Is at Risk

The emphasis EDs must put on efficient care has been strained in recent years because of the higher prevalence of older adults, more complex diagnostic evaluations, and greater boarding of inpatients within the ED.[19] When admitted patients board in the ED, personnel trained and hired to expedite the evaluation and treatment of ED patients are instead used to provide inpatient level of care. These stressors leave clinicians with little time and departments with limited personnel and finances to adequately uncover and address all barriers that hinder ED-to-community care transition success.

Given limited resources, screening instruments have the potential to identify older adults at increased risk of adverse outcomes during the time frame immediately after ED discharge. Screening instruments used in the ED for older patients typically assess activities of daily living and include the Identification of Seniors At Risk (ISAR) tool, the Triage Risk Screening Tool, the Variables Indicative of Placement Risk, and the Inter-RAI ED Screener.[20] Validation studies have shown that no current screening test has optimal test characteristics.[21] The ISAR has been the most frequently assessed tool and has shown only modest predictive accuracy in identifying older adults at high risk of adverse outcomes.[21]

Aside from activities of daily living, emergency clinicians may also consider other tools to screen for factors that impact ED-to-community care transitions including risky medications (AGS Beers Criteria),[22] poor mobility (sit to stand test), and impaired cognition (Brief Alzheimer's Screen or Quick Dementia Rating System).[23,24] Further research is needed to develop screening instruments designed for and validated among ED patients with improved test characteristics that reliably identify older adults in a timely fashion as being at risk during ED-to-community care transitions. In the meantime, emergency clinicians should consider using validated screening tools and engaging a multidisciplinary care team with expertise in geriatric patient care, including case managers, transitional care nurses (TCNs), physical therapists, social workers, and other professionals available locally. Screening questions for emergency clinicians to consider before discharge are shown in **Box 1**.[25]

Discharge Instructions

Older adults discharged from the ED are at particular risk of adverse outcomes, and adherence to ED discharge instructions may mitigate that risk. Suboptimal rates of adherence are present for adults of all ages, with only 68% to 88% filling prescriptions for new medications,[26,27] 51% to 70% following up with primary care providers,[28,29] and 49% having at least a minimal understanding of reasons to return to the ED.[30] Focusing on certain populations may be the most effective use of time at ED discharge, as those of advanced age, with depression, or functional limitations are

---

Box 1
Questions to consider before discharging an older adult from the ED

- Have you accounted for any cognitive deficits or changes in mental status?
- Have you assessed for safe ambulation (if ambulatory)?
- Have you discussed the level of care needed at home and whether carers will be available?
- Do you have any concern for abuse or neglect, even self-neglect?
- Have you double checked any new prescriptions for medication interactions?
- Have you confirmed good understanding of the discharge instructions with the patient and caregiver?
- Does the patient feel comfortable and ready for discharge? Is there anything the patient is worried about?
- Has the plan of care been communicated with the patient's general practitioner?

From Southerland LT, Pearson S, Hullick C, Carpenter CR, Arendts G. Safe to send home? Discharge risk assessment in the emergency department. *Emerg Med Australas.* 2019;31(2):266-270. *With permission.*

---

less likely to recall "red flags" (signs of worsening health requiring further medical attention), and those with limited English proficiency are more likely to have unplanned short-term ED revisits.[31,32] Prior work has shown subsequent hospital revisits may be reduced among older adults by using the limited time at ED discharge to focus on medication adherence, follow-up appointments, and knowledge of clinical warning signs.[33] As part of the discharge instructions, older adults could be provided with a scheduled follow-up primary care visit. Some EDs hire care navigators to schedule these follow-up visits before ED discharge or to help patients establish care if they are new to the area or lack primary care.[34] In broader adult populations, several studies have shown an absolute improvement of approximately 20% in obtaining follow-up care when employing this practice, suggesting the possibility of adapting this practice to the more vulnerable older adult population.[35]

Several health systems have also adopted the "4 Ms" model to enhance geriatric care, including the ED discharge process. Developed by the John A. Hartford Foundation and the Institute for Healthcare Improvement, the Age-Friendly Health Systems' initiative ensures a patient-centered and evidence-based approach is used for older adults through the "4 Ms" model—What Matters, Medication, Mentation, and Mobility.[36] Addressing "What Matters" has proven feasible (3 minutes on average) within the ED setting to gain valuable information from older adults regarding their fears/concerns as well as their desired outcomes (**Box 2**).[37] This structured framework has the potential to facilitate ED clinicians in obtaining valuable information regarding initial and possible future care-seeking behaviors among older adults that may be incorporated within discharge instructions. Components of the Age-Friendly Health Systems initiative and "4 Ms" model have been implemented in several EDs with evidence of success.[38]

Existing Interventions to Enhance Care Transitions

Qualitative studies have identified patient and caregiver concerns surrounding the ED-to-community care transition that should be considered when developing care transition interventions.[7,39,40] Themes have been identified regarding barriers experienced during ED-to-community care transitions and root causes for seeking emergency care again in the immediate time period after ED discharge. Motivations to seek

---

Box 2
"What Matters" semi-structured interview guide for older adult patients and their treating clinicians

Questions for older adult patients
1. One question to ascertain fears or concerns about health care in ED.
   a. What concerns you most when you think about your health and about being in the ED today/tonight? or
   b. What fears and worries do you have about your health as you think about what brought you to the ED today/tonight?
2. One question about outcome patients most want from their ED visit
   a. What outcome are you most hoping for from this ED visit? or
   b. What are you most hoping for or looking for from your ED visit?

From Gettel C, Venkatesh A, Dowd H, et al. A qualitative study of "What Matters" to older adults in the emergency department. *West J Emerg Med.* 2022;23(4):579-588. *With permission.*

---

emergency are included that older adults felt confident that they would get needed care within the ED if acutely ill and that their primary care provider (PCP) suggested seeking emergency care. However, many stated that they could not obtain reliable follow-up with their PCP in a timely fashion and that the index ED visit discharge instructions were not clear. These themes showcase perceived needs by older adults that interventions discussed here have addressed.

Adaptations to the Care Transitions Intervention

One example intervention that has shown promise in improving ED-to-community care transitions has been the Coleman Care Transitions Intervention (CTI).[41,42] Originally developed as a hospital-to-home CTI, the modified CTI model uses community paramedics from ambulance-based emergency medical services (EMS) system to follow up with older adults after ED discharge. Community paramedics can be particularly beneficial for older adults with multiple chronic conditions given training on guiding older adults on self-management strategies and coordinating follow-up care with PCPs. In a population of patients aged $\geq$60 years, the modified CTI did not show a reduction in 30-day ED revisits but did result in a significant increase in key care transition behaviors such as outpatient follow-up and red flag knowledge.[43] Within a preplanned subgroup analysis of community-dwelling older adults with cognitive impairment, the modified CTI did result in a significant reduction in the odds of a repeat ED visit within 30 days (odds ratio [OR] 0.25, 95% confidence interval 0.07–0.90).[44] If considered for use locally, the ED-modified CTI model requires collaboration with EMS agencies but offers considerable opportunity to improve patient outcomes as shown by reduced risk of hospital readmission. Aside from the modified CTI model using community paramedics, researchers have also tested the effect of an adapted CTI using home visits and follow-up telephone calls by Area on Aging care coaches to address the four "pillars" of timely follow-up clinician visits, understanding of disease warning signs, medication reconciliation issues, and lack of a personal health record. Compared to usual care, the adapted CTI did not reduce return ED visits or hospitalizations at 60 days (primary outcome); however, a shorter timeline may be more relevant and is more commonly used in ED-based studies.[39]

Emergency Department Navigators

ED-based TCNs have also proven beneficial with regard to certain patient-centered outcomes and lower Medicare expenditures among fee-for-service beneficiaries.[45,46]

By identifying patients with geriatric-specific health-related needs and coordinating their transition from ED to community, TCNs aim to avoid inpatient admissions that may predispose older adults to deconditioning, delirium, and infections. In a 2018 study, individuals exposed to a TCN had a significantly lower risk of inpatient admission during the index ED visit at 3 included hospitals, and for 2 of the 3 hospitals, this decreased risk persisted over the subsequent 30 days.[47]

Similar to the TCN model, assessments by other ED "navigators" have also shown promise, particularly when risk-prediction tools have been used to identify those at the highest risk.[48] In separate studies, referrals to community services placed by these professionals (eg, social worker, nurse, care coordinator, case manager) for the highest risk older adults resulted in fewer return visits to the ED and fewer admissions to nursing homes.[49,50] Without risk stratification, interventions reliant on referrals among a broader older adult population failed to reduce ED revisits, nursing home admissions, or mortality.[51,52] Aside from one-time in-ED engagement strategies, interventions with multiple touchpoints with health care team members offer a potentially more robust approach to ED-to-community care transitions. Inconsistency across outcomes has been noted,[48] yet reductions in hospitalizations at 30 days and ED revisits at 3 months have been reported for coordinated teams that extend beyond the ED.[53,54]

Telephone Follow-up

Aside from incorporating "positive" findings from existing studies on care transition interventions, it is also critical to consider studies with "null" results as this work may inform clinicians, researchers, and administrators where to invest time and resources and also provide information about study strengths, weakness, and modifications to consider for future investigations. Biese and colleagues reported "null" findings for a scripted telephone intervention for older adults discharged from the ED to home.[55] Although Biese and colleagues did not identify a significant difference in risk of the primary composite outcome of ED revisit, subsequent hospitalization, or death within 30 days, a more recent study of adults of all ages by Fruhan and Bills did identify a reduction in 3-day and 7-day ED return visits after an automated follow-up telephone call about remaining questions about discharge instructions 2 days after ED discharge.[56] These varied results suggest that telephone or telehealth (allowing visualization of the patient) follow-up remains a viable possible ED care transition intervention that could prove efficacious in future studies within specific ED populations, including those with functional or cognitive impairments.[57]

Information Exchange to the Outpatient Setting

A recent systematic review of randomized controlled trials evaluated the impact of ED-based interventions supporting ED-to-community care transitions of all adult populations.[58] The authors determined the ED-based care transition interventions did not reduce subsequent ED revisits or hospital admissions but did significantly improve outpatient follow-up rates. Specific to the geriatric population, prompt primary care and subspecialty care follow-up for older adults seen in the ED has been shown to be associated with reduced rates of subsequent, repeat ED visits within 30 days.[59] Alerting PCPs that older adults sought emergency care has also been proposed and tested as a means to improve ED-to-community care transitions and encourage more older adults to seek close outpatient follow-up. Web-based and electronic health record (EHR) alerts have been most commonly used, with studies across all age categories suggesting higher PCP awareness of the visits but no change in the rate of follow-up.[60,61] Especially if trying to automate this process and pragmatically implement at the point of clinical care, logistical issues associated with this practice include reliable identification of the older adult's PCP, provision of relevant ED information (eg, chief complaint, laboratory values, treatment plan) to the PCP, and recommendation of follow-up care needs. Health information technologies, remote data transfer, and clinical informatics represent burgeoning fields that may advance data-sharing efforts between clinicians and across settings.[62]

Considerations for Unique Populations

Social isolation, defined as "a perceived or objective lack of connection to, or support from, social networks," affects a large proportion of older adults and requires specific attention during ED-to-community care transitions. Findings from a recent national study suggest that approximately 25% of community-dwelling older adults are considered socially isolated.[63] Within the older adult population in the ED, estimates have recently found that over 50% actively were experiencing social disconnection, including feelings of being burdensome to others, as if they did not belong, or that people would be better off if they were gone.[6] In addition to poor psychological, cognitive, and physical outcomes,[64] social isolation has been shown to be associated with lower rates of in-person follow-up in the week following ED discharge.[65] Socially isolated older adult populations in the ED may reasonably be the target of future interventions, such as nonemergency medical transportation or coordination with community organizations, given recent calls to build interventions that reduce the health and medical impacts of social isolation in older adults.

Incident functional decline has been noted for older adults discharged from the ED to the community.[11,66] However, older adults seeking emergency care already with functional impairment before the ED visit have been identified as another population that is particularly at risk during ED-to-community care transitions. Lowthian and colleagues discovered that pre-existing functional impairment in activities of daily living (OR 3.21, 95% confidence interval 2.26–4.53) and instrumental activities of daily living (OR 6.69, 95% confidence interval 4.31–10.38) were both strongly associated with new functional decline in the 30 days after an ED visit.[1] Functional assessments, support service incorporation, mobility aids, and instructions on how to use assistive devices correctly have the potential to prevent worsening functional impairments during ED-to-community care transitions among older adults with pre-existing impairments.

Persons living with dementia (PLWD) and their care partners make up a separate population that often requires additional support to ensure successful ED-to-community care transitions. While the majority of PLWD are discharged from the ED,[67] care partners (eg, family, friends) often provide a significant amount of hands-on care and assistance with navigating follow-up care needs despite frequently being untrained. Thirty-day ED revisit rates are higher for those with a diagnosis of dementia,[68] which may be a result of unique ED-to-community care transition barriers experienced by care partners including poor communication and care partner engagement by clinicians during the discharge process, taking on additional responsibilities while aiding during the PLWD's acute illness recovery phase, and difficulty navigating the health-care system for follow-up.[40]

Measuring Success of Emergency Department Care Transitions

ED revisit rates are frequently used as a proxy measure for the quality and success of ED-to-community care transitions. Age, male sex, polypharmacy, and cognitive impairment have been shown to be independent predictors of 30-day ED revisits.[48,69] However, this outcome measure does not account for the condition burden or change in health-related quality of life faced by patients and family caregivers at home after ED discharge and is of limited utility for certain appropriate clinical scenarios that warrant an ED revisit (eg, wound check). The Centers for Medicare & Medicaid Services (CMS) has more recently prioritized the inclusion of the patient experience in the transition away from process measures, such as ED revisit rates, and toward patient-reported outcome measures (PROMs).[70] Focusing on the outcome of a health care experience, PROMs are questionnaires that report the patient's perception and may address health-related quality of life, condition-specific symptom burden, functional disability, or other considerations. PROMs addressing ED care transitions to date have been limited by their attempted translation from the inpatient hospital setting or absence of dedicated focus to the geriatric population.[71] The multidisciplinary Geriatric Emergency care Applied Research (GEAR) 1.0 and 2.0 Networks, respectively, focus on emergency care as experienced by older adults and persons living with cognitive impairment and their caregivers and have determined that developing PROMs addressing ED care transitions represents a critical knowledge gap that researchers should prioritize.[72,73]

Policy and Payment Implications

To improve hospital-to-home care transitions, the Medicare fee-for-service and Medicare Advantage programs currently allow PCPs to be reimbursed for transitional care management (TCM) services to reduce potentially preventable readmissions and errors during the 30 days following discharge from an inpatient hospitalization, an observation status hospitalization, or a skilled nursing facility stay.[74] Several components are required to bill TCM services, with two relevant components being (1) clinical staff contacting the patient or caregiver via phone, email, or face-face to address the patient's status beyond simply scheduling follow-up care and (2) conducting a follow-up visit within 7 or 14 days of discharge, depending on the complexity of the medical decision-making involved. What is not included as a triggering event to allow TCM services being performed are emergency outpatient visits, including all older adults experiencing an ED-to-community care transition.

Expanding this practice, CMS has the opportunity to use policy levers in two ways. Designating emergency outpatient visits as a reimbursable event for TCM services would allow and encourage PCPs to more regularly address the new diagnoses, new medications, and new care plans that commonly result from emergency care. Second, CMS and other payors should consider an analogous TCM service to be implemented for emergency clinicians treating and discharging high-risk older adults to the community.[75] Currently CMS only allows charges by PCPs for this billing code; however, initiatives stemming from ED-based TCM services could proactively set older adults up for success during ED-to-community care transitions. As an example, ED-based TCM services would be similar to Current Procedural Terminology codes 99495 and 99496 in the outpatient setting and could include facilitating referrals, care coordination, and other needed services for older adults that may reduce ED revisits, hospitalizations, and health-care expenditures in the weeks following ED discharge.

However, to truly move the needle regarding ED-to-community care transitions for older adults, meaningful change can come in the way of holding clinicians accountable for a population of patients and their subsequent outcomes through transitioning reimbursement toward value-based care initiatives and away from the United States' current volume-based fee-for-service model. More widespread uptake of accountable care organizations or capitation models that incentivize high-value care for a population rather than an individual may encourage coordinated clinical care and reduce fragmentation between settings and clinicians. ED-to-community care transition programs, models, and interventions stand to be a central component of needed partnerships with inpatient and outpatient colleagues participating in risk-based contracts.[75–77]

SUMMARY

Improving care transitions for older adults across health-care settings and between clinicians is a national priority. Fragmented and suboptimal ED-to-community care transitions can result in repeat ED visits, hospitalizations, and increased health-care costs. Older adults have higher prevalence of risk factors for poor transitions, such as cognitive or functional impairments, social isolation, and reduced comprehension of ED discharge instructions. Efforts to improve patient-centered outcomes in the period immediately after ED visits must be prioritized for older adults through the implementation of effective care transition intervention strategies, the development of clinical practice guidelines, and the expansion of TCM services.

CLINICS CARE POINTS

- Aside from ED revisit rates, more attention has increasingly been placed on patient-reported outcome measures suggesting that emergency clinicians may benefit by discussing condition-specific symptom burden and functional status and quality of life during the discharge instruction process.

- Emergency clinicians should consider using screening tools (eg, ISAR, Quick Dementia Rating System, and so on) and engaging case managers, transition care nurses, physical therapists, social workers, and other multidisciplinary team members before ED discharge.

- As part of the "4 Ms" model, addressing "What Matters" has been proven feasible within the ED and offers a succinct and structured method to identify the fears/concerns and desired outcomes of older adults.

- Older adults experiencing social isolation and impairments in functional status or cognition represent unique populations that are particularly at risk during ED-to-community transitions of care.

FUNDING SOURCES

C.J. Gettel is a Pepper Scholar with support from the Claude D. Pepper Older Americans Independence Center at Yale School of Medicine (P30AG021342), the National Institute on Aging of the National Institutes of Health, United States (R03AG073988), the Alzheimer's Association, United States (ARCOM-22-878456), the NIA, United States Imbedded Pragmatic Alzheimer's and AD-Related Dementias Clinical Trials Collaboratory (NIA IMPACT Collaboratory; U54AG063546), the Society for Academic Emergency Medicine Foundation, and the Emergency Medicine Foundation, United States. S.N. Hastings received support from the Duke Older Americans Independence Center (P30AG028716) and in-kind support from the Center of Innovation to Accelerate Discovery and Practice Transformation (CIN 13-410) at the Durham VA Health Care System. E.M. Goldberg is supported by the NIA (K76 AG059983). The funders had no role in the design and conduct of the study; collection, management, analysis, and interpretation of the data; and preparation or approval of the manuscript.

DISCLOSURE

K.J. Biese serves as an advisor to Third Eye Health, a telehealth provider focused on the postacute care space. None of the other authors have any conflicts to disclose.

REFERENCES

1. Lowthian JA, Straney LD, Brand CA, et al. Predicting functional decline in older emergency patients-the Safe Elderly Emergency Discharge (SEED) project. Age Ageing 2017;46(2):219–25.

2. Centers for Disease Control and Prevention. National Hospital Ambulatory Medical Care Survey: 2019 Emergency Department Summary Tables. Accessed December 15, 2022. https://www.cdc.gov/nchs/data/nhamcs/web_tables/2019-nhamcs-ed-web-tables-508.pdf.

3. Lowthian JA, Curtis AJ, Cameron PA, et al. Systematic review of trends in emergency department attendances: an Australian perspective. Emerg Med J 2011; 28(5):373–7.

4. Hollander JE, Sharma R. The availablists: emergency care without the emergency department. NEJM Catalyst 2021;. https://catalyst.nejm.org/doi/full/10.1056/CAT.21.0310.

5. Kessler C, Williams MC, Moustoukas JN, et al. Transitions of care for the geriatric patient in the emergency department. Clin Geriatr Med 2013;29(1):49–69.

6. Kandasamy D, Platts-Mills TF, Shah MN, et al. Social disconnection among older adults receiving care in the emergency department. West J Emerg Med 2018; 19(6):919–25.

7. Gettel CJ, Serina PT, Uzamere I, et al. Emergency department-to-community care transition barriers: a qualitative study of older adults. J Am Geriatr Soc 2022; 70(11):3152–62.

8. Sun R, Karaca Z, Wong HS. Trends in hospital emergency department visits by age and payer, 2006-2015. Agency for Healthcare Research and Quality; 2018. Available at: https://www.hcup-us.ahrq.gov/reports/statbriefs/sb238-Emergency-Department-Age-Payer-2006-2015.jsp. Accessed December 12, 2022.

9. Hastings SN, Schmader KE, Sloane RJ, et al. Adverse health outcomes after discharge from the emergency department–incidence and risk factors in a veteran population. J Gen Intern Med 2007;22(11):1527–31.

10. Musso MW, Perret JN, Sanders T, et al. Patients' comprehension of their emergency department encounter: a pilot study using physician observers. Ann Emerg Med 2015;65(2):151–5.e4.

11. Nagurney JM, Fleischman W, Han L, et al. Emergency department visits without hospitalization are associated with functional decline in older persons. Ann Emerg Med 2017;69(4):426–33.

12. Hastings SN, Whitson HE, Purser JL, et al. Emergency department discharge diagnosis and adverse health outcomes in older adults. J Am Geriatr Soc 2009;57(10):1856–61.

13. Gabayan GZ, Asch SM, Hsia RY, et al. Factors associated with short-term bounce-back admissions after emergency department discharge. Ann Emerg Med 2013;62(2):136–44.e1.

14. Duseja R, Bardach NS, Lin GA, et al. Revisit rates and associated costs after an emergency department encounter. Ann Intern Med 2015;162(11):750–6.

15. Aminzadeh F, Dalziel WB. Older adults in the emergency department: a systematic review of patterns of use, adverse outcomes, and effectiveness of interventions. Ann Emerg Med 2002;39(3):238–47.

16. Southerland LT, Lo AX, Biese K, et al. Concepts in practice: geriatric emergency departments. Ann Emerg Med 2020;75(2):162–70.

17. Geriatric Emergency Department Accreditation Program. American College of Emergency Physicians. Accessed September 17, 2022. https://www.acep.org/geda/.

18. American College of Emergency Physicians. American geriatrics society, emergency nurses association, society for academic emergency medicine, geriatric emergency department guidelines task force. Geriatric emergency department guidelines. Ann Emerg Med 2014;63(5):e7–25.

19. Kelen GD, Wolfe R, D'Onofrio G, et al. Emergency Department Crowding: The Canary in the Health. NEJM Catalyst. Published online September 28, 2021. https://catalyst.nejm.org/doi/full/10.1056/CAT.21.0217.

20. Carpenter CR, Shelton E, Fowler S, et al. Risk factors and screening instruments to predict adverse outcomes for undifferentiated older emergency department patients: a systematic review and meta-analysis. Acad Emerg Med 2015; 22(1):1–21.

21. Galvin R, Gilleit Y, Wallace E, et al. Adverse outcomes in older adults attending emergency departments: a systematic review and meta-analysis of the Identification of Seniors at Risk (ISAR) screening tool. Age Ageing 2017;46(2):179–86.

22. By the 2019 American Geriatrics Society Beers Criteria® Update Expert Panel. American geriatrics society 2019 updated AGS Beers Criteria® for potentially inappropriate medication use in older adults. J Am Geriatr Soc 2019;67(4): 674–94.

23. Carpenter CR, Bassett ER, Fischer GM, et al. Four sensitive screening tools to detect cognitive dysfunction in geriatric emergency department patients: brief Alzheimer's Screen, Short Blessed Test, Ottawa 3DY, and the caregiver-completed AD8. Acad Emerg Med 2011;18(4):374–84.

24. Galvin JE. The Quick Dementia Rating System (QDRS): a rapid dementia staging tool. Alzheimers Dement 2015;1(2):249–59.

25. Southerland LT, Pearson S, Hullick C, et al. Safe to send home? Discharge risk assessment in the emergency department. Emerg Med Australas 2019;31(2): 266–70.

26. Suffoletto B, Calabria J, Ross A, et al. A mobile phone text message program to measure oral antibiotic use and provide feedback on adherence to patients discharged from the emergency department. Acad Emerg Med 2012;19(8):949–58.

27. Atzema CL, Jackevicius CA, Chong A, et al. Prescribing of oral anticoagulants in the emergency department and subsequent long-term use by older adults with atrial fibrillation. CMAJ (Can Med Assoc J) 2019;191(49):E1345–54.

28. Shah VV, Villaflores CW, Chuong LH, et al. Association between in-person vs telehealth follow-up and rates of repeated hospital visits among patients seen in the emergency department. JAMA Netw Open 2022;5(10):e2237783.

29. Horwitz SM, Busch SH, Balestracci KMB, et al. Intensive intervention improves primary care follow-up for uninsured emergency department patients. Acad Emerg Med 2005;12(7):647–52.

30. Engel KG, Buckley BA, Forth VE, et al. Patient understanding of emergency department discharge instructions: where are knowledge deficits greatest? Acad Emerg Med 2012;19(9):E1035–44.

31. Benjenk I, DuGoff EH, Jacobsohn GC, et al. Predictors of older adult adherence with emergency department discharge instructions. Acad Emerg Med 2021; 28(2):215–25.

32. Ngai KM, Grudzen CR, Lee R, et al. The association between limited English proficiency and unplanned emergency department revisit within 72 hours. Ann Emerg Med 2016;68(2):213–21.

33. Parry C, Coleman EA, Smith JD, et al. The care transitions intervention: a patient-centered approach to ensuring effective transfers between sites of geriatric care. Home Health Care Serv Q 2003;22(3):1–17.

34. Jiang LG, Zhang Y, Greca E, et al. Emergency department patient navigator program demonstrates reduction in emergency department return visits and increase in follow-up appointment adherence. Am J Emerg Med 2022;53:173–9.

35. Sin DD, Bell NR, Man SFP. Effects of increased primary care access on process of care and health outcomes among patients with asthma who frequent emergency departments. Am J Med 2004;117(7):479–83.

36. Fulmer T, Mate KS, Berman A. The age-friendly health system imperative. J Am Geriatr Soc 2018;66(1):22–4.

37. Gettel C, Venkatesh A, Dowd H, et al. A qualitative study of "What Matters" to older adults in the emergency department. West J Emerg Med 2022;23(4):579–88.

38. McQuown CM, Snell KT, Abbate LM, et al. Telehealth for geriatric post emergency department visit to promote age friendly care. Health Serv Res 2022. https://doi.org/10.1111/1475-6773.14058.

39. Schumacher JR, Lutz BJ, Hall AG, et al. Impact of an emergency department-to-home transitional care intervention on health service use in Medicare beneficiaries: a mixed methods study. Med Care 2021;59(1):29–37.

40. Gettel CJ, Serina PT, Uzamere I, et al. Emergency department care transition barriers: a qualitative study of care partners of older adults with cognitive impairment. Alzheimers Dement 2022;8(1):e12355.

41. Costa Jacobsohn G, Maru AP, Green RK, et al. Multimethod process evaluation of a community paramedic delivered care transitions intervention for older emergency department patients. Prehosp Emerg Care 2022;1–10.

42. Shah MN, Hollander MM, Jones CM, et al. Improving the ED-to-home transition: the community paramedic-delivered care transitions intervention-preliminary findings. J Am Geriatr Soc 2018;66(11):2213–20.

43. Jacobsohn GC, Jones CMC, Green RK, et al. Effectiveness of a care transitions intervention for older adults discharged home from the emergency department: a randomized controlled trial. Acad Emerg Med 2022;29(1):51–63.

44. Shah MN, Jacobsohn GC, Jones CM, et al. Care transitions intervention reduces ED revisits in cognitively impaired patients. Alzheimers Dement 2022;8(1):e12261.

45. Hwang U, Dresden SM, Vargas-Torres C, et al. Association of a geriatric emergency department innovation program with cost outcomes among Medicare beneficiaries. JAMA Netw Open 2021;4(3):e2037334.

46. Dresden SM, Hwang U, Garrido MM, et al. Geriatric emergency department innovations: the impact of transitional care nurses on 30-day readmissions for older adults. Acad Emerg Med 2020;27(1):43–53.

47. Hwang U, Dresden SM, Rosenberg MS, et al. Geriatric emergency department innovations: transitional care nurses and hospital use. J Am Geriatr Soc 2018;66(3):459–66.

48. Karam G, Radden Z, Berall LE, et al. Efficacy of emergency department-based interventions designed to reduce repeat visits and other adverse outcomes for older patients after discharge: a systematic review. Geriatr Gerontol Int 2015;15(9):1107–17.

49. Hegney D, Buikstra E, Chamberlain C, et al. Nurse discharge planning in the emergency department: a Toowoomba, Australia, study. J Clin Nurs 2006;15(8):1033–44.

50. Mion LC, Palmer RM, Meldon SW, et al. Case finding and referral model for emergency department elders: a randomized clinical trial. Ann Emerg Med 2003; 41(1):57–68.
51. Guttman A, Afilalo M, Guttman R, et al. An emergency department-based nurse discharge coordinator for elder patients: does it make a difference? Acad Emerg Med 2004;11(12):1318–27.
52. Miller DK, Lewis LM, Nork MJ, et al. Controlled trial of a geriatric case-finding and liaison service in an emergency department. J Am Geriatr Soc 1996;44(5): 513–20.
53. Caplan GA, Williams AJ, Daly B, et al. A randomized, controlled trial of comprehensive geriatric assessment and multidisciplinary intervention after discharge of elderly from the emergency department–the DEED II study. J Am Geriatr Soc 2004;52(9):1417–23.
54. Lee JS, Hurley MJ, Carew D, et al. A randomized clinical trial to assess the impact on an emergency response system on anxiety and health care use among older emergency patients after a fall. Acad Emerg Med 2007;14(4):301–8.
55. Biese KJ, Busby-Whitehead J, Cai J, et al. Telephone follow-up for older adults discharged to home from the emergency department: a pragmatic randomized controlled trial. J Am Geriatr Soc 2018;66(3):452–8.
56. Fruhan S, Bills CB. Association of a callback program with emergency department revisit rates among patients seeking emergency care. JAMA Netw Open 2022;5(5):e2213154.
57. Hwang U, Hastings SN, Ramos K. Improving emergency department discharge care with telephone follow-up. Does it connect? J Am Geriatr Soc 2018;66(3): 436–8.
58. Aghajafari F, Sayed S, Emami N, et al. Optimizing emergency department care transitions to outpatient settings: a systematic review and meta-analysis. Am J Emerg Med 2020;38(12):2667–80.
59. Magidson PD, Huang J, Levitan EB, et al. Prompt outpatient care for older adults discharged from the emergency department reduces recidivism. West J Emerg Med 2020;21(6):198–204.
60. Atzema CL, Maclagan LC. The transition of care between emergency department and primary care: a scoping study. Acad Emerg Med 2017;24(2):201–15.
61. Hunchak C, Tannenbaum D, Roberts M, et al. Closing the circle of care: implementation of a web-based communication tool to improve emergency department discharge communication with family physicians. CJEM 2015;17(2):123–30.
62. Vollbrecht M, Biese K, Hastings SN, et al. Systems-based practice to improve care within and beyond the emergency department. Clin Geriatr Med 2018; 34(3):399–413.
63. Cudjoe TKM, Roth DL, Szanton SL, et al. The epidemiology of social isolation: national health and aging trends study. J Gerontol B Psychol Sci Soc Sci 2020; 75(1):107–13.
64. Vozikaki M, Linardakis M, Philalithis A. Preventive health services utilization in relation to social isolation in older adults. J Public Health 2017;25(5):545–56.
65. Cayenne NA, Jacobsohn GC, Jones CMC, et al. Association between social isolation and outpatient follow-up in older adults following emergency department discharge. Arch Gerontol Geriatr 2021;93:104298.
66. Sirois MJ, Carmichael PH, Daoust R, et al. Functional decline after nonhospitalized injuries in older patients: results from the Canadian emergency team initiative cohort in elders. Ann Emerg Med 2022;80(2):154–64.

67. LaMantia MA, Stump TE, Messina FC, et al. Emergency department use among older adults with dementia. Alzheimer Dis Assoc Disord 2016;30(1):35–40.

68. Kent T, Lesser A, Israni J, et al. 30-Day emergency department revisit rates among older adults with documented dementia. J Am Geriatr Soc 2019;67(11): 2254–9.

69. de Gelder J, Lucke JA, de Groot B, et al. Predictors and outcomes of revisits in older adults discharged from the emergency department. J Am Geriatr Soc 2018; 66(4):735–41.

70. Centers for Medicare & Medicaid Services. Meaningful Measures Initiative. Meaningful Measures Framework. Accessed December 13, 2022. https://www.cms.gov/Medicare/Quality-Initiatives-Patient-Assessment-Instruments/Quality InitiativesGenInfo/CMS-Quality-Strategy.

71. Vaillancourt S, Cullen JD, Dainty KN, et al. PROM-ED: development and testing of a patient-reported outcome measure for emergency department patients who are discharged home. Ann Emerg Med 2020;76(2):219–29.

72. Gettel CJ, Voils CI, Bristol AA, et al. Care transitions and social needs: a Geriatric Emergency care Applied Research (GEAR) Network scoping review and consensus statement. Acad Emerg Med 2021;28(12):1430–9.

73. Gettel CJ, Falvey JR, Gifford A, et al. Emergency department care transitions for patients with cognitive impairment: a scoping review. J Am Med Dir Assoc 2022; 23(8):1313.e1–13.

74. Centers for Medicare & Medicaid Services. Transitional Care Management Services. Medicare Learning Network. Accessed December 11, 2022. https://www.cms.gov/outreach-and-education/medicare-learning-network-mln/mlnproducts/downloads/transitional-care-management-services-fact-sheet-icn908628.pdf.

75. Biese K, Lash TA, Kennedy M. Emergency department care transition programs-value-based care interventions that need system-level support. JAMA Netw Open 2022;5(5):e2213160.

76. Gettel CJ, Tinloy B, Nedza SM, et al. The future of value-based emergency care: development of an emergency medicine MIPS value pathway framework. J Am Coll Emerg Physicians Open 2022;3(2):e12672.

77. Gettel CJ, Ling SM, Wild RE, et al. Centers for Medicare and Medicaid services merit-based incentive payment system value pathways: Opportunities for emergency clinicians to turn policy into practice. Ann Emerg Med 2021;78(5): 599–603.

Diversity, Equity, and Inclusion: Considerations in the Geriatric Emergency Department Patient

Anita N. Chary, MD, PhD[a,b,*], Lauren Cameron-Comasco, MD[c],
Kalpana N. Shankar, MD, MSc, MSHP[d],
Margaret E. Samuels-Kalow, MD, MPhil, MSHP[e]

KEYWORDS

- Diversity • Equity • Inclusion • Structural inequities • Social determinants of health
- Culture • Geriatrics • Emergency medicine

KEY POINTS

- *Social determinants of health* are the conditions in which people are born, live, work, and age that affect their health outcomes. These conditions affect the physiology of aging as well as access to and experiences of health care.
- *Culture* refers to shared beliefs, values, and behaviors that a group of people are socialized to accept as normal. Culture of patients and health care providers alike can impact older adults' expectations and experiences of health care.
- Institutional policies and practices, such as those of a hospital or emergency department, may unintentionally disadvantage older adults. Clinicians must work with institutional leadership to examine local policies for potential negative impacts on older adults and adjust policies to accommodate older adults' unique health care needs.

INTRODUCTION

The concepts of diversity, equity, and inclusion (DEI) are receiving increasing attention in medicine.[1] Numerous recent events and movements—for example, public response to police brutality against Black Americans in the summer of 2020—have

[a] Department of Emergency Medicine, Baylor College of Medicine, 2450 Holcombe Boulevard, Suite 01Y, Houston, TX 77021, USA; [b] Department of Medicine, Section of Health Services Research, Baylor College of Medicine, 2450 Holcombe Boulevard, Suite 01Y, Houston, TX 77021, USA; [c] Department of Emergency Medicine, Beaumont Hospital, 3601 West 13 Mile Road, Royal Oak, MI 48073, USA; [d] Department of Emergency Medicine, Brigham and Women's Hospital, 75 Francis Street, Neville House, Boston, MA 02115, USA; [e] Department of Emergency Medicine, Massachusetts General Hospital, 125 Nashua Street, Suite 9206, Boston, MA 02114, USA
* Corresponding author. 2450 Holcombe Boulevard, Suite 01Y, Houston, TX 77021.
E-mail address: anita.chary@bcm.edu

Clin Geriatr Med 39 (2023) 673–686
https://doi.org/10.1016/j.cger.2023.04.009
0749-0690/23/© 2023 Elsevier Inc. All rights reserved.

sparked political awareness and recognition of longstanding and persistent inequities.[2] In parallel, there has been increased appreciation for how structural and social
forces impact health care access and health outcomes.[3] The goal of this article is to
introduce core concepts from health equity scholarship and illustrate how they apply
to geriatric patients in the emergency department (ED).

Definitions

To start, the authors offer definitions of DEI adapted from the American Medical Association Center for Health Equity:[1]

- *Diversity* refers to the presence of differences in social identities such as race,
  ethnicity, gender, sexual orientation, class, age, and ability.
- *Equity* refers to fairness and justice. *Health equity* refers to the ability for all to
  achieve optimal health and well-being through fair access to opportunities.
  This concept recognizes that power is not distributed evenly within society and
  the differences in health status based on socioeconomic factors are unjust and
  avoidable. *Health inequities* refer to differences in health that are avoidable, unnecessary, and unjust.
- *Inclusion* refers to one's defining social identities being accepted, valued, respected, and supported within a group or organization. In an inclusive environment, individuals can behave authentically.

Table 1 provides the brief examples of the relevance of DEI in geriatric emergency
care.

In this article, the authors outline a socioecological approach to understanding DEI
in geriatric emergency care. The authors highlight structural inequities, culture, and
institutional policies as key DEI considerations in the care of geriatric patients in the
ED. The authors offer how these forces impact aging physiology, medication safety,
communication with older adults, and care of individuals with cognitive impairment.
The authors focus on geriatric patient identities and experience; the social identities
of the health care workforce, whereas an important consideration in DEI scholarship
is beyond the scope of this article.

Structural Inequities

Structural inequities refer to disparities in wealth, health, and other resources and outcomes that result from political and economic systems that privilege some while disadvantaging others.[1] The relationship between structural inequities and health is often
framed through *social determinants of health*, or the conditions in which people are
born, live, work, and age that affect their health outcomes.[4,5] Examples include.

- economic stability
- access to and quality of education
- access to and quality of health care
- neighborhood, social, and community context

Social determinants of health impact the experience and physiologic process of aging. The accumulation of deprivation and stress over the course of an individual's life
can produce *accelerated aging* or the development of early-onset age-associated disease. Chronic exposure to environmental stressors such as food and housing insecurity, exploitative labor conditions, or discrimination is associated with frailty, cognitive
and physical decline, and changes in brain structure; these changes are mediated by
oxidative stress and epigenetics.[6] Accelerated aging has been observed in racial and
ethnic minorities, that is, Blacks, Hispanics, and American Indians, who on average

Table 1
Examples of the relevance of diversity, equity, and inclusion in geriatric emergency care

Key Concept	Example	Sample Responses to Promote DEI
Diversity	Clinicians are trained to think of chest pain as the presenting symptom of myocardial infarction, but older adults may present instead with weakness	• Consider how aging physiology can impact clinical presentation • Describe presentation as "usual for older adults" rather than "atypical" for adults
Health equity and inequity	In stroke care, racial and ethnic minorities have delays in ED presentation, longer ED wait times, and are less likely to receive thrombolytic therapy than white non-Hispanics[58]	• Engage communities about stroke symptoms • Improve access to emergency medical services • Make clinicians and administrators aware of bias in health care delivery • Perform case reviews and analyze and refine stroke care algorithms
Inclusion	Age-related hearing loss (presbycusis) affects more than half of adults aged 75 y and older.[59] EDs often have background noise from monitors, equipment, and conversations, which can make it hard for older adults with hearing impairment to communicate	• Close doors to minimize distracting noises • Elicit preferences about where a clinician should be positioned to best be heard • Provide hearing-assist devices to make the ED environment more inclusive[35]

bear a higher burden of diabetes, hypertension, cardiovascular, and cerebrovascular disease than whites of the same age.[7,8] Black people also bear a disparately higher burden of cancer and have higher mortality and shorter survival than other racial populations.[9] Frailty, a clinical syndrome of age-associated decline in reserve and function leading to increased physiologic vulnerability to stressors is more prevalent in racial and ethnic minorities and those of low socioeconomic status.[10] Although these inequities are multifactorial and disease prevalence may have contributions from genetic factors, they are also due to socioeconomic and environmental disadvantages that racial and ethnic minorities disproportionately face.[7]

To understand disparities in aging, an explanation of race and ethnicity as social categories is helpful. *Race* is a socially constructed way of categorizing humans based on perceived physical traits such as skin color, facial features, and hair texture. In the United States, common racial categories are white, Black, Asian, American Indian or Alaskan Native, and Hawaiian or Pacific Islander, and non-whites are referred to as racial minorities. There is no biological basis to the race that humans are assigned; in fact, there is greater genetic diversity within so-called racial groups than between them. The same racial categories do not apply across societies, and an individual may identify their race differently than the race that society attributes to them.[11] *Ethnicity* is used to connote a group with shared ancestry, nationality, and often language and culture (eg, Afro-Caribbean, Italian, or Telugu, respectively). In medical journals, ethnicity in the United States is often reported in a binary fashion of Hispanic or non-Hispanic, and Hispanics are considered ethnic minorities.[12]

Both race and ethnicity have been used to perpetuate systems that privilege white people while disadvantaging people of color. For example, the "one-drop rule" in the United States considered any individual with Black ancestry as Black, historically excluding them from rights and opportunities such as land ownership, education, and voting. Over generations, such discriminatory policies have had a cumulative effect of marginalizing racial and ethnic minorities both socially and economically.[13] Resulting disparities in wealth and access to health resources contribute to accelerated aging.

CLINICS CARE POINTS

Accelerated aging is important to consider in the geriatric ED patient. Typically, ED policies for geriatric patients and individual clinicians' applications of geriatric medicine are for patients aged 65 and older. However, in certain populations, comorbidity and frailty should be considered at younger ages. Institutions where broadening the definition of geriatric patients at the system level could be beneficial include safety net EDs that primarily serve uninsured or underinsured racial/ethnic minorities. In addition, this action should be considered in EDs that serve large homeless populations, whose chronic disease burden at age 50 years approximates that of adults aged 65 years and over.[10,14,15] In these settings, lower age cutoffs should be considered when developing protocols for.

- Geriatric trauma activations, as those with more comorbidities experience undertriage[16] and those geriatric patients with trauma who are undertriaged are likelier to die[17]
- Screening for geriatric syndromes, such as ED delirium or falls, which is currently recommended for all adults aged 65 years and over[18]
- Consulting geriatric care coordination teams from the ED, which perform geriatric assessments and screen patients for targeted interventions (eg, occupational therapy, pharmacy consultation) to improve multidisciplinary inpatient care and facilitate patients' access to outpatient resources[19–21]

Example: Medication Safety

Medication safety is a core topic in geriatrics and geriatric emergency medicine, as management of chronic diseases can result in polypharmacy and initiation of high-risk medications. Social determinants of health can heavily influence older adults' experiences with medication management. Consider an 80-year-old Mexican female with hypertension, hyperlipidemia, diabetes, heart failure, and atrial fibrillation. As she recently relocated to the United States with grandchildren, she is not eligible for Medicare. She has repeated presentations to the ED due to hyperglycemia and fluid overload. **Table 2** offers the examples of how social determinants of health impact her medication management and the context of her ED utilization.

Pharmacoequity has been defined as the goal of ensuring that all individuals, regardless of resource availability, socioeconomic status, or social identity, can access the highest quality medications to manage their health needs.[22] Some ED strategies that can be used to promote pharmacoequity specifically for geriatric patients include.

- Expand medication histories to elicit any barriers to medication access. If elicited, work with the hospital pharmacy to deliver essential medications to

Table 2
Examples of how social determinants of health impact medication safety in an older adult in the emergency department

Social Determinant of Health	Example of Impacts on Medication Safety
Economic factors	Patient has no insurance and is unable to regularly afford out-of-pocket costs for multiple prescriptions
Education access and quality	Patient had limited formal schooling and is illiterate, has a hard time keeping pills straight and distinguishing medicines
Health care access and quality	Patient visits a free clinic on an ad hoc basis for prescription refills; no access to regular primary care
Neighborhood context	Patient lives in low-income area with no pharmacy as businesses have not invested in the area Nearest pharmacy is independent and has higher retail drug prices
Community context	Friends and relatives intermittently send her medications and vitamin supplements from Mexico Grandchildren as social support and cultural and linguistic brokers to assist with health care

bedside before discharging a patient. Prior ED-based programs have identified socially vulnerable patients to receive free prepackaged medications for common acute conditions[23,24] with one study showing a 50% decrease in ED return visits.[24]

- Couple screening for polypharmacy, as recommended in the geriatric ED guidelines, with pharmacy consults or interdisciplinary assessments.[18] Although these evaluations have been used for deprescribing,[25] they could also be used to substitute more affordable options (eg, generic for brand name or combination medications) and identify resources for patients such as nearest pharmacies or medication mailing services.
- Perform medication discharge teaching verbally and offer written instructions in a patient's preferred language and at an appropriate reading level. Work with interpreters to confirm understanding before a patient leaves the ED.[26]

CULTURE

Culture refers to shared beliefs, values, and behaviors that a group of people are socialized to accept as normal. The term has historically been and is commonly used to describe the lifeways of particular ethnic groups or people with a shared nationality. Culture includes.

- codes of manners
- rituals
- language
- dress
- family structure
- religion and spirituality

Culture—both of patients and health care providers—affects experiences and delivery of health care for older adults in numerous ways. The following are two common examples from emergency practice.

Communication About Critical Illness

Emergency clinicians must often lead conversations about serious illness that guide decisions about resuscitation, intubation, and end-of-life care—sometimes directly with patients and other times with their relatives or caregivers.[27] Such conversations may also include informing patients and/or loved ones about a poor prognosis, as only one-third of older adults survive hospitalization after ED intubation.[28]

Culture influences the extent to which individuals feel comfortable directly communicating with a clinician about serious illness and dying.[29] As one example, studies with older adults in Japan have demonstrated preferences to defer to a physician's judgment rather than actively discussing end-of-life decision-making.[30,31] As another example, an ethnographic account of cancer care in Guatemala has described familial preferences to exclude patients from prognostic conversations with physicians, due in part to local understandings that such information can lead to emotional distress that itself provokes the death of a patient.[32]

Cultural values shape where and how people would hope to die. For example, in Thailand, where reincarnation is a common framework for understanding life and death, dying at home is thought to produce a higher quality of rebirth compared with dying in the hospital. The home offers a rich moral environment for death, given its energy from prior ceremonies and familial relationships, in comparison to the hospital, which has no ceremonial history and is haunted by spirits. As such, families may rush critically ill patients home from the hospital by ambulance, hoping to withdraw life support and facilitate death in an ethical place.[33]

Culturally-defined family relationships also influence which individuals make decisions on behalf of a critically ill patient. The Western biomedical and legal concepts of a health care proxy and power of attorney assume a single surrogate decision-maker. However, such concepts may not neatly overlay onto multigenerational households where multiple family members are involved in an older adult's care, where no single individual has assumed an authoritative legal designation, and where caregivers may not agree about goals of care. **Box 1** offers a case that exemplifies these considerations.

CLINICS CARE POINTS

Developing awareness of sociocultural dynamics that inform decision-making during serious illness can help emergency clinicians refine their approach to communication with older adult patients and caregivers. Culturally-sensitive strategies include:[27]

- Ask for permission to speak with a patient about their serious illness.
- Assess a patient's understanding of their own situation.
- Ask which caregivers and/or family members a patient wants involved in the conversation.
- If unable to speak directly with a patient, ask available care partners who else should be involved and included in decisions about the patient's care.
- Respect that a family may need to come to consensus and may not be able to provide a decision in the ED.

Ultimately, these actions can facilitate a clinician's recommendation of a course of action that aligns with what matters most to patients and care partners.

Elderspeak and Ageism

Culture can be shared by distinct professional groups or organizations, such as health care providers, who through training or a work environment are socialized to think and

> **Box 1**
> **Case: An example of how cultural context impacts serious illness conversations in the emergency department**
>
> Mr Singh is a 76-year-old Hindi-speaking man with dementia, diabetes, hypertension, and benign prostatic hypertrophy with an indwelling Foley catheter who presents to the ED with altered mental status and vomiting. Owing to COVID-19-related infection control measures and crowding of the ED with boarding patients, his family members are not allowed to enter. The ED team finds Mr Singh is febrile and hypotensive and has cloudy urine concerning for urosepsis. The emergency physician speaks with Mr Singh's wife to obtain history and is told that Mr Singh is full code. After administering fluids, antibiotics, and starting pressors, he shows minimal improvement and groans to ED staff that he is ready to die. The emergency physician calls the same phone number, but this time reaches the patient's son, who states that he is the primary decision-maker in his father's medical care. However, his son has not been legally or formally designated as such in the medical record and is unsure about what care his father would want in this situation. The patient's wife does not have her own phone and has returned to her own home for the night.

act similarly. Within a cultural group or organization, people may be socialized to associate negative values with aging. *Ageism* refers to stereotypes (how we think), prejudice (how we feel), and discrimination (how we behave) by a person's age.[34]

Ageist attitudes trickle into medical environments, where aging is commonly equated with disease, disability, and dependence on others.[35] One common manifestation of ageism in medical culture is *elderspeak.* Elderspeak is a form of communication overaccommodation used with older adults. It arises from ageist stereotypes and is characterized by the use of inappropriately juvenile word choices and intonation. Examples in medicine include clinicians using terms of endearment such as "honey" or "dear" to address older people, using a high pitch or overly nurturing voice and exaggerating smiles and nods. Nonverbal features include speaking loudly or yelling into an older patient's ear, patting an older patient on the head, or preferentially speaking about a patient in the third person with their loved one while in front of the patient.[36] Clinicians may engage in elderspeak unknowingly once they perceive old age cues—for example, gray hair, wrinkles—which provokes assumptions about the patient's abilities and triggers automatic speech and behavioral adjustments. These in turn reinforce age-based stereotypes.[37] In this way, elderspeak is an example of *implicit bias* or automatic and unconscious assumptions that affect judgments about others.

The intention behind elderspeak may be to express care or facilitate understanding, but the impact on patients and on the patient–clinician relationship can be negative. Elderspeak makes older adults feel impaired and incapable and leads them to perceive their health care team as patronizing and disrespectful.[36] Among persons living with dementia, elderspeak can lead to resistiveness to care or behaviors that prevent caregivers from performing or assisting with activities of daily living. In a nursing home-based study, persons living with dementia were twice as likely to resist care when health care workers used elderspeak compared with speaking normally.[38] Communication training to reduce elderspeak in nursing homes has been shown to reduce resistiveness to care among persons living with dementia.[39]

CLINICS CARE POINTS

In the ED, clinicians can use several strategies to avoid elderspeak, optimize communication, and create an inclusive care environment with older adults:[35]

- When interviewing a patient, turn on lights and minimize noise from stimuli such as intravenous (IV) pumps or TVs.
- Help patients retrieve their reading glasses or hearing aids from their belongings when speaking with them. Offer sensory assist devices such as hearing aids or reading glasses if available in your ED.[40]
- Help patients find a comfortable position in a chair or stretcher, allowing them to fully engage in conversation.
- Address patients by their stated preferred name.
- Acknowledge care partners at bedside, but also speak to and look directly at their older patients.

Institutional Policies

Inequities can be produced through institutions such as schools, workplaces, or in health care, through clinics and hospitals. Institutional policies and practices can lead to disparate access to resources and inequitable outcomes based on social identities. Often, institutional policies are not intended to disadvantage particular individuals, but do so inadvertently.

An important example of inequality mediated by institutions is reflected by the experiences of older adults with cognitive impairment who sought emergency care early in the COVID-19 pandemic. The prevalence of cognitive impairment increases with age. Older adults with cognitive impairment may not be able to accurately relay the history of a present illness, engage with a health care team, or fully understand testing or treatment plans on their own.[41] Often, to navigate medical visits, they rely on caregivers or care partners.[42] During initial surges of the COVID-19 pandemic, hospitals developed visitor restriction policies as an infection control measure. Such policies generally classify caregivers as visitors, but caregivers' roles more accurately involve helping patients engage in health care, advocating for patient comfort, and providing context for medical decision-making.[43] In a survey of over 350 hospitals in the United States conducted in 2020, only a minority of hospitals (39%) and EDs (29%) reported exceptions to visitor restriction policies for caregivers of persons with cognitive impairment.[44]

Visitor restriction policies are generally intended to benefit patients, visitors, and hospital staff by minimizing exposure to and spread of COVID-19. However, they can negatively impact people with cognitive impairment, who depend on care partners to communicate with a care team and advocate for their comfort. Such policies can have profound implications for patient safety: one study found that hospitals with visitor restrictions had increased in-hospital fall and sepsis rates for older adults.[45] Another study found that without caregivers at bedside during the pandemic, emergency clinicians had a harder time evaluating patients with cognitive dysfunction and were more likely to perform broader testing and hospitalize them.[46]

The existence of exceptions to visitor restriction policies for caregivers of persons with cognitive impairment is a step forward. However, various social factors can affect individuals' abilities to navigate such exceptions. Information about patient accompaniment and visitation policies may be listed on a hospital's Website, which may be inaccessible to caregivers with limited Internet or technological skills. In the above-mentioned survey, only 12% of hospitals with visitor restriction policies had telephone or Web-based information available in non-English languages.[44] Consider a caregiver arriving with a person with cognitive impairment to ED triage. If the caregiver knows about visitor policy exceptions policies, they may advocate entering the ED. However, if the individual is a racial or ethnic minority who primarily speaks a non-English

> **Box 2**
> **Case: The concept of intersectionality**
>
> The concept of *intersectionality* is helpful in understanding how multiple social factors can converge in ways that disproportionately disadvantage some individuals. Intersectionality posits that the experience of inequalities based on marginalized social identities is synergistic, rather than simply additive.[47] Imagine an older Vietnamese-speaking man with dementia and deafness who presents to the ED with hip pain after a fall. The challenges of hearing impairment, cognitive impairment, language barriers, and absence of a bedside caregiver to help engage the care team all amplify each other to lead to undesirable outcomes such as delayed administration of pain medications and development of delirium.

language and is socialized to defer to authorities, they may not inquire about exceptions if a triage clinician informs them in English that they may not enter. **Boxes 2–4** offer the additional examples of how institutional policies and practices can adversely impact older adults in the ED.

CLINICS CARE POINTS

> - Consider the impact of all ED policies on patients with diverse social identities and abilities. Work with administrators and leadership to adjust policies as needed.
> - Distinguish between care partners of older adults and visitors. The former plays crucial roles in communication, advocacy, and navigating health care.
> - For patients whose primary language is not the language of health care delivery, work with in-person interpreters, rather than remote interpreters, to promote patients' engagement with the care team.

DISCUSSION

Accounting for structural, cultural, and institutional factors in geriatric emergency care can seem complex and overwhelming, particularly given time pressures and high-acuity situations that clinicians face in the ED. However, recognition of the broader structures that shape clinical interactions can encourage clinicians to imagine innovations, advocate for vulnerable patients, and implement interventions. This has been referred to as developing *structural competency*.[56] Structural competency has been used as a guiding principle to develop medical education curricula that frame patient encounters in structural, rather than individualistic terms. Recently, within emergency medicine, a framework has been developed to help researchers, as well, to

> **Box 3**
> **Case: Emergency department crowding: Negative impacts on older adults**
>
> ED crowding occurs when the need for emergency services exceeds available ED and hospital resources. Studies have shown that how institutional policies and practices related to ED crowding can disproportionately impact older adults. As one example, one study found that an ED census 120% greater than bed capacity was associated with longer time to pain assessment and delays in pain treatment of older adults with hip fracture.[48] As another example, a common institutional response to boarding, or a lack of inpatient beds, is to deliver ED care in hallways.[49] Importantly, a study found that hallway care is associated with increased ED delirium in older adults.[50]

Box 4
Considering equity implications of geriatric emergency department accreditation

Geriatric ED accreditation is a process that encourages EDs to use evidence-based strategies to systematically tailor emergency care to the unique clinical needs of older adults. Adoption of the geriatric ED guidelines—which includes recommendations for practices such as geriatric screenings and management of Foley catheters—allows institutions to apply for formal external recognition of their geriatric initiatives.[18] Geriatric ED accreditation can help make emergency care more inclusive of older adults. There are important considerations for health equity associated with geriatric ED accreditation. On the one hand, geriatric ED accreditation requires institutions to have multiple types of resources, such as those for patients (eg, 24/7 access to food and drink) and those to support training of designated care team members in geriatrics. Geriatric ED accreditation also requires institutional infrastructure to support monitoring of adopted processes. These requirements, along with the application fee that ranges by accreditation level from $2500 to $15,000, may be prohibitive for low-resource institutions such as public safety net hospitals. Indeed, most of the geriatric EDs are in urban areas, and hospitals with academic affiliations and a large population of privately insured patients may have greater capability of meeting accreditation requirements.[51] As such, geriatric ED accreditation could widen gaps between institutions that can afford to provide quality geriatric care through evidence-guided principles and staffing and those that cannot. On the other hand, adoption of processes outlined in the geriatric ED guidelines has the potential to help mitigate some types of health inequities. As one example, Black and Hispanic populations more often have a missed or delayed dementia diagnosis when compared with white populations.[52] Black and Hispanic populations also have higher ED utilization for routine or usual care.[53,54] The adoption of dementia screenings in the ED, when paired with robust referral mechanisms for outpatient neurocognitive testing, has the potential to mitigate disparities in early dementia detection. However, sites adopting dementia screening must consider that certain screening tests such as the Mini Mental Status Exam are unreliable in individuals with low literacy.[55]

---

understand and incorporate into their work structural forces that produce health inequities.[57]

Simultaneously, clinicians can strive to engage in *cultural humility*, a longitudinal process of developing skills to respectfully approach and treat a patient of any cultural background at any time. The process focuses on coming to common understanding and building a therapeutic partnership based on openness to a patient's cultural values. Cultural humility also emphasizes the clinician's introspection on their own values with specific attention to recognizing and reducing power differences inherent to the clinician–patient relationship.[1]

SUMMARY

DEI is important considerations in the emergency care of geriatric patients who have multiple social identities beyond their age. Cultivating awareness of structural, cultural, and institutional influences on geriatric acute care is a first step toward promoting equitable emergency care.

DISCLOSURE

The authors have no commercial or financial conflicts of interest. A.N. Chary receives support from the HVA HSR&D C for Innovations in Quality, Effectiveness, and Safety (CIN13-413).

REFERENCES

1. American Medical Association, American Association of Medical Colleges Center for Justice. Advancing Health Equity: A Guide to Language, Narrative and Concepts. Available at: https://www.ama-assn.org/system/files/ama-aamc-equity-guide.pdf. Accessed January 4, 2023.
2. Salles A, Arora VM, Mitchell KA. Everyone must address Anti-black racism in health care: steps for non-black health care professionals to take. JAMA 2021; 326(7):601–2.
3. Franks NM, Gipson K, Kaltiso SA, et al. The time is now: racism and the responsibility of emergency medicine to Be Antiracist. Ann Emerg Med 2021;78(5): 577–86.
4. World Health Organization. Social determinants of health. Published 2023. Available at: https://www.who.int/health-topics/social-determinants-of-health. Accessed 9 January, 2023.
5. Office of Disease Prevention and Health Promotion, U.S. Department of Health and Human Services. Social Determinants of Health - Healthy People 2030 | health.gov. Published 2023 Available at: https://health.gov/healthypeople/priority-areas/social-determinants-health. Accessed January 9, 2023.
6. Guidi J, Lucente M, Sonino N, et al. Allostatic load and its impact on health: a systematic review. Psychother Psychosom 2021;90(1):11–27.
7. Noren Hooten N, Pacheco NL, Smith JT, et al. The accelerated aging phenotype: the role of race and social determinants of health on aging. Ageing Res Rev 2022; 73:101536.
8. Manson SM, Buchwald DS. Aging and health of American Indians and Alaska natives: contributions from the native investigator development program. J Aging Health 2021;33(7–8 Suppl):3S–9S.
9. American Cancer Society, Cancer facts & figures for african Americans 2019-2021, 2019, American Cancer Society, Inc., Available at: https://www.cancer.org/content/dam/cancer-org/research/cancer-facts-and-statistics/cancer-facts-and-figures-for-african-americans/cancer-facts-and-figures-for-african-americans-2019-2021.pdf. Accessed January 15, 2023.
10. Bandeen-Roche K, Seplaki CL, Huang J, et al. Frailty in older adults: a nationally representative profile in the United States. J Gerontol A Biol Sci Med Sci 2015; 70(11):1427–34.
11. American Anthropological Association. AAA Statement on Race. Published May 17, 1998. Available at: https://www.americananthro.org/ConnectWithAAA/Content.aspx?ItemNumber=2583. Accessed December 4, 2020.
12. Flanagin A, Frey T, Christiansen SL. AMA manual of style committee. Updated guidance on the reporting of race and ethnicity in medical and science journals. JAMA 2021;326(7):621–7.
13. Jones CP. Levels of racism: a theoretic framework and a gardener's tale. Am J Public Health 2000;90(8):1212–5.
14. Gelberg L, Linn LS, Mayer-Oakes SA. Differences in health status between older and younger homeless adults. J Am Geriatr Soc 1990;38(11):1220–9.
15. Garibaldi B, Conde-Martel A, O'Toole TP. Self-reported comorbidities, perceived needs, and sources for usual care for older and younger homeless adults. J Gen Intern Med 2005;20(8):726–30.
16. Anantha RV, Painter MD, Diaz-Garelli F, et al. Undertriage despite use of geriatric-specific trauma team activation guidelines: who are we missing? Am Surg 2021; 87(3):419–26.

17. Rogers A, Rogers F, Bradburn E, et al. Old and undertriaged: a lethal combination. Am Surg 2012;78(6):711–5.
18. American College of Emergency Physicians, American Geriatrics Society, Emergency Nurses Association, Society for Academic Emergency Medicine. Geriatric emergency department guidelines. Ann Emerg Med 2014;63(5):e7–25.
19. Keene SE, Cameron-Comasco L. Implementation of a geriatric emergency medicine assessment team decreases hospital length of stay. Am J Emerg Med 2022; 55:45–50.
20. Huded JM, Lee A, Song S, et al. Association of a geriatric emergency department program with healthcare outcomes among veterans. J Am Geriatr Soc 2022; 70(2):601–8.
21. Aldeen AZ, Courtney DM, Lindquist LA, et al. Geriatric emergency department innovations: preliminary data for the geriatric nurse liaison model. J Am Geriatr Soc 2014;62(9):1781–5.
22. Essien UR, Dusetzina SB, Gellad WF. A policy prescription for reducing health disparities—Achieving pharmacoequity. JAMA 2021;326(18):1793–4.
23. Molina MF, Chary AN, Baugh JJ, et al. To-go medications as a means to treat discharged emergency department patients during COVID-19. Am J Emerg Med 2021;41:239–40.
24. Hayes BD, Zaharna L, Winters ME, et al. To-Go medications for decreasing ED return visits. Am J Emerg Med 2012;30(9):2011–4.
25. Houlind MB, Andersen AL, Treldal C, et al. A collaborative medication review including deprescribing for older patients in an emergency department: a longitudinal feasibility study. J Clin Med 2020;9(2):348.
26. Samuels-Kalow ME, Stack AM, Porter SC. Effective discharge communication in the emergency department. Ann Emerg Med 2012;60(2):152–9.
27. Ouchi K, George N, Schuur JD, et al. Goals-of-Care conversations for older adults with serious illness in the emergency department: challenges and opportunities. Ann Emerg Med 2019;74(2):276–84.
28. Ouchi K, Jambaulikar GD, Hohmann S, et al. Prognosis after emergency department intubation to inform shared decision-making. J Am Geriatr Soc 2018;66(7): 1377–81.
29. Krikorian A, Maldonado C, Pastrana T. Patient's perspectives on the notion of a good death: a systematic review of the literature. J Pain Symptom Manage 2020;59(1):152–64.
30. Hirai K, Miyashita M, Morita T, et al. Good death in Japanese cancer care: a qualitative study. J Pain Symptom Manage 2006;31(2):140–7.
31. Akechi T, Miyashita M, Morita T, et al. Good death in elderly adults with cancer in Japan based on perspectives of the general population. J Am Geriatr Soc 2012; 60(2):271–6.
32. Chary A. A poor woman's disease": an ethnography of cervical cancer and global health in Guatemala [PhD dissertation]. St. Louis: Washington University; 2015.
33. Stonington SD. On ethical locations: the good death in Thailand, where ethics sit in places. Soc Sci Med 2012;75(5):836–44.
34. World Health Organization. Ageing: Ageism. Published March 18, 2021. Available at: https://www.who.int/news-room/questions-and-answers/item/ageing-ageism. Accessed March 2, 2022.
35. Chary A, Cameron-Comasco L, Rohra A, et al. Strategies to combat ageism in emergency medicine. J Geriatr Emerg Med 2022;3(2):1–4.
36. Shaw CA, Gordon JK. Understanding elderspeak: an evolutionary concept Analysis. Innov Aging 2021;5(3):igab023.

77a w7

37. Ryan EB, Giles H, Bartolucci G, et al. Psycholinguistic and social psychological components of communication by and with the elderly. Lang Commun 1986;6(1):1–24.
38. Williams KN, Herman R, Gajewski B, et al. Elderspeak communication: impact on dementia care. Am J Alzheimers Dis Other Demen 2009;24(1):11–20.
39. Williams KN, Perkhounkova Y, Herman R, et al. A communication intervention to reduce resistiveness in dementia care: a cluster randomized controlled trial. Gerontol 2017;57(4):707–18.
40. Fareed N, Southerland LT, Rao BM, et al. Geriatric assistive devices improve older patient engagement and clinical care in an emergency department. Am J Emerg Med 2020. https://doi.org/10.1016/j.ajem.2020.07.073.
41. Carpenter CR, Leggett J, Bellolio F, et al. Emergency department communication in persons living with dementia and care partners: a scoping review. J Am Med Dir Assoc 2022;23(8):1313.e15–46.
42. Dresden SM, Taylor Z, Serina P, et al. Optimal emergency department care practices for persons living with dementia: a scoping review. J Am Med Dir Assoc 2022;23(8):1314.e1–29.
43. Chary AN, Naik AD, Kennedy M. Visitor policies and health equity in emergency care of older adults. J Am Geriatr Soc 2022;70(2):376–8.
44. Lo AX, Wedel LK, Liu SW, et al. COVID-19 hospital and emergency department visitor policies in the United States: impact on persons with cognitive or physical impairment or receiving end-of-life care. J Am Coll Emerg Physicians Open 2022;3(1):e12622.
45. Silvera GA, Wolf JA, Stanowski A, et al. The influence of COVID-19 visitation restrictions on patient experience and safety outcomes: a critical role for subjective advocates. Patient Exp J 2021;8(1):30–9.
46. Chary AN, Castilla-Ojo N, Joshi C, et al. Evaluating older adults with cognitive dysfunction: a qualitative study with emergency clinicians. J Am Geriatr Soc 2022;70(2):341–51.
47. Crenshaw KW. Beyond racism and misogyny: Black feminism and 2 live crew. In: Meyers DT, editor. Feminist social thought: a reader. London: Routledge; 1997. p. 245–63.
48. Hwang U, Richardson LD, Sonuyi TO, et al. The effect of emergency department crowding on the management of pain in older adults with hip fracture. J Am Geriatr Soc 2006;54(2):270–5.
49. Feldman JA. When the Aberrant becomes the accepted: the rise of hallway care in emergency medicine. Acad Emerg Med 2020;27(3):256–8.
50. van Loveren K, Singla A, Sinvani L, et al. Increased emergency department hallway length of stay is associated with development of delirium. West J Emerg Med 2021;22(3):726–35.
51. Kennedy M, Lesser A, Israni J, et al. Reach and adoption of a geriatric emergency department accreditation program in the United States. Ann Emerg Med 2022;79(4):367–73.
52. Lin PJ, Daly AT, Olchanski N, et al. Dementia diagnosis disparities by race and ethnicity. Med Care 2021;59(8):679.
53. Walls CA, Rhodes KV, Kennedy JJ. The emergency department as usual source of medical care: estimates from the 1998 national health interview survey. Acad Emerg Med 2002;9(11):1140–5.
54. Hong R, Baumann BM, Boudreaux ED. The emergency department for routine healthcare: race/ethnicity, socioeconomic status, and perceptual factors. J Emerg Med 2007;32(2):149–58.

55. Pellicer-Espinosa I, Díaz-Orueta U. Cognitive screening instruments for older adults with low educational and literacy levels: a systematic review. J Appl Gerontol 2022;41(4):1222–31.
56. Metzl JM, Hansen H. Structural competency: theorizing a new medical engagement with stigma and inequality. Soc Sci Med 2014;103:126–33.
57. Zeidan A, Salhi B, Backster A, et al. A structural competency framework for emergency medicine Research: results from a scoping review and consensus conference. West J Emerg Med 2022;23(5):650–9.
58. Cruz-Flores S, Rabinstein A, Biller J, et al. Racial-ethnic disparities in stroke care: the American experience: a statement for healthcare professionals from the American Heart Association/American Stroke Association. Stroke 2011;42(7):2091–116.
59. National Institute on Deafness and Other Communication Disorders. Age-Related Hearing Loss (Presbycusis): Causes and Treatment. Age-Related Hearing Loss (Presbycusis): Causes and Treatment. Published March 16, 2022. Available at: https://www.nidcd.nih.gov/health/age-related-hearing-loss. Accessed January 26, 2023.

1. Publication Title	2. Publication Number	3. Filing Date
CLINICS IN GERIATRIC MEDICINE	000 – 704	9/18/2023

4. Issue Frequency	5. Number of Issues Published Annually	6. Annual Subscription Price
FEB, MAY, AUG, NOV	4	$312.00

7. Complete Mailing Address of Known Office of Publication *(Not printer) (Street, city, county, state, and ZIP+4®)*

ELSEVIER INC.
230 Park Avenue, Suite 800
New York, NY 10169

Contact Person
Malathi Samayan

Telephone *(Include area code)*
91-44-4299-4507

8. Complete Mailing Address of Headquarters or General Business Office of Publisher *(Not printer)*

ELSEVIER INC.
230 Park Avenue, Suite 800
New York, NY 10169

9. Full Names and Complete Mailing Addresses of Publisher, Editor, and Managing Editor *(Do not leave blank)*

Publisher *(Name and complete mailing address)*

Dolores Meloni, ELSEVIER INC.
1600 JOHN F KENNEDY BLVD. SUITE 1600
PHILADELPHIA, PA 19103-2899

Editor *(Name and complete mailing address)*

JOANNA COLLETT, ELSEVIER INC.
1600 JOHN F KENNEDY BLVD. SUITE 1600
PHILADELPHIA, PA 19103-2899

Managing Editor *(Name and complete mailing address)*

PATRICK MANLEY, ELSEVIER INC.
1600 JOHN F KENNEDY BLVD. SUITE 1600
PHILADELPHIA, PA 19103-2899

10. Owner *(Do not leave blank. If the publication is owned by a corporation, give the name and address of the corporation immediately followed by the names and addresses of all stockholders owning or holding 1 percent or more of the total amount of stock. If not owned by a corporation, give the names and addresses of the individual owners. If owned by a partnership or other unincorporated firm, give its name and address as well as those of each individual owner. If the publication is published by a nonprofit organization, give its name and address.)*

Full Name	Complete Mailing Address
WHOLLY OWNED SUBSIDIARY OF REED/ELSEVIER, US HOLDINGS	1600 JOHN F KENNEDY BLVD. SUITE 1600 PHILADELPHIA, PA 19103-2899

11. Known Bondholders, Mortgagees, and Other Security Holders Owning or Holding 1 Percent or More of Total Amount of Bonds, Mortgages, or Other Securities. If none, check box. ▶ ☐ None

Full Name	Complete Mailing Address
N/A	

12. Tax Status *(For completion by nonprofit organizations authorized to mail at nonprofit rates) (Check one)*
The purpose, function, and nonprofit status of this organization and the exempt status for federal income tax purposes:
☒ Has Not Changed During Preceding 12 Months
☐ Has Changed During Preceding 12 Months *(Publisher must submit explanation of change with this statement)*

PS Form **3526**, July 2014 *[Page 1 of 4 (see instructions page 4)]* PSN: 7530-01-000-9931   PRIVACY NOTICE: See our privacy policy on www.usps.com.

---

13. Publication Title	14. Issue Date for Circulation Data Below
CLINICS IN GERIATRIC MEDICINE	AUGUST 2023

15. Extent and Nature of Circulation			Average No. Copies Each Issue During Preceding 12 Months	No. Copies of Single Issue Published Nearest to Filing Date
a. Total Number of Copies *(Net press run)*			87	82
b. Paid Circulation *(By Mail and Outside the Mail)*	(1)	Mailed Outside-County Paid Subscriptions Stated on PS Form 3541 (Include paid distribution above nominal rate, advertiser's proof copies, and exchange copies)	54	51
	(2)	Mailed In-County Paid Subscriptions Stated on PS Form 3541 (Include paid distribution above nominal rate, advertiser's proof copies, and exchange copies)	0	0
	(3)	Paid Distribution Outside the Mails Including Sales Through Dealers and Carriers, Street Vendors, Counter Sales, and Other Paid Distribution Outside USPS®	23	24
	(4)	Paid Distribution by Other Classes of Mail Through the USPS (e.g., First-Class Mail®)	9	6
c. Total Paid Distribution *(Sum of 15b (1), (2), (3), and (4))* ▶			86	81
d. Free or Nominal Rate Distribution *(By Mail and Outside the Mail)*	(1)	Free or Nominal Rate Outside-County Copies included on PS Form 3541	0	0
	(2)	Free or Nominal Rate In-County Copies Included on PS Form 3541	0	0
	(3)	Free or Nominal Rate Copies Mailed at Other Classes Through the USPS (e.g., First-Class Mail)	0	0
	(4)	Free or Nominal Rate Distribution Outside the Mail (Carriers or other means)	1	1
e. Total Free or Nominal Rate Distribution *(Sum of 15d (1), (2), (3) and (4))* ▶			1	1
f. Total Distribution *(Sum of 15c and 15e)* ▶			87	82
g. Copies not Distributed *(See Instructions to Publishers #4 (page 83))* ▶			0	0
h. Total *(Sum of 15f and g)* ▶			87	82
i. Percent Paid *(15c divided by 15f times 100)* ▶			98.85%	98.78%

* If you are claiming electronic copies, go to line 16 on page 3. If you are not claiming electronic copies, skip to line 17 on page 3.

PS Form **3526**, July 2014 (Page 2 of 4)

16. Electronic Copy Circulation	Average No. Copies Each Issue During Preceding 12 Months	No. Copies of Single Issue Published Nearest to Filing Date
a. Paid Electronic Copies ▶		
b. Total Paid Print Copies (Line 15c) + Paid Electronic Copies (Line 16a) ▶		
c. Total Print Distribution (Line 15f) + Paid Electronic Copies (Line 16a) ▶		
d. Percent Paid (Both Print & Electronic Copies) (16b divided by 16c × 100) ▶		

☒ I certify that 50% of all my distributed copies (electronic and print) are paid above a nominal price.

17. Publication of Statement of Ownership

☒ If the publication is a general publication, publication of this statement is required. Will be printed
in the **NOVEMBER 2023** issue of this publication.

☐ Publication not required.

18. Signature and Title of Editor, Publisher, Business Manager, or Owner

Malathi Samayan   Date 9/18/2023

Malathi Samayan - Distribution Controller

I certify that all information furnished on this form is true and complete. I understand that anyone who furnishes false or misleading information on this form or who omits material or information requested on the form may be subject to criminal sanctions (including fines and imprisonment) and/or civil sanctions (including civil penalties).

PS Form **3526**, July 2014 (Page 3 of 4)   PRIVACY NOTICE: See our privacy policy on www.usps.com.

Printed and bound by CPI Group (UK) Ltd, Croydon, CR0 4YY

03/10/2024

01040466-0002